Pharmacogenomics in Drug Discovery and Development

Pharmacogenomics in Drug Discovery and Development

Editor: Karoline Hodge

MURPHY & MOORE
www.murphy-moorepublishing.com

www.murphy-moorepublishing.com

MURPHY & MOORE

Cataloging-in-Publication Data

Pharmacogenomics in drug discovery and development / edited by Karoline Hodge.
p. cm.
Includes bibliographical references and index.
ISBN 978-1-63987-781-2
1. Pharmacogenomics. 2. Drug development. 3. Drugs--Effectiveness.
4. Drugs--Design. 5. Pharmacokinetics. I. Hodge, Karoline.
RM301.3.G45 P43 2023
615.7--dc23

Murphy & Moore Publishing
1 Rockefeller Plaza,
New York City,
NY 10020, USA

ISBN 978-1-63987-781-2

Contents

Preface

Pharmacogenomics refers to the study of the influence of genes in an individual's response to drugs. This field draws from two fields, namely, pharmacology and genomics. It aims at developing safe and effective medications that can be prescribed based on an individual's genetic makeup. Pharmacogenomics involves the use of genetics to reduce unfavorable drug responses, enhance drug therapies and increase drug efficacy. The use of pharmacogenomics in drug development is expected to eliminate the unpredictable response of drug treatments that occurs due to genetic polymorphisms, which affect metabolism, tolerance and clearance. Pharmacogenomics can potentially be used to create tailored drugs for treating a variety of health issues such as Alzheimer's disease, asthma, cardiovascular disease, and cancer. This book aims to shed light on the role of pharmacogenomics in drug discovery and development. It covers in detail some existent theories and innovative concepts revolving around this domain. Those in search of information to further their knowledge will be greatly assisted by this book.

All of the data presented henceforth, was collaborated in the wake of recent advancements in the field. The aim of this book is to present the diversified developments from across the globe in a comprehensible manner. The opinions expressed in each chapter belong solely to the contributing authors. Their interpretations of the topics are the integral part of this book, which I have carefully compiled for a better understanding of the readers.

At the end, I would like to thank all those who dedicated their time and efforts for the successful completion of this book. I also wish to convey my gratitude towards my friends and family who supported me at every step.

Editor

1

Structure of *N*-Terminal Sequence Asp-Ala-Glu-Phe-Arg-His-Asp-Ser of Aβ-Peptide with Phospholipase A_2 from Venom of Andaman Cobra Sub-Species *Naja naja sagittifera* at 2.0 Å Resolution

Zeenat Mirza [1,2,*], Vikram Gopalakrishna Pillai [2,3] and Wei-Zhu Zhong [4]

1 Proteomics and Structural Biology Unit, Fundamental and Applied Biology Group, King Fahd Medical Research Center, King Abdulaziz University, P.O. Box 80216, Jeddah 21589, Saudi Arabia

2 Department of Biophysics, All India Institute of Medical Sciences, New Delhi 110029, India; E-Mail: vikgopal@gmail.com

3 Children's Hospital of Philadelphia, Philadelphia, PA 19104, USA

4 Gordon Life Science Institute, Boston, MA 02478, USA; E-Mail: wzzhong@gordonlifescience.org

* Author to whom correspondence should be addressed; E-Mail: zmirza1@kau.edu.sa or zeenat_mirza@rediffmail.com

---

Abstract: Alzheimer's disease (AD) is one of the most significant social and health burdens of the present century. Plaques formed by extracellular deposits of amyloid β (Aβ) are the prime player of AD's neuropathology. Studies have implicated the varied role of phospholipase A_2 (PLA_2) in brain where it contributes to neuronal growth and inflammatory response. Overall contour and chemical nature of the substrate-binding channel in the low molecular weight PLA_2s are similar. This study involves the reductionist fragment-based approach to understand the structure adopted by *N*-terminal fragment of Alzheimer's Aβ peptide in its complex with PLA_2. In the current communication, we report the structure determined by X-ray crystallography of *N*-terminal sequence Asp-Ala-Glu-Phe-Arg-His-Asp-Ser (DAEFRHDS) of Aβ-peptide with a Group I PLA_2 purified from venom of Andaman Cobra sub-species *Naja naja sagittifera* at 2.0 Å resolution (Protein Data Bank (PDB) Code: 3JQ5). This is probably the first attempt to structurally establish interaction between amyloid-β peptide fragment and hydrophobic substrate binding site of PLA_2 involving H bond and van der Waals interactions.

We speculate that higher affinity between Aβ and PLA_2 has the therapeutic potential of decreasing the Aβ–Aβ interaction, thereby reducing the amyloid aggregation and plaque formation in AD.

Keywords: cobra venom; phospholipase A_2; co-crystallization; Alzheimer's disease; neuroinflammation; DAEFRHDS

---

1. Introduction

An estimated 36 million people globally are suffering from Alzheimer's disease (AD), which causes irreversible neurodegeneration and usually strikes in the later years of life. According to the World Health Organization, this figure is anticipated to rise to 65.7 million by 2030 and may increase to 115.4 million by 2050 [1]. Dementia is the most frequent type of neurodegenerative disease and it is rarely detected before symptoms develop; no drugs presently exist for its therapy [2,3]. The characteristic disease landmarks include neurofibrillary tangles [4] and amyloid plaques, surrounded by reactive astrocytes, activated microglial cells causing neuroinflammatory responses and dystrophic neuritis. Although the neuroinflammation mechanism in AD brain is not apparent, there is ample data suggesting a role for specific forms of amyloid beta peptide (Aβ) in inducing release of pro-inflammatory cytokines by microglia and astrocytes. Hence, identifying the modulating mechanisms of neuroinflammatory responses and neuronal degeneration will unravel vital aspects to develop new therapeutic strategies [5,6]. Developing chemical interventions for AD is exigent and has proceeded in a virtual vacuum due to lack of tertiary structural information of amyloid-β peptide [7], which is cleaved via the β/γ-secretase pathway from the membrane-bound amyloid precursor protein (APP) [8]. β-secretase generates the *N*-terminus of Aβ by cleaving β-APP within the Glu-Val-Lys-Met-↓-Asp-Ala sequence or by cleaving the Swedish mutant β-APP_{SW} within the Glu-Val-Asn-Leu-↓-Asp-Ala sequence. In addition, cleavage has been reported to occur within the Aβ sequence Asp-Ser-Gly-Tyr^{10}-Glu^{11}-Val, generating $A\beta_{11-40/42}$ [9]. Solubility may be modulated in a pH-dependent manner by the charged *N*-terminal sequence [10].

The phospholipase A_2 (PLA_2) is a lipolytic enzyme commonly expressed in several types of mammalian cells [11]. Two most notable forms of PLA_2 are the secretory PLA_2 ($sPLA_2$) and the calcium-dependent cytosolic PLA_2 ($cPLA_2$). In healthy brain cells, equilibrium between arachidonic acid conversion into proinflammatory mediators and arachidonic acid reincorporation into the membrane is maintained by PLA_2 regulation. Unregulated PLA_2 activity causes production of an inconsistent amount of proinflammatory mediators, leading to oxidative stress and neuroinflammation as seen in neurological diseases such as AD, epilepsy, and multiple sclerosis. The most common and extensively studied PLA_2s belong to group I and II. $sPLA_2$-IIA mRNA is up-regulated in AD brains as compared to non-demented elderly brains, and a higher percentage of $sPLA_2$-IIA-immunoreactive astrocytes associated with Aβ plaques have been reported in the AD hippocampus and inferior temporal gyrus [12]. Increased $sPLA_2$ activity is observed in the cerebrospinal fluid of humans with AD and multiple sclerosis, and can perhaps be a marker of permeability increases of the blood–cerebrospinal fluid barrier [13]. Also, other types of $sPLA_2$ bearing a similar structure—e.g., groups 1B, IIE, V and

X—are present in distinct brain regions [14]. A feature identified for the design of tight PLA_2 inhibitors is the presence of the OH group on the aromatic framework, which may be extended in the opposite direction with the hydrophobic moiety [15].

A series of recent studies have indicated that much useful information for drug development can be obtained in a timely manner by conducting various studies, either experimentally or theoretically. However, different targets would need different approaches. For instance, to reveal the molecular mechanism of Alzheimer's disease [16–18] and find useful clues for developing drugs against Alzheimer's disease [19,20], the structural bioinformatics tools [21] were adopted. On the other hand, as is well known, X-ray crystallography and high-resolusion NMR (see, e.g., [22–24]) are two very powerful tools for structure-based drug design. Although it is time-consuming and expensive to use these facilities, the results thus acquired are usually more reliable and dependable. Our primary goal is to determine the possibility of a direct interaction between Aβ peptide and PLA_2 and the structure adopted by the peptide that may in the future pave the way for novel approaches for better understanding AD and its therapeutics.

2. Results

2.1. Quality of the Final Model

The final model consists of 909 protein atoms, 68 atoms of peptide molecule, one calcium ion and 99 water molecules. The final $|2F_o - F_c|$ electron density map is continuous and well defined for both the backbone and the side chains of the protein. The final model has a good overall geometry with the r.m.s. deviations in bond lengths and angles are 0.009 Å and 1.1°, respectively. The Ramachandran plot calculated using PROCHECK [25], indicates that 89.1% of the residues are present in the most favourable regions, 10.0% were observed in the additionally allowed regions, while the remaining 0.9% residues were observed in the generously allowed regions of the Ramachandran plot [26] (Figure 1). The results of data collection and processing are given in Table 1 and the refinement statistics are given in Table 2.

2.2. Overall Structure

The general structure of PLA_2 contains an *N*-terminal helix, H1 (residues: 2–12), a calcium-binding loop (residues: 25–35), a second α-helix, H2 (residues: 40–55), a short two-stranded antiparallel β-sheet (residues: 75–78 and 81–84), referred to as the β-wing and a third α-helix, H3 (residues: 90–108). There are two helical short turns involving residues 19–22 (SH4) and 113–115 (SH5) (Figure 2). The two antiparallel helices H2 and H3 form the core of the protein structure. The hydrophobic residues on the inner surface of the helix H1 are highly conserved and form one wall of the hydrophobic channel, which provides access to the catalytic site (Figure 3). Additional contributions to the hydrophobic channel include amino acid 19, which is located in the short turn following the helix H1, amino acid 30, 31 and 32 located within the calcium-binding loop and amino acid 69 located before the first strand of the β-wing. The structure is in accordance with previously reported structures [27].

Figure 1. A Ramachandran plot of the main chain torsion angles (φ,ψ) for the final refined model. The plot was calculated with the program PROCHECK [25]; non-glycine residues are identified by squares.

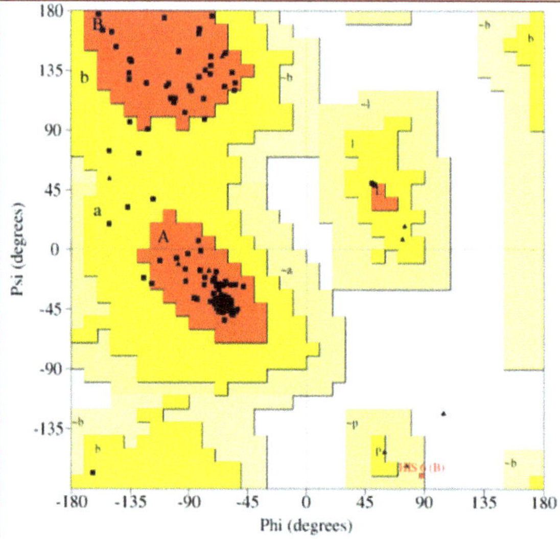

Plot statistics

Residues in most favoured regions [A,B,L]	98	89.1%
Residues in additional allowed regions [a,b,l,p]	11	10.0 %
Residues in generously allowed regions [~a,~b,~l,~p]	1	0.9 %
Residues in disallowed regions	0	0.0 %
Number of non-glycine and non-proline residues	110	100.0 %
Number of end-residues (excl. Gly and Pro)	4	
Number of glycine residues (shown as triangles)	9	
Number of proline residues	4	
Total number of residues	127	

Table 1. Data collection statistics.

Space group	**$P4_1$**
System	Tetragonal
Unit-cell parameters (Å)	
a = b	42.7
c	65.8
V_m ($Å^3$/Da)	2.3
Solvent Content (%)	46.7
Resolution range (Å)	20.0–2.0
No. of observed reflections	33,510
No. of unique reflections	7735
Overall completeness (%)	98.7
Completeness in the highest shell (2.06–2.03 Å) (%)	87.7
Overall R_{sym} (%)	7.0
R_{sym} in the highest shell (2.06–2.03 Å) (%)	18.8
Overall I/σ(I)	11.1
I/σ(I) in the highest shell (2.06–2.03 Å)	2.3

Table 2. Refinement statistics.

PDB code	3JQ5
Resolution range (Å)	20.0–2.0
Number of reflections	7735
R_{Cryst} (for all data) (%)	18.1
R_{Free} (5% data) (%)	22.0
Number of protein atoms	909
Number of peptide atoms	68
Number of Water Molecules	99
Number of calcium atoms	1
R.m.s. deviations	
Bond length ($Å^2$)	0.009
Bond angles (°)	1.1
Dihedral angles (°)	14.4
Overall *G* factor	0.05
Mean B factor ($Å^2$)	
Main chain atoms	22.0
Side chains and water molecules	27.3
Overall	24.8
Ramachandran plot statistics	
Residues in the most allowed region (%)	89.1
Residues in the additionally allowed region (%)	10.0
Residues in the generously allowed region (%)	0.9

Figure 2. A ribbon diagram showing the overall structure of PLA_2: helical segment is shown in red, β strands colored yellow and disulfide links shown in ball and stick, colored green and yellow. The three main helices are indicated as H1, H2 and H3, while two short helices are designated as SH4 and SH5. β wing, calcium-binding loop and disulfide linkages are also indicated.

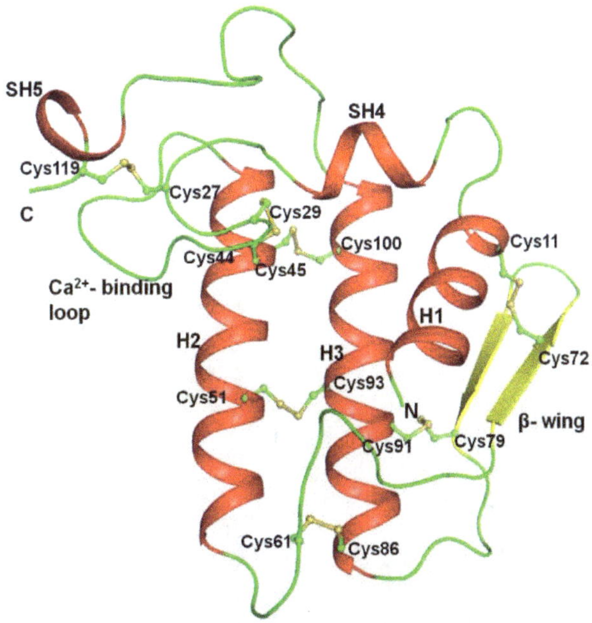

Figure 3. The $|F_o - F_c|$ electron density map contoured at 2.0 σ showing the electron density for the peptide Asp-Ala-Glu-Phe-Arg-His-Asp-Ser.

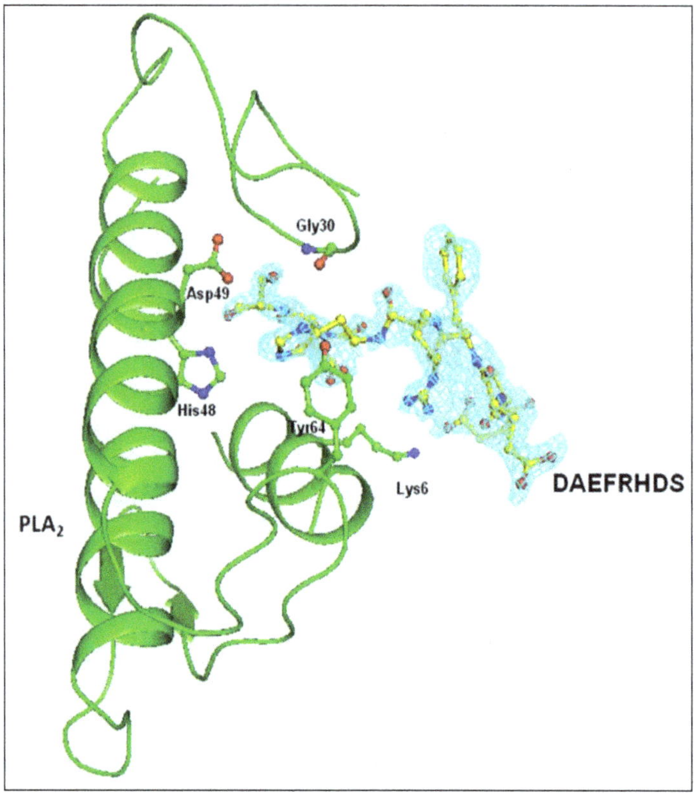

The overall folding of PLA_2 observed in the complex with peptide is essentially similar to that of native PLA_2 (1MF4) with an r.m.s. shift of 0.2 Å for the C^α positions. One milli molar $CaCl_2$ was added in the protein drops that were used for crystallization and the structure revealed the presence of Ca^{2+} ion in the so-called calcium-binding loop. The Ca^{2+} ion is considered generally essential for catalytic activities of secretory PLA_2s [28,29]. In the present structure, the Ca^{2+} ion stabilizes the conformation of the calcium-binding loop (Figure 4).

Figure 4. Difference $|F_o - F_c|$ electron density for the calcium ion drawn at 2σ. Calcium coordinated interactions are indicated by dotted lines. Ser8 of peptide is shown in green.

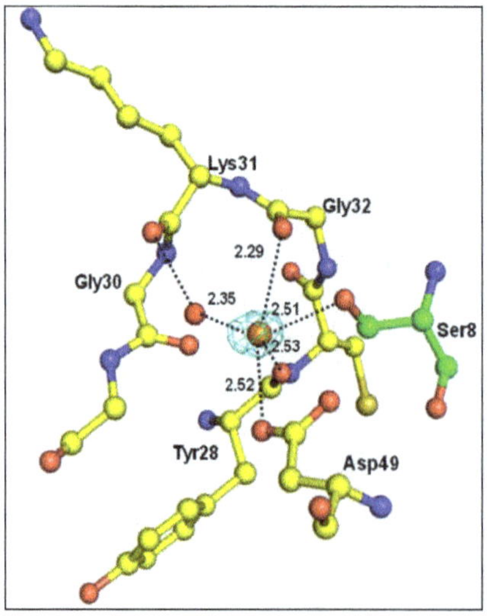

2.3. Structure of Peptide

The structure of PLA_2 in the complex remains unchanged from its native structure. All the eight residues of the peptide can be traced from their electron densities (Figure 3). The interaction of the peptide with the protein is depicted in Figure 5. Half of the peptide residue's torsional angles are in the most favoured region of the Ramachandran plot, although none were observed in the disallowed region. The structure of the peptide is given in Figure 6.

Figure 5. Interactions between PLA_2 and the peptide Asp-Ala-Glu-Phe-Arg-His-Asp-Ser. The peptide residues are colored yellow. The critical interactions between peptide and protein are shown by the dotted line.

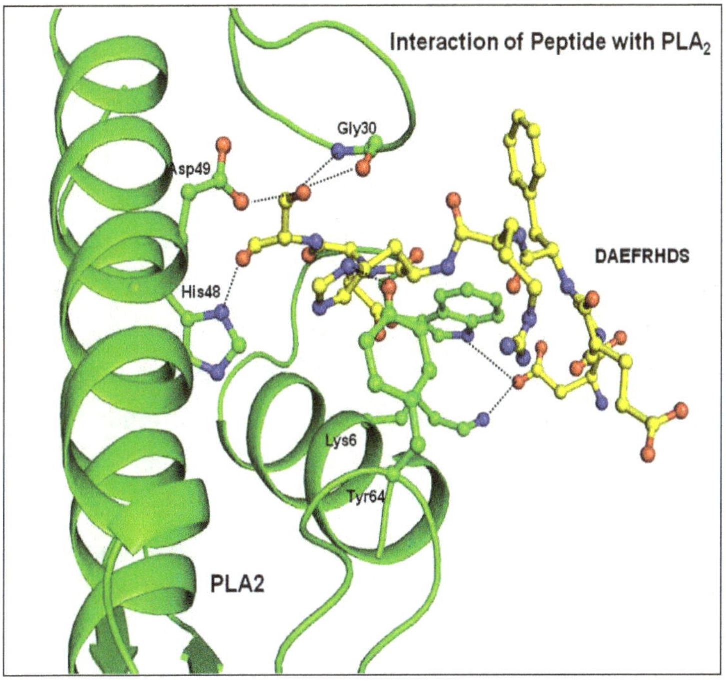

Figure 6. The structure of peptide Asp-Ala-Glu-Phe-Arg-His-Asp-Ser in complex with PLA_2.

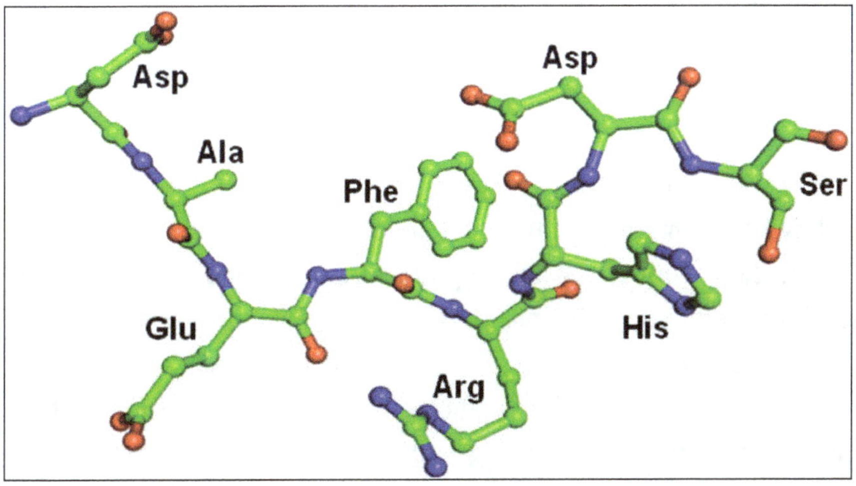

3. Discussion

We have attempted the fragment assembly approach to elucidate the structure of Aβ. The fragment assembly and global optimization method has been established and extensively used in computational biology [30,31]. This work may be the first design of experiments following this approach. However, reductionist methods are common in protein crystallography. There are vast numbers of entries in PDB that are exclusively the domains, or even a small fragment of proteins. Most of the time, the intact protein is not amenable to crystallization, such as the beta-amyloid precursor protein. The co-crystallization method is another useful method of crystallography. Hundreds of Fab–Ag complexes are available to corroborate this fact. Co-crystallization of complete Aβ with mitochondrial alcohol dehydrogenase has been attempted [32]. The presence of Aβ in the crystal has been established by SDS-PAGE and *N*-terminal sequencing of the washed crystal in this study. However, no electron density corresponding to Aβ could be observed in the determined structure. This suggests the Aβ in this complex is flexible. The only instance where the Aβ molecule is seen in the crystal is the structure of the complex between Aβ and insulin-degrading enzyme (IDE). The Aβ is seen as a cleaved substrate. The complete molecule is not observed—only residues 1–3 and 17–22 are same [33].

There are many NMR studies describing the structures of partial and complete abeta molecule (3BAE, 1BA6, 1BA4, 2BEG). The results are generally combined with molecular modelling calculations. From all these studies, the following structural properties for the aggregating abeta is proposed—the central region $A\beta_{16-21}$ and *C*-terminal region $A\beta_{33-40(42)}$ are in β-strand conformation; $A\beta_{25-29}$ is in loop conformation, and the rest of the molecule is in random conformation. This is also corroborated by X-ray fiber—diffraction of the fibrils while the attempts to crystallize or co-crystallize the $A\beta_{17-21}$ and $A\beta_{35-40}/A\beta_{37-42}$ have been described and the peptides are observed in β-conformation. Apparently, the nature of binding sites of the protein influences the conformation of the Aβ peptide. The large space available in IDE accommodated the intact Aβ molecule. In 2OTK, [34], $A\beta_{17-36}$ is seen in β-sheet conformation with residues 25–29 forming the loop. In their studies, Lustbader *et al.* could not view the Aβ molecule even though it was in the crystal. One conclusive aspect of crystal structures are that the peptides, $A\beta_{17-21}$, $A\beta_{35-42}$ and $A\beta_{17-36}$ are in β conformation. This is in contrast to the solution studies that report all conformational possibilities. The same peptide has been observed in different conformations in different studies. Most of the studies report helical or coil conformation [35–38]. These results may be due to the variable solvent conditions used in these studies. Solvent conditions vary from completely polar to non-polar. The conformation of Aβ is highly dependent on the environmental conditions. Solvent polarity, temperature, pH and additives influence the solubility and aggregation behaviour of Aβ [39,40].

An electron density was observed in the difference Fourier $|F_o - F_c|$ map in the complex structure (Figure 3), which allowed the interpretation of one molecule of the octa-peptide, as well as the detailed description of its interactions with PLA_2. The peptide was positioned well in the hydrophobic channel (Figure 7) and was fitted well in the substrate binding site of enzyme. Peptide interacts with active site residues through a series of hydrogen bonds and hydrophobic interactions. The *N*-terminal part of the peptide lies towards the opening of the hydrophobic channel at the protein surface. The *C*-terminal serine residue is involved in hydrogen bonding with the active site residues. The rest of the peptide aligned in the hydrophobic channel makes a series of van der Waals contacts with protein atoms. The oxygen atom Oγ of Ser8 of peptide is hydrogen bonded with active site residue Asp49 Oδ1 and also with backbone atoms of Gly30 of the calcium-binding loop. The backbone oxygen atom of Ser8 is directly hydrogen bonded to His48 Nδ1. Thus the peptide interacts with the active site residues through direct hydrogen bonds (Table 3). The peptide also interacts with important residues of the hydrophobic channel like Asp1 residue of peptide interacts with Lys6 and Trp19 residue of protein and His6 residue of peptide interacts with Gly30 and Tyr64. Additionally the peptide is involved in van der Waals interaction with most of the residues lining the substrate-binding hydrophobic channel (Table 4).

Figure 7. Surface diagram representation of the binding cavity and the hydrophobic channel with the peptide DAEFRHDS going inside the pocket.

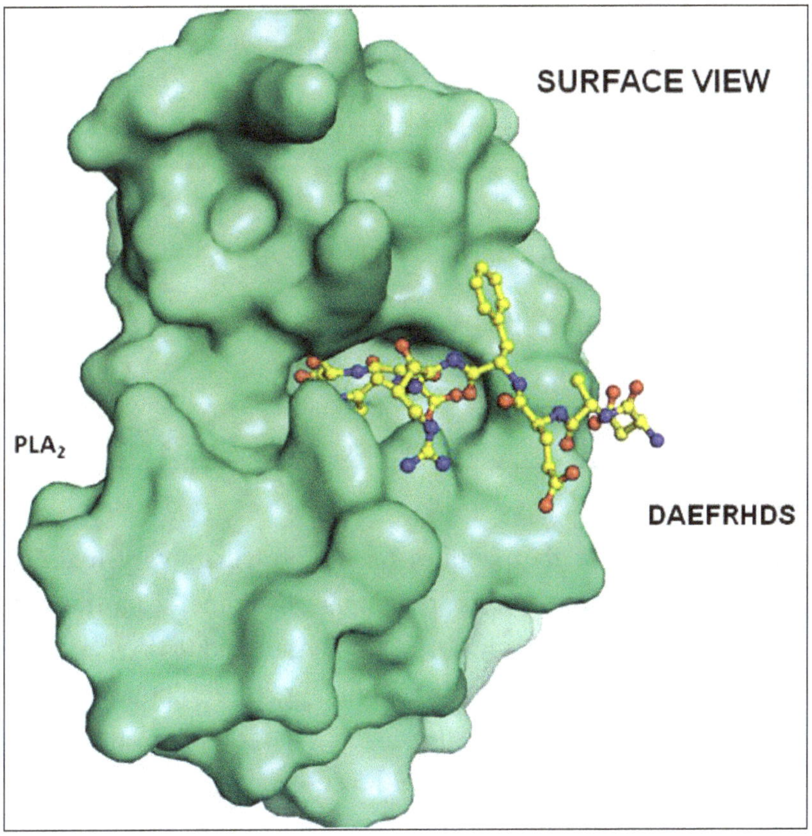

Table 3. Hydrogen bonds between PLA_2 and peptide DAEFRHDS.

Atoms of peptide	Protein atoms	Distance (Å)
Asp1 Oδ2	Lys6 Nζ	3.35
	Trp19 Nε1	2.64
His6 Nδ1	Gly30 O	3.43
	Tyr64 OH	2.78
Ser8 Oγ	Gly30 N	3.22
	Gly30 O	2.62
	Tyr28 O	3.35
	Asp49 Oδ1	2.95
Ser8 O	His48 Nδ1	2.80

Table 4. Van der Waal interactions between PLA_2 and peptide DAEFRHDS.

Atoms of peptide	Protein atoms	Distance (Å)
Asp1 Cγ	Trp19 Cε2	3.79
	Trp19 Cζ2	3.48
Ala2 Cβ	Trp19 CH2	3.73
	Trp19 Cζ2	3.97
Phe4 Cδ1	Ala23 Cβ	3.91
Arg5 Cζ	Leu2 Cδ2	3.53
His6 Cα	Leu2 Cδ2	3.69
His6 Cβ	Gly30 Cα	3.63
	Gly30 C	3.68
His6 Cε1	Tyr64 Cζ	3.75
Asp7 Cα	Ala23 Cα	3.75
Asp7 Cβ	Ile9 Cδ1	3.78
	Phe5 Cε2	3.97
Asp7 C	Phe5 Cε2	3.92
Ser8 Cβ	Tyr28 C	3.90
	Cys29 Cα	3.51
	Cys29 C	3.64
	Gly30 Cα	3.76
Ser8 C	Phe101 Cζ	3.92
	His48 Cγ	3.98
	Cys45 Cβ	3.81

In our studies, the binding site of the peptides on the protein is very hydrophobic. The binding cavity of PLA_2 is lined with residues such as tryptophan, histidine, aspartic acid, and glycine. The non-polar surface extends from the molecule to the catalytic residues Aspartate and histidine at the other end. We expect that the non-polar nature of the binding site could have influenced the folding of the Aβ peptide fragment. This is possible given the fact that the folding of the Aβ molecule is mediated and stabilized by non-polar interactions. Moreover, the co-crystallization experiments were carried at 35% ethanol concentrations. Organic solvents (mostly alcohols have been studied), generally induce a random conformation in Aβ molecule as seen from the experiments. The peptide in our co-crystallization experiment strongly interacted with the non-polar binding-cavity residues of PLA_2. The only interaction arginine displays in DAEFRHDS is non-polar (Table 3). Even though this peptide is polar it has more non-polar interactions than polar interactions (Tables 3 and 4). The observed conformation of the peptide in our result must have been dictated by the protein–ligand interactions. Though our aim of fragment assembly has not been achieved, the observations made by us are nevertheless interesting in their own right, exemplifying the strength of the interactions of the protein and ligand on one hand, and their effect on the conformation of the ligand on the other.

4. Experimental Section

4.1. Purification of Monomeric PLA_2

The lyophilized samples of crude cobra venom of *Naja naja sagittifera* were obtained from Irula Snake Catchers Industrial Cooperative Society, Chennai, India. The crude venom was dissolved in 50 mM Tris-HCl, 100 mM NaCl, pH 7.0 at 100 mg/mL concentration and centrifuged at 12,000× *g* for 10 min to remove insoluble material. The collected supernatant was size fractionated on Sephadex G-100 column (100 × 2 cm) pre-equilibrated with 50 mM Tris-HCl, 100 mM NaCl, pH 7.0. The column was eluted with the same buffer at a flow rate of 6 mL/h. The peak corresponding to molecular weight of 14 kDa on SDS-PAGE and showing PLA_2 activity was pooled for further purification. The pooled fractions were desalted and dialysed against 50 mM Tris-HCl, pH 7.0 and loaded on CM Sephadex C-50 column (Pharmacia, Uppsala, Sweden). The column was washed with the above buffer. The unbound fractions were pooled and dialysed against ammonium acetate buffer, pH 6.0. The diluted sample was loaded on a pre-equilibrated column with same buffer containing Affi-gel Cibacron blue F3GA. The column was washed with 50 mM ammonium acetate buffer pH 6.0 to remove unbound fractions. The column was eluted with 50 mM ammonium bicarbonate buffer pH 8.0. These fractions showed PLA_2 activity and indicated a molecular weight of 14 kDa on SDS-PAGE. The samples were pooled, desalted by ultrafiltration using a 3 kDa cutoff membrane and lyophilized, and their purity was checked by matrix-assisted laser desorption-ionization–time of flight (MALDI-TOF) (Kratos, Shimadzu, Kyoto, Japan) and by activity measurements. On MALDI-TOF it showed a molecular weight of 13,401.99 Da. The protein samples were blotted on a polyvinyl difluoride (PVDF) membrane (Sigma-Aldrich, St. Louis, MO, USA) and were subjected to the *N*-terminal sequencing using an automated protein sequencer PPSQ-21A (Shimadzu, Japan). The *N*-terminal sequence of the first 15 residues was determined. It was found identical to the sequence of PLA_2 whose structure was reported earlier [41].

4.2. Enzymatic Assay and Inhibition Studies

The purified enzyme was used for kinetic studies done using a PLA_2 Assay Kit (Cayman Chemical Company, Ann Arbor, MI, USA). The enzymatic chromogenic assay utilized the conversion of arachidonoyl thio-phosphocholine into sulfahydryl molecule by PLA_2. Arachidonoyl thio-PC is a synthetic substrate used to detect phospholipase activity [42]. Hydrolysis of the arachidonoyl thioester bound at the *sn*-2 position by PLA_2 releases free thiol, colorimetrically detected by Ellman's reagent [5,5'-dithiobis (2-nitrobenzoic acid) (DTNB)], which results in yellow colour along with the released sulfahydryl product. Stock concentration at 1.5 mM of PC-substrate and 0.1 mM of PLA_2 were used for the assay. Ten μL of colouring agent (DTNB) was added in each assay reaction. Peptide inhibitors (GenScript Corporation, Piscataway, NJ, USA) were dissolved in dimethyl sulfoxide and only 5 μL added to the assay. Peptide concentrations of 0.10, 0.20, 0.30 and 0.40 mM were taken for studying PLA_2 inhibition reactions. Bee venom PLA_2 was taken as positive control. The assay included a 30 min pre-incubation of enzyme with peptide and a further incubation of 60 min at room temperature after the addition of 200 μL substrate solution. The absorbance was measured at 414 nm wavelength on a plate reader and measurements were repeated thrice. Two wells were designated as non-enzyme controls and their absorbance was subtracted from the absorbance measured in the sample wells. Significant decrease in enzyme activity was seen in the presence of an inhibitor.

4.3. Crystallization

The purified samples of PLA_2 were dissolved in 10 mM sodium phosphate buffer pH 6.0 containing 1 mM $CaCl_2$ to a final concentration of 2.5 mg/mL. Peptide was dissolved in the above buffer, containing 10% acetonitrile and added to the protein solution at 10-fold high molar concentration. The solution was incubated for 3 h, mixed well, centrifuged and kept for crystallization trials using hanging drop vapor diffusion method. The 10 μL drops of the above mixture were equilibrated against the same buffer containing 30% ethanol in the reservoir. The crystals grew to a size of $0.4 \times 0.2 \times 0.2$ mm^3 after two weeks.

4.4. Data Collection and Data Processing

The crystals of the complex formed between PLA_2 and the *N*-terminus fragment DAEFRHDS were used for data collection at low temperature. A single crystal was mounted in a nylon loop and flash-frozen in a stream of nitrogen gas at 100 K. The data were collected on a 345 mm diameter MAR research scanner with 1.54 Å radiation generated by a Rigaku RU-300 rotating anode X-ray Generator filled with Osmic mirrors (Rigaku USA, Woodlands, TX, USA). The data were processed with DENZO and SCALEPACK from HKL package [43]. The final data set was complete to 87.7% up to 2.0 Å resolution. The crystals belong to the tetragonal space group $P4_1$ with unit cell dimensions a = b = 42.7 Å, c = 65.8 Å. The presence of one molecule per asymmetric unit gave a crystal volume per protein mass (V_m) of 2.3 $Å^3Da^{-1}$ corresponding to a solvent content of 46.7%. The final data show an overall completeness of 98.7% with a R_{sym} of 7.0% to 2.0 Å resolution (Tables 1 and 2).

4.5. Structure Determination and Refinement

The crystal structure was determined with molecular replacement method using auto-AMoRe [44] from the CCP4 software suit (Collaborative Computational Project, Number 4, 1994). The coordinates of a native PLA_2 structure (PDB code: 1MF4) were used as a search model. The rotation and translation functions calculated with data in the resolution range, 12.0–3.5 Å yielded a unique solution with the first peak being very distinct. The stacking arrangement of the molecules in the unit cell for this solution yielded no unfavourable intermolecular contacts in space group $P4_1$, thus confirming it as the correct space group. The coordinates were transformed using AMoRe and were then subjected to 20 cycles of rigid-body refinement with REFMAC5 [45]. This reduced the R_{cryst} and R_{free} factors to 18.1% and 22.0%, respectively. Of the reflections, 2% were used for the calculation of R_{free}, and were not included in the refinement. The manual model building of the protein using Fourier $|2F_o - F_c|$ and difference Fourier $|F_o - F_c|$ maps was carried out with the Graphics Program "O" [46] on a Silicon Graphics O_2 Workstation (Figure 2). A continuous non-protein electron density at 2.0 σ cut off was observed in the proximity of the active site that extended in a direction parallel to helix H_2. The ligand was only included because it was well defined by unbiased difference Fourier (*i.e.*, before inclusion of any ligand) $|F_o - F_c|$ map. The coordinates of the peptide structure were fitted into the characteristic electron density (Figure 3). Water molecules were then added using ARP/WARP [45]. The presence of calcium ions was detected from the difference Fourier $|F_o - F_c|$ maps (Figure 4). Further refinement was carried out after adding the coordinates of the peptide molecule, one calcium ion and 99 water molecules. The final R_{cryst} and R_{free} factors for the complete data in the resolution range of 20.0–2.03 Å were 0.188 and 0.202, respectively (Table 2). A portion of the electron density indicating the quality of the structure at 2.03 Å resolution is shown in Figure 3. The atomic coordinates of this structure have been deposited to protein data bank (PDB) with an accession code of 3JQ5.

5. Conclusions

This is likely the first attempt to structurally establish the interaction between the amyloid-β peptide fragment and PLA_2 peptide to the hydrophobic substrate binding site of PLA_2 involving at least nine H bond and several van der Waals interactions. Higher affinity between Aβ and PLA_2 decreases the Aβ–Aβ interaction probability, thereby reducing the aggregation and subsequent plaque formation. In conclusion, this study is a step towards understanding the mechanism behind the Aβ and PLA_2 interaction that may facilitate the development of novel therapeutic strategies to inhibit inflammatory responses to retard many diseases.

Acknowledgments

Authors acknowledge the help and support of all the faculties and the facilities of Department of Biophysics, All India Institute of Medical Sciences, New Delhi, India. ZM was recipient of Junior and Senior Research Fellowship from Council of Scientific and Industrial Research, Govt. of India. We would also like to acknowledge Deanship of Scientific Research (DSR) and King Fahd Medical Research Center (KFMRC), King Abdulaziz University (Jeddah, Saudi Arabia) for providing the necessary research and support facilities.

Author Contributions

Zeenat Mirza is the corresponding author and designed research project conception, development of overall research plan, and study oversight. Zeenat Mirza and Vikram Gopalakrishna Pillai were involved in hands-on conduct of the experiments, data collection and analysis. Zeenat Mirza was involved in writing of the manuscript. Wei-Zhu Zhong is the senior author and helped in revising and significantly improving the final content of this paper.

References

1. Pouryamout, L.; Dams, J.; Wasem, J.; Dodel, R.; Neumann, A. Economic evaluation of treatment options in patients with Alzheimer's disease: A systematic review of cost-effectiveness analyses. *Drugs* **2012**, *72*, 789–802.
2. Israel, M.A.; Yuan, S.H.; Bardy, C.; Reyna, S.M.; Mu, Y.; Herrera, C.; Hefferan, M.P.; van Gorp, S.; Nazor, K.L.; Boscolo, F.S.; *et al.* Probing sporadic and familial Alzheimer's disease using induced pluripotent stem cells. *Nature* **2012**, *482*, 216–220.

3. Young, J.E.; Goldstein, L.S. Alzheimer's disease in a dish: Promises and challenges of human stem cell models. *Hum. Mol. Genet.* **2012**, *21*, R82–R89.
4. Silvestrelli, G.; Lanari, A.; Parnetti, L.; Tomassoni, D.; Amenta, F. Treatment of Alzheimer's disease: From pharmacology to a better understanding of disease pathophysiology. *Mech. Ageing Dev.* **2006**, *127*, 148–157.
5. Craft, J.M.; Watterson, D.M.; van Eldik, L.J. Human amyloid beta-induced neuroinflammation is an early event in neurodegeneration. *Glia* **2006**, *53*, 484–490.
6. Stuchbury, G.; Munch, G. Alzheimer's associated inflammation, potential drug targets and future therapies. *J. Neural Transm.* **2005**, *112*, 429–453.
7. Landau, M.; Sawaya, M.R.; Faull, K.F.; Laganowsky, A.; Jiang, L.; Sievers, S.A.; Liu, J.; Barrio, J.R.; Eisenberg, D. Towards a pharmacophore for amyloid. *PLoS Biol.* **2011**, *9*, e1001080.
8. Querfurth, H.W.; LaFerla, F.M. Alzheimer's disease. *N. Engl. J. Med.* **2010**, *362*, 329–344.
9. Vassar, R.; Bennett, B.D.; Babu-Khan, S.; Kahn, S.; Mendiaz, E.A.; Denis, P.; Teplow, D.B.; Ross, S.; Amarante, P.; Loeloff, R.; *et al.* Beta-secretase cleavage of Alzheimer's amyloid precursor protein by the transmembrane aspartic protease BACE. *Science* **1999**, *286*, 735–741.
10. Jarrett, J.T.; Berger, E.P.; Lansbury, P.T., Jr. The carboxy terminus of the beta amyloid protein is critical for the seeding of amyloid formation: Implications for the pathogenesis of Alzheimer's disease. *Biochemistry* **1993**, *32*, 4693–4697.
11. Murakami, M.; Kudo, I. Phospholipase A2. *J. Biochem.* **2002**, *131*, 285–292.
12. Moses, G.S.; Jensen, M.D.; Lue, L.F.; Walker, D.G.; Sun, A.Y.; Simonyi, A.; Sun, G.Y. Secretory PLA2-IIA: A new inflammatory factor for Alzheimer's disease. *J. Neuroinflamm.* **2006**, *3*, 28.
13. Chalbot, S.; Zetterberg, H.; Blennow, K.; Fladby, T.; Andreasen, N.; Grundke-Iqbal, I.; Iqbal, K. Blood-cerebrospinal fluid barrier permeability in Alzheimer's disease. *J. Alzheimers Dis.* **2011**, *25*, 505–515.
14. Kolko, M.; Christoffersen, N.R.; Barreiro, S.G.; Miller, M.L.; Pizza, A.J.; Bazan, N.G. Characterization and location of secretory phospholipase A2 groups IIE, V, and X in the rat brain. *J. Neurosci. Res.* **2006**, *83*, 874–882.
15. Singh, R.K.; Singh, N.; Jabeen, T.; Sharma, S.; Dey, S.; Singh, T.P. Crystal structure of the complex of group I PLA2 with a group II-specific peptide Leu-Ala-Ile-Tyr-Ser (LAIYS) at 2.6 Å resolution. *J. Drug Target.* **2005**, *13*, 367–374.
16. Carter, D.B.; Chou, K.C. A model for structure dependent binding of Congo Red to Alzeheimer beta-amyloid fibrils. *Neurobiol. Aging* **1998**, *19*, 37–40.
17. Chou, K.C. Insights from modelling the tertiary structure of BACE2. *J. Proteome Res.* **2004**, *3*, 1069–1072.
18. Chou, K.C.; Howe, W.J. Prediction of the tertiary structure of the beta-secretase zymogen. *Biochem. Biophys. Res. Commun.* **2002**, *292*, 702–708.
19. Gu, R.X.; Gu, H.; Xie, Z.Y.; Wang, J.F.; Arias, H.R.; Wei, D.Q.; Chou, K.C. Possible drug candidates for Alzheimer's disease deduced from studying their binding interactions with alpha7 nicotinic acetylcholine receptor. *Med. Chem.* **2009**, *5*, 250–262.
20. Zheng, H.; Wei, D.Q.; Zhang, R.; Wang, C.; Wei, H.; Chou, K.C. Screening for new agonists against Alzheimer's disease. *Med. Chem.* **2007**, *3*, 488–493.
21. Chou, K.C. Review: Structural bioinformatics and its impact to biomedical science. *Curr. Med. Chem.* **2004**, *11*, 2105–2134.

22. Berardi, M.J.; Shih, W.M.; Harrison, S.C.; Chou, J.J. Mitochondrial uncoupling protein 2 structure determined by NMR molecular fragment searching. *Nature* **2011**, *476*, 109–113.
23. OuYang, B.; Xie, S.; Berardi, M.J.; Zhao, X.M.; Dev, J.; Yu, W.; Sun, B.; Chou, J.J. Unusual architecture of the p7 channel from hepatitis C virus. *Nature* **2013**, *498*, 521–525.
24. Schnell, J.R.; Chou, J.J. Structure and mechanism of the M2 proton channel of influenza A virus. *Nature* **2008**, *451*, 591–595.
25. Laskowski, R.; Macarthur, M.; Moss, D.; Thornton, J. PROCHECK: A program to check the stereochemical quality of protein structures. *J. Appl. Crystallogr.* **1993**, *26*, 283–290.
26. Ramachandran, G.N.; Sasisekharan, V. Conformation of polypeptides and proteins. *Adv. Protein Chem.* **1968**, *23*, 283–438.
27. Singh, N.; Kumar, R.P.; Kumar, S.; Sharma, S.; Mir, R.; Kaur, P.; Srinivasan, A.; Singh, T.P. Simultaneous inhibition of anti-coagulation and inflammation: Crystal structure of phospholipase A2 complexed with indomethacin at 1.4 Å resolution reveals the presence of the new common ligand-binding site. *J. Mol. Recognit.* **2009**, *22*, 437–445.
28. Berg, O.G.; Yu, B.Z.; Rogers, J.; Jain, M.K. Interfacial catalysis by phospholipase A2: Determination of the interfacial kinetic rate constants. *Biochemistry* **1991**, *30*, 7283–7297.
29. Yu, B.Z.; Berg, O.G.; Jain, M.K. The divalent cation is obligatory for the binding of ligands to the catalytic site of secreted phospholipase A2. *Biochemistry* **1993**, *32*, 6485–6492.
30. Jones, D.T. Predicting novel protein folds by using FRAGFOLD. *Proteins* **2001**, *45*, 127–132.
31. Hegler, J.A.; Latzer, J.; Shehu, A.; Clementi, C.; Wolynes, P.G. Restriction versus guidance in protein structure prediction. *Proc. Natl. Acad. Sci. USA* **2009**, *106*, 15302–15307.
32. Lustbader, J.W.; Cirilli, M.; Lin, C.; Xu, H.W.; Takuma, K.; Wang, N.; Caspersen, C.; Chen, X.; Pollak, S.; Chaney, M.; *et al.* ABAD directly links Abeta to mitochondrial toxicity in Alzheimer's disease. *Science* **2004**, *304*, 448–452.
33. Shen, Y.; Joachimiak, A.; Rosner, M.R.; Tang, W.J. Structures of human insulin-degrading enzyme reveal a new substrate recognition mechanism. *Nature* **2006**, *443*, 870–874.
34. Hoyer, W.; Hard, T. Interaction of Alzheimer's A beta peptide with an engineered binding protein—Thermodynamics and kinetics of coupled folding-binding. *J. Mol. Biol.* **2008**, *378*, 398–411.
35. Luhrs, T.; Ritter, C.; Adrian, M.; Riek-Loher, D.; Bohrmann, B.; Dobeli, H.; Schubert, D.; Riek, R. 3D structure of Alzheimer's amyloid-beta(1–42) fibrils. *Proc. Natl. Acad. Sci. USA* **2005**, *102*, 17342–17347.
36. Miles, L.A.; Wun, K.S.; Crespi, G.A.; Fodero-Tavoletti, M.T.; Galatis, D.; Bagley, C.J.; Beyreuther, K.; Masters, C.L.; Cappai, R.; McKinstry, W.J.; *et al.* Amyloid-beta-anti-amyloid-beta complex structure reveals an extended conformation in the immunodominant B-cell epitope. *J. Mol. Biol.* **2008**, *377*, 181–192.
37. Watson, A.A.; Fairlie, D.P.; Craik, D.J. Solution structure of methionine-oxidized amyloid beta-peptide (1–40). Does oxidation affect conformational switching? *Biochemistry* **1998**, *37*, 12700–12706.
38. Coles, M.; Bicknell, W.; Watson, A.A.; Fairlie, D.P.; Craik, D.J. Solution structure of amyloid beta-peptide(1–40) in a water-micelle environment. Is the membrane-spanning domain where we think it is? *Biochemistry* **1998**, *37*, 11064–11077.
39. Castelletto, V.; Hamley, I.W.; Harris, P.J.; Olsson, U.; Spencer, N. Influence of the solvent on the

self-assembly of a modified amyloid beta peptide fragment. I. Morphological investigation. *J. Phys. Chem. B* **2009**, *113*, 9978–9987.

40. Davis, C.H.; Berkowitz, M.L. Structure of the amyloid-beta (1–42) monomer absorbed to model phospholipid bilayers: A molecular dynamics study. *J. Phys. Chem. B* **2009**, *113*, 14480–14486.
41. Singh, R.K.; Vikram, P.; Makker, J.; Jabeen, T.; Sharma, S.; Dey, S.; Kaur, P.; Srinivasan, A.; Singh, T.P. Design of specific peptide inhibitors for group I phospholipase A2: Structure of a complex formed between phospholipase A2 from Naja naja sagittifera (group I) and a designed peptide inhibitor Val-Ala-Phe-Arg-Ser (VAFRS) at 1.9 Å resolution reveals unique features. *Biochemistry* **2003**, *42*, 11701–11706.
42. Reynolds, L.J.; Hughes, L.L.; Yu, L.; Dennis, E.A. 1-Hexadecyl-2-arachidonoylthio-2-deoxy-*sn*-glycero-3-phosphorylcholine as a substrate for the microtiterplate assay of human cytosolic phospholipase A2. *Anal. Biochem.* **1994**, *217*, 25–32.
43. Otwinowski, Z.; Minor, W. Processing of X-ray diffraction data collected in oscillation mode. *Methods Enzymol.* **1997**, *276*, 307–326.
44. Navaza, J. AmoRe: An automated package for molecular replacement. *Acta Crystallogr. A* **1994**, *50*, 157–163.
45. Murshudov, G.N.; Dodson, E.J. Simplified error estimation *a la* Cruickshank in macromolecular crystallography. *CCP4 Newslett. Protein Crystallogr.* **1997**, *33*, 31–39.
46. Jones, T.A.; Zou, J.Y.; Cowan, S.W.; Kjeldgaard, M. Improved methods for building protein models in electron density maps and the location of errors in these models. *Acta Crystallogr. A* **1991**, *47*, 110–119.

2

Synthesis, Preliminary Bioevaluation and Computational Analysis of Caffeic Acid Analogues

Zhiqian Liu [1], Jianjun Fu [2], Lei Shan [1], Qingyan Sun [1] and Weidong Zhang [1,*]

[1] Department of Phytochemistry, School of Pharmacy, School of Pharmacy, Second Military Medical University, 325 Guo He Road, Shanghai 200433, China; E-Mails: qian12@yeah.net (Z.L.); shanleicn@126.com (L.S.); sqy_2000@163.com (Q.S.)
[2] Shanghai Key Laboratory of New Drug Design, School of Pharmacy, East China University of Science and Technology, 130 Mei Long Road, Shanghai 200237, China; E-Mail: ivanliu2012@hotmail.com

* Author to whom correspondence should be addressed; E-Mail: wdzhangy@hotmail.com

---

Abstract: A series of caffeic acid amides were designed, synthesized and evaluated for anti-inflammatory activity. Most of them exhibited promising anti-inflammatory activity against nitric oxide (NO) generation in murine macrophage RAW264.7 cells. A 3D pharmacophore model was created based on the biological results for further structural optimization. Moreover, predication of the potential targets was also carried out by the PharmMapper server. These amide analogues represent a promising class of anti-inflammatory scaffold for further exploration and target identification.

Keywords: anti-inflammatory; caffeic acid amides; synthesis; pharmacophore; target predication

---

1. Introduction

Inflammation is a hallmark of many diseases, which may lead to various diseases including sepsis, arthritis, atherosclerosis, diabetes and even cancer [1,2]. Nowadays, several steroidal anti-inflammatory drugs (SAID) and nonsteroidal anti-inflammatory drugs (NSAID) have been developed. However, they still have some unexpected side effects and the inflammation mechanism is not exactly clear.

Currently, the most important targets are attracting a great deal of interest in contemporary anti-inflammatory drug design and discovery, including signal transducers and activators of transcription (STAT) [3], interleukin (IL) [4], stem cell factor (SCF) [5], macrophage migration inhibitory factor (MIF) [6], Annexin-1 [7], CC chemokine receptor (CCR) [8], Adenosine A2A receptor (A2A-R) [9], melanocortin receptor (MC-R) [10] and NF-κB signaling [11]. Very recently, our group has identified that 5-lipoxygenase was a potential target of (+)-2-(1-hydroxyl-4-oxocyclohexyl) ethyl caffeate [12].

Caffeic acid, a common natural product from *Eucalyptus globulus* [13], *Salvinia molesta* [14], *Phellinus linteus* [15] and coffee, was reported to possess promising *in vitro* and *in vivo* anti-inflammatory properties [16]. The caffeic acid is usually found as various simple derivatives including amides, esters, sugar esters and glycosides [17]. Yuu Osanai's group showed that caffeic acids with the ester functional group had good anti-inflammatory activity but with high cyctoxicity [18] (Figure 1). These findings prompted us to look for new caffeic acid amides with different substituent against inflammation while reducing cyctoxicity. In this report, 20 caffeic acid aimdes were rationally designed, synthesized and evaluated the inhibition of no production in murine macrophage RAW 264.7 cells. Based on the biological result, a 3D pharmacophore model was generated by using the seven active compounds with HipHop approach, which has been recognized as a time-saving and cost-effective technique for discovering new active compounds [19,20]. Furthermore, potential drug target predication was then carried out using pharmacophore-mapping approach [21]. The biological validation is ongoing now.

Figure 1. Structure of (**A**) ester; (**B**) amide; and (**C**) ketone derivatives of caffeic acid.

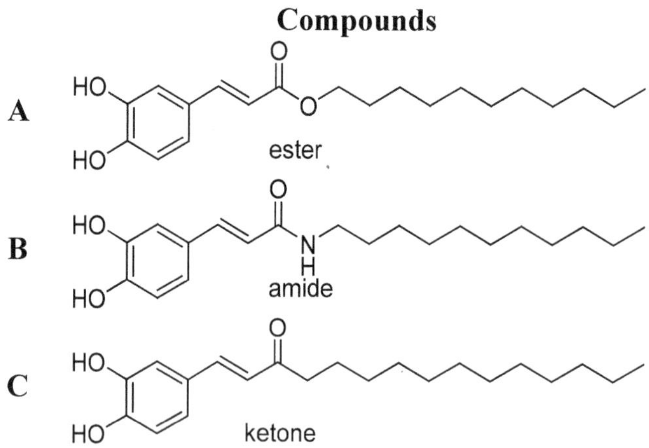

2. Results and Discussion

2.1. Biological Studies

A series of caffeic acid amides was synthesized according to general procedure [22] (Scheme 1). Firstly, R_1 and R_2 were first replaced with different alkyl groups (Compounds **3a–3f**). Unfortunately, only the *n*-Butyl derivative showed moderate nitric oxide (NO) inhibition with an IC_{50} value of 6.1 μM. The other alkyl derivatives with cyclic or di-substituted groups were completely inactive in the *in vitro* inhibition assay at 10 μM, probably due to the limited binding space (Table 1). Then, aromatic groups (Compounds **3g–3r**) were introduced and four compounds demonstrated good inhibitory activity. Structure–activity relationship (SAR) analysis identified that the type and position of the substituents were important for the inhibitory activity. Substituents on the 3 (Compound **3i**, IC_{50} = 7.9 μM) and 4 (Compound **3j**, IC_{50} = 5.2 μM and Compound **3k**, IC_{50} = 3.7 μM) positions of the benzene ring were favorable for the inhibition of NO production but not suitable for 3-chloro (Compound **3n**) and bromo (Compound **3o**) derivatives. Similarly, the derivatives with 2-substituents (Compounds **3l**, **3m** and **3q**) were absolutely inactive. Interestingly, the compounds with 3,5-difluorophenylo group (Compound **3h**, IC_{50} = 4.1 μM) and the 3,5-bis(trifluoromethyl)phenyl group (Compound **3g**, IC_{50} > 10 μM) were totally different. Encouraged by the above results, privileged bioactive structures with aromatic ring, such as indol (Compound **3s**) and piperonyl (Compound **3t**), were then synthesized. Both of them showed promising inhibitory activity with the IC_{50} of 6.7 and 5.0 μM, respectively, which can be taken as lead structures for further exploration. To our delight, the amides were much better than the original caffeic acid, which only had an IC_{50} value of 165 μM.

Scheme 1. Synthetic route of the caffic acid amides.

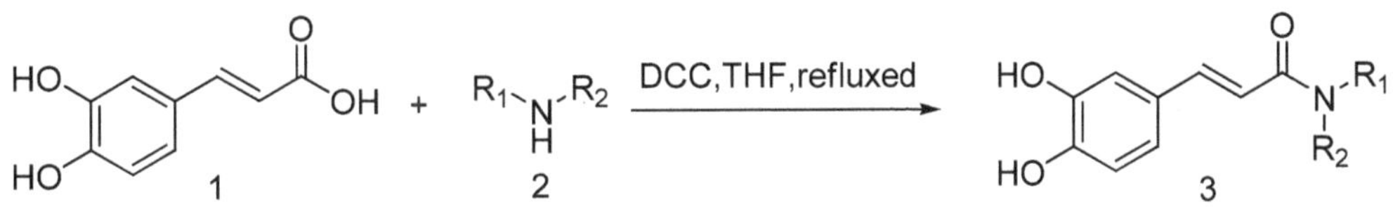

Table 1. Synthesis of caffeic acid amide (**3a**–**3t**) and inhibitory effect of caffeic acid amides on Lipopolysaccharide (LPS) induced nitrite production.

Compounds	R_1	R_2	Nitric Oxide Inhibition/IC_{50} (μM)
f	*n*-butyl	H	6.1
3b	cyclopropylmethanyl	H	>10
3c	–$CH_2)_5$–	–$(CH_2)_5$–	>10
3d	–$(CH_2)_4$–	–$(CH_2)_4$–	>10
3e	–$(CH_2)_2$–	–$(CH_2)_2$–	>10
3f	*n*-butyl	*n*-butyl	>10
3g	3,5-bis(trifluoromethyl)phenyl	H	>10
3h	3,5-difluorophenyl	H	4.1
3i	3-(trifluoromethyl)phenyl	H	7.9
3j	4-methoxyphenyl	H	5.2
3k	4-fluorophenyl	H	3.7
3l	2-(hydroxymethyl)phenyl	H	>10
3m	2-acetylphenyl	H	>10
3n	3-chlorophenyl	H	>10
3o	3-bromophenyl	H	>10
3p	4-methanylphenyl	H	>10
3q	2-methanylphenyl	H	>10
3r	phenylmethanyl	H	>10
3s	2-(1H-indol-3-yl)ethyl	H	6.7
3t	2-(benzo[d][1,3]dioxol-5-yl)ethyl	H	5.0
caffeic acid	-	-	165 [a]

[a] data from the reference [2].

2.2. Pharmacophore Model

A set of the seven most potent Compounds **3a**, **3h**–**3k**, **3s** and **3t** was selected as a training set to generate the 3D pharmacophore model. The common feature pharmacophore generation run resulted in 10 pharmacophore models. All the 10 models were generated with three pharmacophoric features, along with good ranking scores ranging from 117.3 to 119.49. As all pharmacophore models didn't have much difference in their 3D distance constraints, the best model was chosen based on the ranking score of a pharmacophore model and the fit values of the training set compounds. As a result, "Hypo 1" was selected with best ranking score of 119.49 and good fit values from the mapping of the training set compounds upon the chemical features. The pharmacophore model "Hypo 1" containing three hydrophobic (HY), two hydrogen bond acceptor (HBA) and two hydrogen bond donor (HBD) features are shown in Figure 2. The best pharmacophore model, Hypo1, was predicted using seven active compounds. It can map all seven active compounds (Figures S1–S7). The above results mimicked the 3D model of the newly synthesized active small molecules and guided further design strategy of structural optimization.

Figure 2. Pharmacophore model of seven active compounds. Three-dimensional spatial arrangement of the best pharmacophore hypothesis "Hypo 1". Green color represents hydrogen bond acceptor (HBA), magenta represents hydrogen bond donor (HDB) and cyan represents hydrophobic (HY) features.

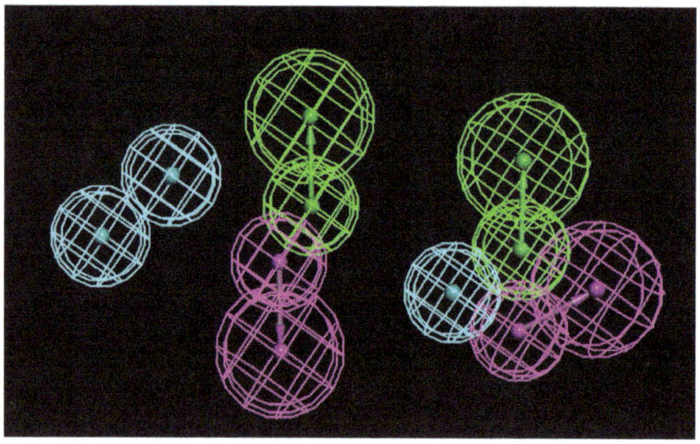

2.3. Target Predication and Molecular Docking

Despite our synthesized compounds showed promising inhibition of NO production, the exact molecular mechanism by which exerts their effects is not yet clearly understood. Potential drug target predication was then carried out using pharmacophore-mapping approach [21]. Binding properties for Compounds **3a**, **3g**, **3h**–**3k**, **3s** and **3t** on potential targets were estimated by a reverse pharmacophore mapping server [23]. These compounds were divided into three categories: aliphatic group (Compound **3a**), aromatic group (Compounds **3h**–**3k**) and heterocyclic group (Compounds **3s** and **3t**). All the predicted targets of these three groups were ranked by the fit score. Among the top 0.3% of the predicted target candidates, there were three common targets (GTPase HRas, Chorismate synthase and Orotidine 5-phosphate decarboxylase), indicating that above compounds may target different proteins comparing with the published caffeic acid ester. Further molecular docking revealed a good interaction between the ligands and the protein active site. Compound **3k** has formed hydrogen interactions with Ser17 and Thr35 (Figure 3). In the second potential protein, it has participated in hydrogen bonds interaction with the amino acids Ala133, Asn251, Asp399 and Thr315 (Figure 4). The active site of 5-phosphate decarboxylase surrounds and binds **3k** with hydrogen bonds at Val1182 and Asp1020 (Figure 5). These three docking models supported the significance of the hydroxyl group of **3k**.

Figure 3. The proposed binding mode of Compound **3k** within the active site of GTPase HRas (PDB code: 5P21).

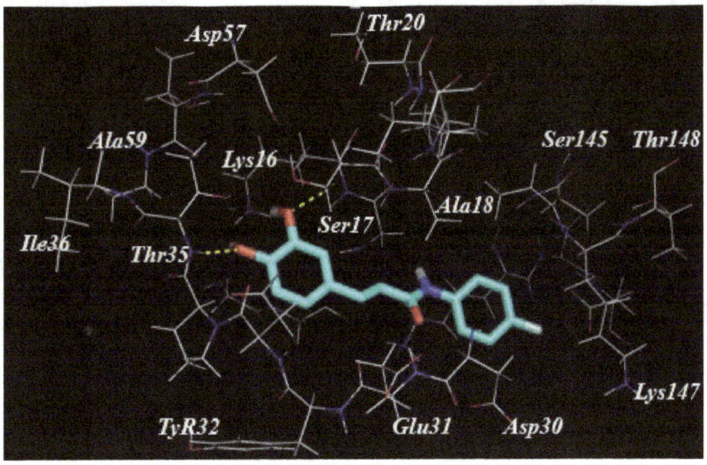

Figure 4. The proposed binding mode of Compound **3k** within the active site of Chorismate synthase (PDB code: 1QOX).

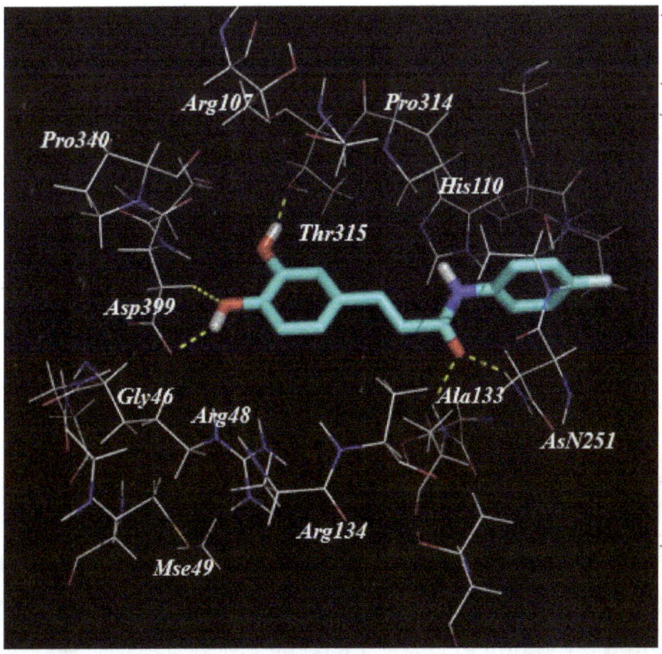

Figure 5. The proposed binding mode of Compound **3k** within the active site of Orotidine 5-phosphate decarboxylase (PDB code: 1LOS) and the proposed binding mode of compound **3k** within the active site of Orotidine 5-phosphate decarboxylase (PDB code: 1LOS).

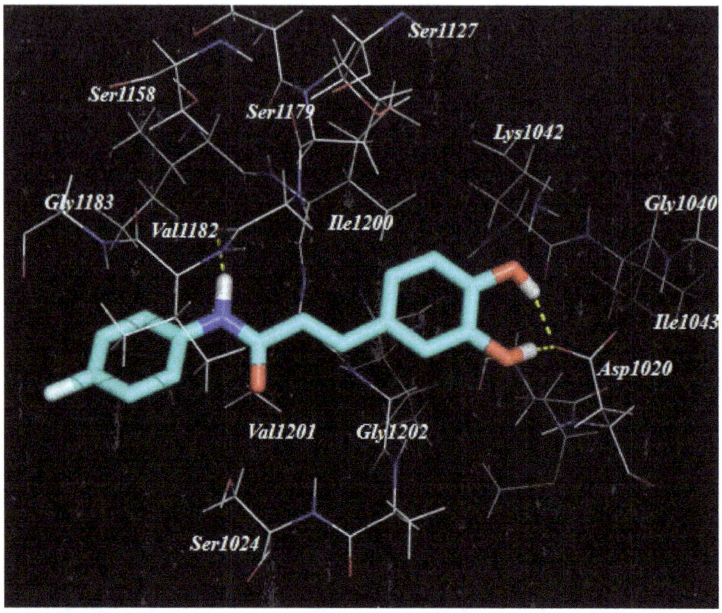

3. Experimental Section

3.1. Chemistry

All other commercial reagents and solvents were used as received without further purification. Anhydrous solvent and reagents were analytical pure and dried through routine protocols. The reactions were monitored using analytical thin layer chromatography (TLC) with Merck silica gel 60, F-254 precoated plates (0.25 mm thickness). And the TLC plates were detected under UV light. Flash column chromatography was performed with Merck silica gel 60 (Merck KGaA, Darmstadt, Germany) (200–400 mesh) or the crude product was purified by precipitation from dichloromethane with diethyl ether. ^{1}H NMR and ^{13}C NMR spectra were recorded on Bruker DRX 400 (Bruker Co., Bruker, Germany) at 400, 500 and 100 MHz, using TMS as an internal standard and DMSO-d_6 (Sigma-Aldrich Co., St. Louis, MO, USA) as solvents. Chemical shifts (δ values) and coupling constants (*J* values) are given in ppm and Hz, respectively. ESI-MS (Agilent Technologies, Palo Alto, CA, USA) was recorded on a Waters ZQ 4000 LC-MS (Waters, Milford, MA, USA) spectrometer. The purity of the final compounds was determined using CH_3CN/H_2O (85:15) with 0.1% triethylamine as the mobile phase with a flow rate of 1.0 mL/min on a C_{18} column.

3.1.1. General Procedure for the Preparation of Amine (**3a–3t**)

A solution of the caffeic acid (180 mg, 1 mmol), the dicyclohexyl carbodiimide (DCC, 206 mg, 1 mmol) and amide (1 mmol) was refluxed in THF and the progress of the reaction was monitored by TLC. The solvent was removed under vacuum. The residue was purified by flash chromatography using dichloromethane with diethyl ether (2:1–1:1) as the eluent [18].

(E)-N-Butyl-3-(3,4-dihydroxyphenyl)acrylamide (**3a**). Yield: 65%; ^{1}H NMR (DMSO-d_6, 500 MHz) δ: 9.30 (s, 1H), 9.07 (s, 1H), 7.90 (t, J = 5.6 Hz, 1H), 7.19 (d, J = 15.7 Hz, 1H), 6.91 (d, J = 2.0 Hz, 1H), 6.80 (dd, J = 8.1, 1.9 Hz, 1H), 6.71 (d, J = 8.1 Hz, 1H), 6.29 (d, J = 15.7 Hz, 1H), 3.30 (s, 2H), 3.12 (dd, J = 12.8, 6.8 Hz, 2H), 1.97 (s, 2H), 1.48–1.36 (m, 2H), 1.36–1.16 (m, 2H), 0.90–0.81 (m, 3H). ^{13}C NMR (126 MHz, DMSO) δ: 165.6, 139.2, 126.8, 120.6, 119.0, 116.14, 114.18, 38.66, 31.75, 20.04, 14.09. ESI-MS (*m*/*z*): 236.12 [M + 1]. High performace liquid chromatograph (HPLC) purity: 97%. Anal. calcd for $C_{13}H_{17}NO_3$: C 66.36, H 7.28, N 5.95, O 20.40, found: C 66.27, H 7.18, N 5.90.

(E)-N-(Cyclopropylmethyl)-3-(3,4-dihydroxyphenyl)acrylamide (**3b**). Yield: 55%; ^{1}H NMR (DMSO-d_6, 400 MHz) δ: 9.36 (s, 1H), 9.13 (s, 1H), 8.05–8.08 (m, 1H), 7.22 (d, J = 16 Hz, 1H), 6.94 (s, 1H), 6.83 (d, J = 8.0 Hz, 1H), 6.74 (d, J = 8.4 Hz, 1H), 6.35 (d, J = 16.0 Hz, 1H), 3.04 (t, J = 6.0 Hz, 2H), 0.40–0.44 (m, 2H), 0.16–0.19 (m, 2H). ESI-MS (*m*/*z*): 234.11 [M + 1]. HPLC purity: 96.5%.

(E)-3-(3,4-Dihydroxyphenyl)-1-(piperidin-1-yl)prop-2-en-1-one (**3c**). Yield: 35%; ^{1}H NMR (DMSO-d_6, 400 MHz) δ: 9.42 (s, 1H), 8.97 (s, 1H), 7.3 (d, J = 15.2 Hz, 1H), 7.08 (s, 1H), 6.89–6.98 (m, 2H), 6.73 (d, J = 15.2 Hz, 1H), 3.51–3.59 (m, br, 4H), 1.48–1.60 (m, 6H). ESI-MS (*m*/*z*): 248.02 [M + 1]. HPLC purity: 98%.

(E)-3-(3,4-Dihydroxyphenyl)-1-(pyrrolidin-1-yl)prop-2-en-1-one (**3d**). Yield: 45%; ^{1}H NMR (DMSO-d_6, 400 MHz) δ: 9.47 (s, 1H), 9.10 (s, 1H), 7.29 (d, J = 15.2 Hz, 1H), 7.05 (s, 1H), 6.96 (d, J = 8.0 Hz, 1H), 6.74 (d, J = 7.6 Hz, 1H), 6.64 (d, J = 15.2 Hz, 1H), 3.59 (t, J = 6.0 Hz, 2H), 3.67 (t, J = 6.0 Hz, 2H), 1.90 (m, 2H), 1.79 (m, 2H). ESI-MS (*m*/*z*): 234.1 [M + 1]. HPLC purity: 97%.

(E)-1-(Aziridin-1-yl)-3-(3,4-dihydroxyphenyl)prop-2-en-1-one (**3e**). Yield: 69%; ^{1}H NMR (DMSO-d_6, 400 MHz) δ: 9.37 (s, 1H), 9.14 (s, 1H), 7.22 (d, J = 15.6 Hz, 1H), 6.92 (s, 1H), 6.82 (d, J = 8.0 Hz, 1H), 6.73 (d, J = 8.0 Hz, 1H), 6.23 (d, J = 15.6 Hz, 1H), 0.64–0.67 (m, 2H), 0.42–0.43 (m, 2H). ESI-MS (*m*/*z*): 206.07 [M + 1]. HPLC purity: 97.2%.

(E)-N,N-Dibutyl-3-(3,4-dihydroxyphenyl)acrylamide (**3f**). Yield: 57%; ^{1}H NMR (DMSO-d_6, 400 MHz) δ: 9.41 (s, 1H), 9.04 (s, 1H), 7.30 (d, J = 15.2 Hz, 1H), 7.04 (s, 1H), 6.94 (d, J = 8.0 Hz, 1H), 6.73–6.77 (m, 2H), 3.41 (t, J = 7.2 Hz, 2H), 3.30(t, J = 7.2 Hz, 2H), 1.0–1.5 (m, 8H), 0.87–0.94 (m, 6H). ESI-MS (*m*/*z*): 292.02 [M + 1]. HPLC purity: 98%.

(E)-N-(3,5-Bis(trifluoromethyl)phenyl)-3-(3,4-dihydroxyphenyl)acrylamide (**3g**). Yield: 90%; 1H NMR (DMSO-d_6, 400 MHz) δ: 10.46 (s, 1H), 9.50 (s, 1H), 9.24 (s, 1H), 7.39–7.48 (m, 3H), 7.02 (s, 1H), 6.88–6.94 (m, 2H), 6.78 (d, J = 8.0 Hz, 1H), 6.47 (d, J = 15.2 Hz, 1H). ESI-MS (*m*/*z*): 392.06 [M + 1]. HPLC purity: 96%.

(E)-N-(3,5-Difluorophenyl)-3-(3,4-dihydroxyphenyl)acrylamide (**3h**). Yield: 71%; ^{1}H NMR (DMSO-d_6, 500 MHz) δ: 7.46–7.22 (m, 3H), 7.00 (d, J = 1.7 Hz, 1H), 6.95–6.80 (m, 2H), 6.76 (d, J = 8.1 Hz, 1H), 6.45 (d, J = 15.6 Hz, 1H). ^{13}C NMR (126 MHz, DMSO) δ: 164.9, 163.7, 161.9, 148.5, 146.0, 142.4, 126.2, 121.5, 116.2, 114.4, 102.2. ESI-MS (*m*/*z*): 292.07 [M + 1]. HPLC purity: 97.2%. Anal. calcd for $C_{15}H_{11}F_2NO_3$: C 61.86, H 3.81, F 13.05, N 4.81, O 16.48, found: C 61.76, H 3.80, F 13.00, N 4.69, O 16.27.

(E)-3-(3,4-Dihydroxyphenyl)-N-(3-(trifluoromethyl)phenyl)acrylamide (**3i**). Yield: 59%; ^{1}H NMR (DMSO-d_6, 500 MHz) δ: 8.18 (s, 1H), 7.83 (d, *J* = 8.4 Hz, 1H), 7.53 (dd, *J* = 14.6, 6.6 Hz, 1H), 7.43 (d, *J* = 15.6 Hz, 1H), 7.37 (d, *J* = 7.7 Hz, 1H), 7.00 (d, *J* = 1.9 Hz, 1H), 6.91 (d, *J* = 8.2, 2.0 Hz, 1H), 6.76 (d, *J* = 8.1 Hz, 1H), 6.50 (d, *J* = 15.6 Hz, 1H). ^{13}C NMR (126 MHz, DMSO) δ: 164.91, 148.38, 146.06, 142.00, 140.66, 130.40, 126.38, 122.99, 121.45, 119.73, 118.14–117.25, 116.24, 115.50, 114.43. ESI-MS (*m*/*z*): 324.08 [M + 1]. HPLC purity: 98%. Anal. calcd for $C_{16}H_{12}F_3NO_3$:C 59.45, H 3.74, F 17.63, N 4.33, O 14.85, found: C59.35, H 3.50, F 17.53, N 4.31, O 14.65.

(E)-3-(3,4-Dihydroxyphenyl)-N-(4-methoxyphenyl)acrylamide (**3j**). Yield: 78%; ^{1}H NMR (DMSO-d_6, 500 MHz) δ: 9.90 (s, 1H), 7.58 (d, *J* = 9.0 Hz, 2H), 7.35 (d, *J* = 15.6 Hz, 1H), 6.98 (d, *J* = 1.8 Hz, 1H), 6.90–6.82 (m, 3H), 6.75 (d, *J* = 8.1 Hz, 1H), 6.49 (d, *J* = 15.6 Hz, 1H), 3.71 (s, 3H). ^{13}C NMR (DMSO-d$_6$, 126 MHz,) δ: 163.9, 155.5, 147.9, 146.0, 140.6, 133.1, 126.7, 121.0, 118.99 (s, 3H), 116.2, 114.3, 55.5. ESI-MS (*m*/*z*): 286.1 [M + 1]. HPLC purity: 96.6%. Anal. calcd for $C_{15}H_{16}NO_4$: C 67.36, H 5.34, N 4.91, O 22.43, found: C 67.20, H 5.22, N 4.90. O 22.25.

(E)-3-(3,4-Dihydroxyphenyl)-N-(4-fluorophenyl)acrylamide (**3k**). Yield: 61%; ^{1}H NMR (DMSO-d_6, 500 MHz) δ: 10.09 (s, 1H), 9.33 (br, 2H), 7.68 (d, *J* = 14.1 Hz, 2H), 7.38 (d, *J* = 15.6 Hz, 1H), 7.13 (d, *J* = 15.6 Hz, 2H), 6.98 (s, 1H), 6.88 (dt, *J* = 15.2, 7.6 Hz, 1H), 6.75 (d, *J* = 8.1 Hz, 1H), 6.48 (d, *J* = 6.0 Hz, 1H). ^{13}C NMR (DMSO-d_6, 126 MHz) δ: 164.3, 159.2, 157.3, 146.0, 141.2, 121.2, 118.6, 116.2, 115.83, 115.7, 114.3. ESI-MS (*m*/*z*): 274.08 [M + 1]. HPLC purity: 97.4%. Anal. calcd for $C_{15}H_{12}FNO_3$:C 65.93, H 4.43, F 6.95, N 5.13, O 17.57, found: C 65.65, H 4.35, F 6.72, N 5.05, O 17.37.

(E)-3-(3,4-Dihydroxyphenyl)-N-(2-(hydroxymethyl)phenyl)acrylamide (**3l**). Yield: 63%; ^{1}H NMR (DMSO-d_6, 400 MHz) δ: 9.48 (s, 1H), 9.46 (s, 1H), 9.17 (s, 1H), 7.76 (d, *J* = 4.0 Hz, 1H), 7.36–7.43 (m, 2H), 7.25 (t, *J* = 8.0 Hz, 1H), 7.15 (t, *J* = 8.0 Hz, 1H), 7.03 (s, 1H), 6.92 (d, *J* = 8.8 Hz, 1H), 6.77 (d, *J* = 8.4 Hz, 1H), 6.60 (d, *J* = 15.2 Hz, 1H), 4.53 (s, 2H). ESI-MS (*m*/*z*): 286.1 [M + 1]. HPLC purity: 97.6%.

(E)-N-(2-Acetylphenyl)-3-(3,4-dihydroxyphenyl)acrylamide (**3m**). Yield: 53%; ^{1}H NMR (DMSO-d_6, 400 MHz) δ: 11.39 (s, 1H), 9.55 (s, 1H), 9.16 (s, 1H), 8.42 (d, *J* = 8.0 Hz, 1H), 8.00 (d, *J* = 8.0 Hz, 1H), 7.62 (t, *J* = 7.6 Hz, 2H), 7.44 (d, *J* = 15.2 Hz, 1H), 7.22 (t, *J* = 7.6 Hz, 1H), 7.09 (s, 1H), 7.01 (d, *J* = 8.0 Hz, 1H), 6.78 (d, 2H, *J* = 8.0 Hz), 6.53 (d, *J* = 15.2 Hz, 1H), 2.64 (s, 3H). ESI-MS (*m*/*z*): 298.1 [M + 1]. HPLC purity: 97.8%.

(E)-N-(3-Chlorophenyl)-3-(3,4-dihydroxyphenyl)acrylamide (**3n**). Yield: 72%; ^{1}H NMR (DMSO-d_6, 400 MHz) δ: 10.27 (s, 1H), 9.51 (s, 1H), 9.23 (s, 1H), 7.93 (s, 1H), 7.51 (d, *J* = 8.0 Hz, 1H), 7.42 (d, *J* = 15.2 Hz, 1H), 7.36 (t, *J* = 8.0 Hz, 1H), 7.10 (d, *J* = 8.0 Hz, 1H), 7.01 (s, 1H), 6.92 (d, *J* = 8.0 Hz, 1H), 6.78 (d, *J* = 8.0 Hz, 1H), 6.50 (d, *J* = 15.2 Hz, 1H). ESI-MS (*m*/*z*): 290.02 [M + 1]. HPLC purity: 97.9%.

(E)-N-(3-Bromophenyl)-3-(3,4-dihydroxyphenyl)acrylamide (**3o**). Yield: 67%; ^{1}H NMR (DMSO-d_6, 400 MHz) δ: 10.24 (s, 1H), 9.51 (s, 1H), 9.22 (s, 1H), 8.06 (s, 1H), 7.55 (d, *J* = 8.0 Hz, 1H), 7.42 (d, *J* = 15.2 Hz, 1H), 7.22–7.30 (m, 2H), 7.01 (s, 1H), 6.92 (d, *J* = 8.0 Hz, 1H), 6.77 (d, *J* = 8.0 Hz, 1H), 6.50 (d, *J* = 15.2 Hz, 1H). ESI-MS (*m*/*z*): 334.16 [M + 1]. HPLC purity: 97.6%.

(E)-3-(3,4-Dihydroxyphenyl)-N-p-tolylacrylamide (**3p**). Yield: 76%; ^{1}H NMR (DMSO-d_6, 400 MHz) δ: 9.98 (s, 1H), 9.44 (s, 1H), 9.20 (s, 1H), 7.57 (d, J = 6.8 Hz, 2H), 7.38 (d, J = 15.2 Hz, 1H), 7.20 (d, J = 6.8 Hz, 2H), 7.00 (s, 1H), 6.90 (d, J = 8.0 Hz, 1H), 6.77 (d, J = 8.0 Hz, 1H), 6.52 (d, J = 15.2 Hz, 1H), 2.26 (s, 3H). ESI-MS (*m/z*): 270.11 [M + 1]. HPLC purity: 97.3%.

(E)-3-(3,4-Dihydroxyphenyl)-N-o-tolylacrylamide (**3q**). Yield: 68%; ^{1}H NMR (DMSO-d_6, 400 MHz) δ: 9.45 (s, 1H), 9.32 (s, 1H), 9.17 (s, 1H), 7.58 (d, J = 8.0 Hz, 1H), 7.38 (d, J = 15.2 Hz, 1H), 7.16–7.23 (m, 2H), 7.01–7.08 (m, 2H), 6.91 (d, J = 8.0 Hz, 1H), 6.77 (d, J = 8.0 Hz, 1H), 6.68 (d, J = 15.2 Hz, 1H), 2.24 (s, 3H). ESI-MS (*m/z*): 270.1 [M + 1]. HPLC purity: 96%.

(E)-N-Benzyl-3-(3,4-dihydroxyphenyl)-N-methylacrylamide (**3r**). Yield: 64%; ^{1}H NMR (DMSO-d_6, 400 MHz) δ: 9.41 (s, 1H), 9.00 (s, 1H), 7.21–7.40 (m, 6H), 6.89–7.01 (m, 3H), 6.71–6.76 (m, 1H), 4.69 (s, 2H), 2.98 (s, 3H). ESI-MS (*m/z*): 284.12 [M + 1]. HPLC purity: 97%.

(E)-N-(2-(1H-Indol-3-yl)ethyl)-3-(3,4-dihydroxyphenyl)acrylamide (**3s**). Yield: 91%; ^{1}H NMR (DMSO-d_6, 500 MHz) δ: 10.78 (s, 1H), 9.20 (d, J = 101.6 Hz, 2H), 8.07 (t, J = 5.7 Hz, 1H), 7.54 (d, J = 7.9 Hz, 1H), 7.32 (d, J = 8.1 Hz, 1H), 7.23 (d, J = 15.6 Hz, 1H), 7.14 (s, 1H), 7.04 (dd, J = 11.1, 4.0 Hz, 1H), 7.00–6.88 (m, 2H), 6.81 (dd, J = 8.2, 1.9 Hz, 1H), 6.73 (d, J = 8.1 Hz, 1H), 6.32 (d, J = 15.7 Hz, 1H), 3.44 (d, J = 13.4, 7.1 Hz, 2H), 2.86 (t, J = 7.4 Hz, 2H). ^{13}C NMR (DMSO-d_6, 126 MHz) δ: 165.7, 147.6, 145.9, 139.3, 136.6, 127.6, 126.8, 123.0, 121.3, 120.7, 119.1, 118.6, 116.1, 114.2, 112.2, 111.7, 31.0, 25.7. ESI-MS (*m/z*): 323.13 [M + 1]. HPLC purity: 98%. Anal. calcd for $C_{20}H_{20}N_2O_3$: C 71.41, H 5.99, N 8.33, O 14.24, found: C 71.26, H 5.55, N 8.12, O 14.17.

(E)-N-(2-(Benzo[d][1,3]dioxol-5-yl)ethyl)-3-(3,4-dihydroxyphenyl)acrylamide (**3t**). Yield: 52%; ^{1}H NMR (DMSO-d_6, 500 MHz) δ: 9.37 (s, 1H), 9.14 (s, 1H), 8.03 (t, J = 5.5 Hz, 1H), 7.22 (d, J = 15.7 Hz, 1H), 6.93 (s, 1H), 6.82 (d, J = 7.9 Hz, 3H), 6.73 (d, J = 8.1 Hz, 1H), 6.67 (d, J = 8.0 Hz, 1H), 6.31 (d, J = 15.7 Hz, 1H), 5.96 (s, 2H), 3.37–3.29 (m, 4H), 2.69 (dd, J = 18.5, 11.2 Hz, 2H). ^{13}C NMR (DMSO-d_6, 126 MHz) δ: 165.7, 161.3, 147.5, 145.9, 139.3, 133.5, 126.8, 121.9, 120.7, 118.9, 116.1, 114.2, 109.4, 108.5, 101.0, 35.2, 35.0. ESI-MS (*m/z*): 228.3 [M + 1]. HPLC purity: 97.7%. Anal. calcd for $C_{18}H_{17}NO_5$: C 66.05, H 5.23, N 4.28, O 24.44, found: C 65.95, H 5.13, N 4.15, O 24.26.

3.2. Biology

3.2.1. Cell Culture

RAW 264.7 murine macrophages were obtained from the Shanghai Institute of Cell Biology, Chinese Academy of Sciences (Shanghai, China) and maintained in DMEM recommended by the suppliers, supplemented with 10% fetal bovine serum (Gibco, Paisley, UK), penicillin (100 U/mL) and streptomycin (100 mg/mL) in a humidified 5% CO_2 atmosphere at 37 °C.

3.2.2. Measurement of Nitric Oxide

The amount of NO was assessed by determining the nitrite concentration with Griess reagent. Briefly, in the experiment to assess NO in culture supernatants, RAW 264.7 macrophages were seeded into 48-well plates (2 × 10^6 cells per mL) for 18 h. Then, the cells were pretreated each sample, aminoguanidine or vehicle solution for 20 min, then stimulated with LPS (1 μg/mL) for 18 h. Samples of supernatants (100 mL) were incubated with 50 mL 1% sulfanilamide, then 50 mL of 0.1% naphthylethylenediamine in 2.5% phosphoric acid solution. The absorbance at 570 nm was read and referred to a standard curve of sodium nitrite solution to determine the nitrite concentration. In the other experiment to determine the NO concentration of exudates from rat air pouches, the exudates (50 mL) were incubated with nitrate reductase solution (200 mL; Jiancheng Bioengineering Institute, Nanjing, China) at 37 °C for 1 h. Nitrate was converted into nitrite. After centrifugation, the nitrite concentration in the cell-free supernatants was assessed with Griess reagent as described above [24].

3.3. Computational Protocols

3.3.1. Pharmacophore Generation

All the studies were carried out using Discovery Studio (DS) 2.5 unless it is mentioned. Seven most active compounds as shown in Figure 2 were selected as a training set to generate qualitative pharmacophore models to be used in future database screening to identify new scaffolds for drug discovery. The 2D chemical structures of the training set compounds were built using ChemSketch program version 12, and subsequently converted into 3D structures using DS. All compounds in the training set were given a Principal value of 2 and a Maximum Omitted Feature value of 0 to make sure that all the features of these compounds are considered during pharmacophore generation. Diverse conformational models for every training set compound were generated to cover the flexibility of their chemical nature using polling algorithm. All the compounds were energetically minimized using CHARMM force field implemented in DS. Diverse Conformation Generation protocol with BEST flexible search option implemented in DS was employed with the default value of generating maximum of 250 conformers within the energy range of 20 kcal/mol, with respect to the global minimum. Feature mapping protocol was employed prior to the original pharmacophore generation calculation to identify the chemical features present in the training set compounds. The chemical features such as hydrogen bond acceptor (HBA), hydrogen bond donor (HBD) and hydrophobic (HY) features were used during pharmacophore generation. These chemical features were selected based on the feature mapping results and the possible interaction points. All the other parameters were maintained at their default settings. The seven compounds in the training set along with the generated conformational models were used in pharmacophore model generation. Common feature pharmacophore models, generally, are developed by comparing a set of conformational models and a number of 3D configurations of chemical features shared among the training set compounds. Common Feature Pharmacophore Model Generation protocol implemented in DS was used to generate pharmacophore models. Minimum interfeature distance was 0.5. The other parameters were default.

3.3.2. Molecular Docking Study

All the molecular docking studies were performed by GOLD 5.1 program with ChemPLP function score (Cambridge Crystallographic Data Center, London, UK). X-ray crystal structures (PDB ID:

1LOS, PDB ID: 1QXO, PDB ID: 5P21) were used to define the binding site for molecular docking studies. The radius of 12 Å around the active compound was defined to form the active site of the protein.

4. Conclusions

In summary, we rationally designed a series of caffeic acid amide analogues. The preliminary biological evaluations revealed that this class of compounds possessed moderate to good anti-inflammatory activity. A 3D pharmacophore model was then generated based on the biological activity and the better understanding of this feature could provide meaningful insights for further optimization. Potential targets were also predicted by the PharmMapper server. A further study of the structural modification and biological target validation are in process in our laboratory and will be reported elsewhere.

Acknowledgments

The work was supported by programfor New Century Excellent Talents in University Foundation, National Natural Science Foundation of China (81230090), partially supported by Global Research Network for Medicinal Plants (GRNMP) and King Saud University, Shanghai Leading Academic Discipline Project (B906), Key laboratory of drug research for special environments, PLA, Shanghai Engineering Research Center for the Preparation of Bioactive Natural Products (10DZ2251300), the Scientific Foundation of Shanghai China (12401900801,09DZ1975700, 09DZ1971500, 10DZ1971700), National Major Project of China (2011ZX09307-002-03), and National Key Technology R&D Program of China (2012BAI29B06).

Author Contributions

Zhiqian Liu: acquisition of data; analysis and interpretation of data; and drafting of the manuscript; Jianjun Fu, Lei Shan and Qingyan Sun funding obtained and study supervision. All authors read and approved the final manuscript. Weidong Zhang administrative support; and study supervision; and review of the manuscript.

References

1. Hu, J.; Wang, Y.; Wei, X.; Wu, X.; Chen, G.; Cao, G.; Shen, X.; Zhang, X.; Tang, Q.; Liang, G.; *et al.* Synthesis and biological evaluation of novel thiazolidinone derivatives as potential anti-inflammatory agents. *Eur. J. Med. Chem.* **2013**, *64*, 292–301.
2. Uwai, K.; Osanai, Y.; Imaizumi, T.; Kanno, S.; Takeshita, M.; Ishikawa, M. Inhibitory effect of the alkyl side chain of caffeic acid analogues on lipopolysaccharide-induced nitric oxide production in RAW264.7 macrophages. *Bioorg. Med. Chem.* **2008**, *16*, 7795–7803.
3. O'Sullivan, L.A.; Liongue, C.; Lewis, R.S.; Stephenson, S.E.; Ward, A.C. Cytokine receptor signaling through the Jak-Stat-Socs pathway in disease. *Mol. Immunol.* **2007**, *44*, 2497–2506.

4. Jacques, C.; Gosset, M.; Berenbaum, F. The role of IL-1 and IL-1Ra in joint inflammation and cartilage degradation. *Vitam. Horm.* **2006**, *74*, 371–403.
5. Reber, L.; da Silva, C.A.; Frossard, N. Stem cell factor and its receptor c-Kit as targets for inflammatory diseases. *Eur. J. Pharmacol.* **2006**, *533*, 327–340.
6. Flaster, H.; Bernhagen, J.; Calandra, T.; Bucala, R. The macrophage migration inhibitory factor-glucocorticoid dyad: Regulation of inflammation and immunity. *Mol. Endocrinol.* **2007**, *21*, 1267–1280.
7. Dalli, J.; Norling, L.V.; Renshaw, D.; Cooper, D.; Leung, K.Y.; Perretti, M. Annexin 1 mediates the rapid anti-inflammatory effects of neutrophil-derived microparticles. *Blood* **2008**, *112*, 2512–2519.
8. De Lucca, G.V. Recent developments in CCR3 antagonists. *Curr. Opin. Drug Discov. Devel.* **2006**, *9*, 516–524.
9. Chen, J.F.; Pedata, F. Modulation of ischemic brain injury and neuroin-flammation by adenosine A2A receptors. *Curr. Pharm. Des.* **2008**, *14*, 1490–1499.
10. Luger, T.A.; Brzoska, T. Alpha-MSH related peptides: A new class of anti-inflammatory and immunomodulating drugs. *Ann. Rheum. Dis.* **2007**, *66*, 52–55.
11. Ghosh, S.; May, M.J.; Kopp, E.B. NF-kappa B and Rel proteins: evolutionarily conserved mediators of immune responses. *Annu. Rev. Immunol.* **1998**, *16*, 225–260.
12. Li, L.; Zeng, H.W.; Liu, F.; Zhang, J.G.; Yue, R.C.; Lu, W.Q.; Yuan, X.; Dai, W.X.; Yuan, H.; Sun Q.Y.; *et al.* Target identification and validation of (+)-2-(1-hydroxyl-4-oxocyclohexyl) ethyl caffeate, An anti-inflammatory natural product. *Eur. J. Inflamm.* **2012**, *10*, 297–309.
13. Santos, S.A.; Freire, C.S.; Domingues, M.R.; Silvestre, A.J.; Pascoal, N.C. Characterization of phenolic components in polar extracts of *Eucalyptus globulus* Labill bark by high-performance liquid chromatography-mass spectrometry. *J. Agric. Food Chem.* **2011**, *59*, 9386–9393.
14. Choudhary, M.I.; Naheed, N.; Abbaskhan, A.; Musharraf, S.G.; Siddiqui, H.; Atta-Ur-Rahman. Phenolic and other constituents of fresh water fern Salvinia molesta. *Phytochemistry* **2008**, *69*, 1018–1023.
15. Lee., Y.S.; Kang, Y.H.; Jung, J.Y.; Lee, S.; Ohuchi, K.; Shin, KH.; Kang, I.J.; Park, J.H.; Shin, H.K.; Lim, S.S. Protein Glycation Inhibitors from the Fruiting Body of *Phellinus linteus*. *Biol. Pharm. Bull.* **2008**, *31*, 1968–1972.
16. Nagaoka, T.; Banskota, A.H.; Tezuka, Y.; Midorikawa, K. Caffeic acid phenethyl ester (CAPE) analogues: Potent nitric oxide inhibitors from the Netherlands propolis. *Biol. Pharm. Bull.* **2003**, *26*, 487–491.
17. Sherif, Y.E.; Fu, J.; Lotfy, M.; Zhu, H.L. QSAR study for newly caffeic acid amides with prominent antibacterial and antifungal activity. *Der Pharma Chem.* **2010**, *2*, 105.
18. Fu, J.; Cheng, K.; Zhang, Z.M.; Fang, R.Q.; Zhu, H.L. Synthesis, structure and structure–activity relationship analysis of caffeic acid amides as potential antimicrobials. *Eur. J. Med. Chem.* **2010**, *45*, 2638–2643.
19. Lyne, P.D. Structure-based virtual screening: An overview. *Drug Discov. Today* **2002**, *7*, 1047–1055.
20. Nagarajan, S.; Choo, H.; Cho, Y.S.; Oh, K.S.; Lee, B.H.; Shin, K.J.; Pae, A.N. IKKbeta inhibitors identification part II: Ligand and structure-based virtual screening. *Bioorg. Med. Chem.* **2010**, *18*, 3951–3960.

21. Liu, X.; Ouyang, S.; Yu, B.; Liu, Y.; Huang, K.; Gong, J.; Zheng, S.; Li, Z.; Li, H.; Jiang, H. PharmMapper server: A Web server for potential drug target identification using pharmacophore mapping approach. *Nucleic. Acids Res.* **2010**, *38*, 609–614.
22. Hung, C.C.; Tsai, W.J.; Kuo, L.M.; Kuo, Y.H. Evaluation of caffeic acid amide analogues as anti-platelet aggregation and anti-oxidative agents. *Bioorg. Med. Chem.* **2005**, *13*, 1791–1797.
23. Pharmmapper. Available online: http://59.78.96.61/pharmmapper/index.php (access on 23 June 2013).
24. Zeng, H.; Liu, X.; Dou, S.; Xu, W.; Li, N.; Liu, X., Zhang, W.; Hu, Z.; Liu, R. Huang-Lian-Jie-Du-Tang exerts anti-inflammatory effects in rats through inhibition of nitric oxide production and eicosanoid biosynthesis via the lipoxygenase pathway. *J. Pharm. Pharmacol.* **2009**, *61*, 1699–707.

3

Synthesis, Characterization and Anti-Breast Cancer Activity of New 4-Aminoantipyrine-Based Heterocycles

Mostafa M. Ghorab [1,*], Marwa G. El-Gazzar [2] and Mansour S. Alsaid [1]

1 Department of Pharmacognosy, College of Pharmacy, King Saud University, P.O. Box 2457, Riyadh 11451, Saudi Arabia; E-Mail: msalsaid@ksu.edu.sa

2 Department of Drug Radiation Research, National Center for Radiation Research and Technology, Nasr City, Cairo 113701, Egypt; E-Mail: marwagalalgazzar@yahoo.com

* Author to whom correspondence should be addressed; E-Mail: mmsghorab@yahoo.com

---

Abstract: 4-Aminoantipyrine was utilized as key intermediate for the synthesis of pyrazolone derivatives bearing biologically active moieties. The newly synthesized compounds were characterized by IR, ^{1}H- and ^{13}C-NMR spectral and microanalytical studies. The compounds were screened as anticancer agents against a human tumor breast cancer cell line MCF7, and the results showed that (*Z*)-4-((3-amino-5-imino-1-phenyl-1*H*-pyrazol-4(5*H*)-ylidene)methylamino)-1,5-dimethyl-2-phenyl-1,2-dihydropyrazol-3-one **5**, 3-(4-bromophenyl) -1-(1,5-dimethyl-3-oxo-2-phenyl-2,3-dihydro-1*H*-pyrazol-4-yl)-4-oxo-2-thioxo-1,2,3,4-tetrahydropyrimidine-5-carbonitrile **13**, 1-(1,5-dimethyl-3-oxo-2-phenyl-2,3-dihydro-1*H*-pyrazol-4-yl)-3-(4-iodophenyl)-4-oxo-2-thioxo-1,2,3,4-tetrahydropyrimidine-5-carbonitrile **14**, 3,3′-(4,4′-sulfonylbis(4,1-phenylene))bis(1-(1,5-dimethyl-3-oxo-2-phenyl-2,3-dihydro-1*H*-pyrazol-4-yl)-4-oxo-2-thioxo-1,2,3,4-tetrahydropyrimidine-5-carbonitrile) **16**, (*Z*)-1-(1,5-dimethyl-3-oxo-2-phenyl-2,3-dihydro-1*H*-pyrazol-4-yl)-2-hydrazono-4-oxo-3-phenyl-1,2,3,4-tetrahydropyrimidine-5-carbonitrile **17**, (*Z*)-1-(1,5-dimethyl-3-oxo-2-phenyl-2,3-dihydro-1*H*-pyrazol-4-yl)-4-oxo-3-phenyl-2-(2-phenylhydrazono)-1,2,3,4-tetrahydro pyrimidine-5-carbonitrile **18**, and (*Z*)-4-(3-amino-6-hydrazono-7-phenyl-6,7-dihydro pyrazolo[3,4-*d*]pyrimidin-5-yl)-1,5-dimethyl-2-phenyl-1,2-dihydropyrazol-3-one **19** were the most active compounds with IC_{50} values ranging from 30.68 to 60.72 μM compared with Doxorubicin as positive control with the IC_{50} value 71.8 μM.

Keywords: pyrazoles; sulfonamides; anti-breast cancer

1. Introduction

Pyrazolone derivatives such as antipyrine, aminopyrine, and dipyrone are well known compounds used mainly as analgesic and antipyretic drugs and their pharmacological molecular mechanism has been widely surveyed [1,2]. One of the best known antipyrine derivatives is 4-aminoantipyrine which is used for the protection against oxidative stress as well as prophylactic of some diseases including cancer, and these are important directions in medical applications [3]. Several derivatives of antipyrine were also biologically evaluated, and analgesic [4], anti-inflammatory [5], antimicrobial [6], and anticancer activity [7–9] have been reported. Antipyrine derivatives are strong inhibitors of cycloxygenase isoenzymes, platelet tromboxane synthesis, and prostanoids synthesis [10], which catalyze the rate-limiting step of prostaglandin synthesis. Pyrazolones are also a well-known elicitor of hypersensitivity [11]. Recently, Al-Haiza *et al.* [12] synthesized a new compound with pyrazolone moiety with antimicrobial and antifungal activities. In the last decade, several pyrazole derivatives proved to have potent anticancer action by the inhibition of the cyclindependent kinases (CDKs) which are members of the large family of protein kinases and are responsible for the eukaryotic cell cycle regulation; they are intensively studied for their cancer implication [13]. Based on the above information and due to our interest in pyrazole as a biologically active pharmacophore [14–18], we synthesized a new series of heterocycles incorporating antipyrine moiety starting from 4-aminoantipyrine to be evaluated for their anticancer activity against human tumor breast cell line (MCF7).

2. Results and Discussion

2.1. Chemistry

The starting key reagent 4-aminoantipyrine was purchased from Sigma-Aldrich chemical company (St. Louis, MO, USA). In this work, the reactivity of 4-aminoantipyrine with active methylene containing compounds (malononitrile, 2-(ethoxymethylene)malononitrile, ethylcyanoacetate, (ethoxymethylene)ethylcyanoacetate and acetylacetone) was studied and the reaction proceeded in the presence of triethylorthoformate in methanol containing catalytic amounts of acetic acid following the reported reaction condition [19]. The obtained pyrazolone derivatives **2**–**4**, respectively, were identified by elemental and spectral data. Due to the biological importance of pyrazole, pyrrole and pyrimidine rings as anticancer agents [20–22], the pyrazolone derivative **2** was reacted with different nucleophiles in order to obtain biologically active pyrazole **5**, pyrrole **6**–**8** and pyrimidine **9**–**16** derivatives bearing pyrazolone moieties. Thus, interaction of compound **2** with phenyl hydrazine yielded the corresponding pyrazole derivative **5**. On the other hand, interaction of compound **2** with 2-chloroacetonitrile, ethylbromoacetate or 2-chloroacetamide in dioxane containing a catalytic amount of triethylamine yielded the corresponding pyrrole derivatives **6**–**8**, respectively. Reaction of compound **2** with thiourea in refluxing ethanol containing sodium ethoxide gave the corresponding pyrimidine derivative **9** (Scheme 1). The reactivity of compound **2** towards different aryl isothiocyanates/NaOH was studied and the reaction proceeded via an addition reaction onto the isothiocyanato group followed by intramolecular cyclization to produce the pyrimidine ring as in compounds **10–15**. Similarly, the bis-compound **16** was obtained expectedly via the reaction of one mole of 1-(4-isothio cyanatophenylsulfonyl)-4-isothiocyanatobenzene with two moles of compound **2** in ethanol containing sodium ethoxide (Scheme 2). The hydrazono pyrimidine derivatives **17**, **18** were synthesized from compound **10** through reaction with either hydrazine hydrate or phenyl hydrazine, respectively, and the reaction proceeded via elimination of H_2S which was detected by a lead acetate paper. On the other hand, double cyclization took place when one mole of compound **10** was reacted with two moles of hydrazine hydrate to yield the corresponding pyrazolo[3,4-d]pyrimidine **19** (Scheme 3). Finally, treatment of 4-aminoantipyrine **1** with either triethylorthoformate or acetate in acetic anhydride resulted in the formation of compounds **20**, **21**, respectively (Scheme 4). The structures of compounds were proved by microanalytical and spectral data and were consistent with the proposed structures.

Scheme 1. Synthetic pathways for compounds **2–9**.

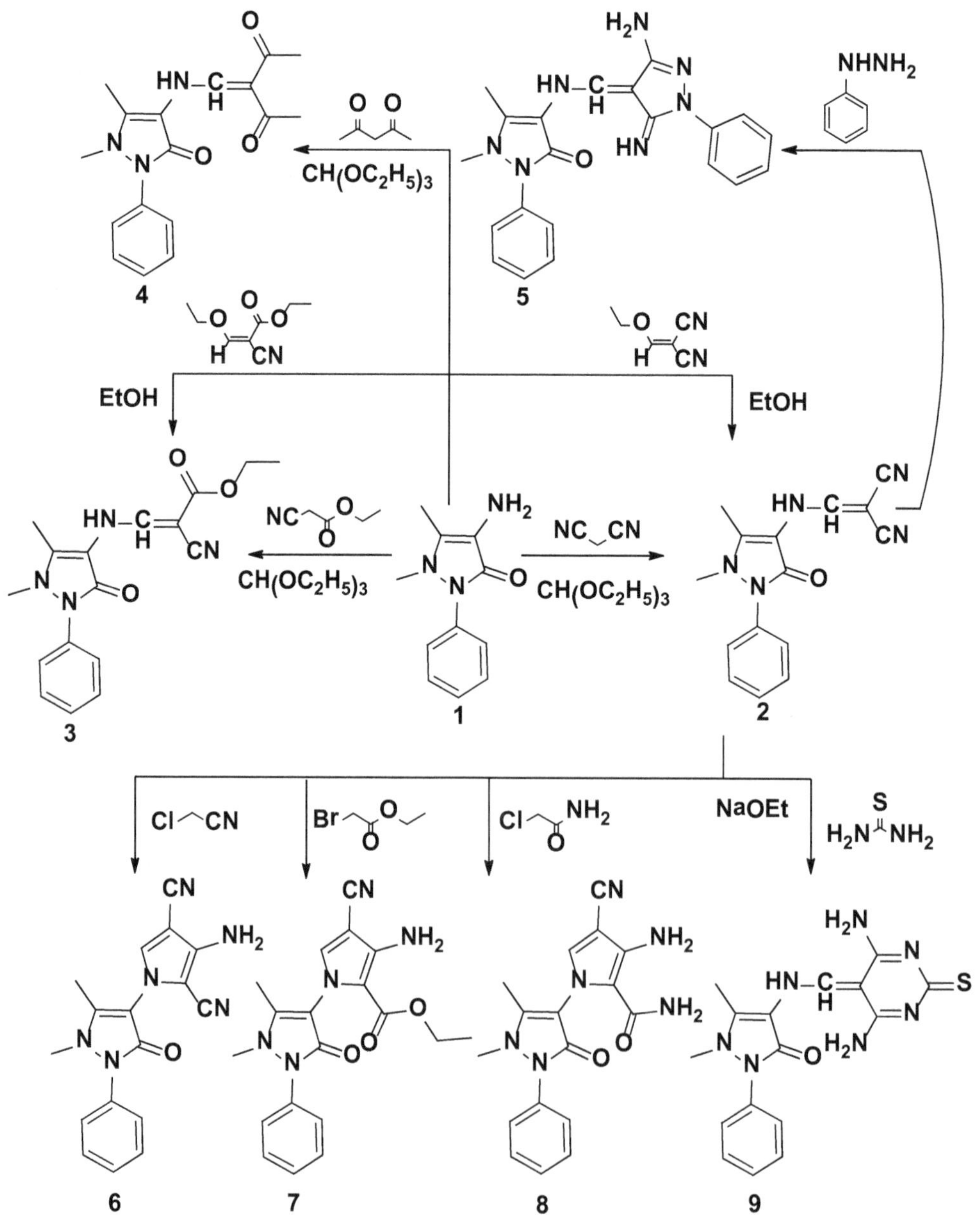

Scheme 2. Synthetic pathways for compounds **10–16**.

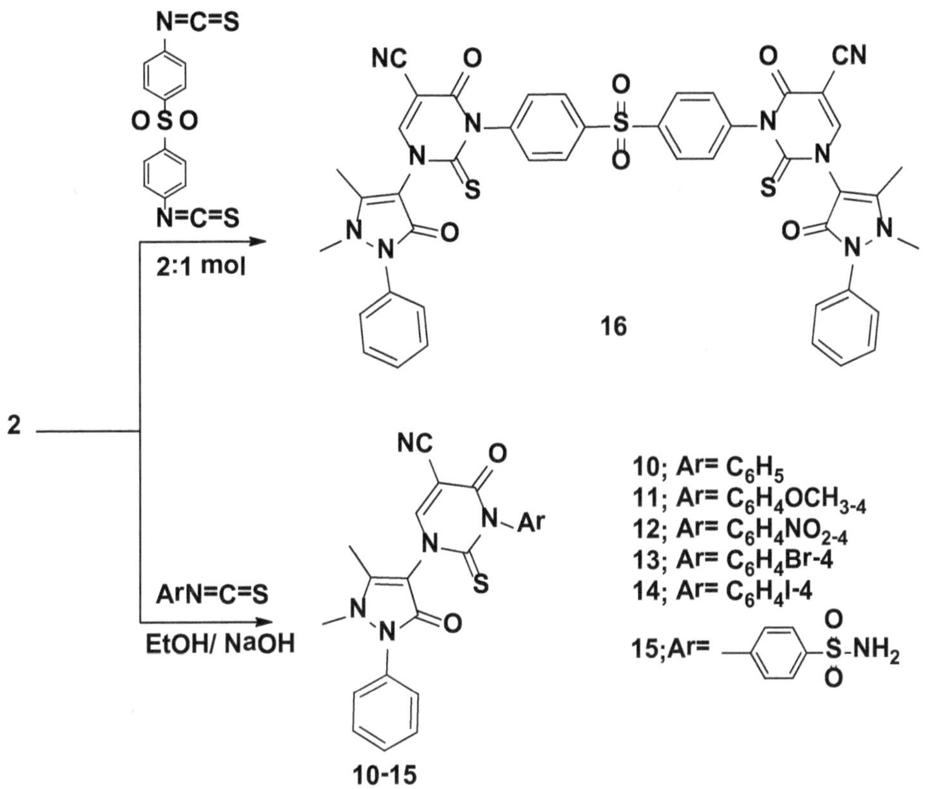

Scheme 3. Synthetic pathways for compounds **17–19**.

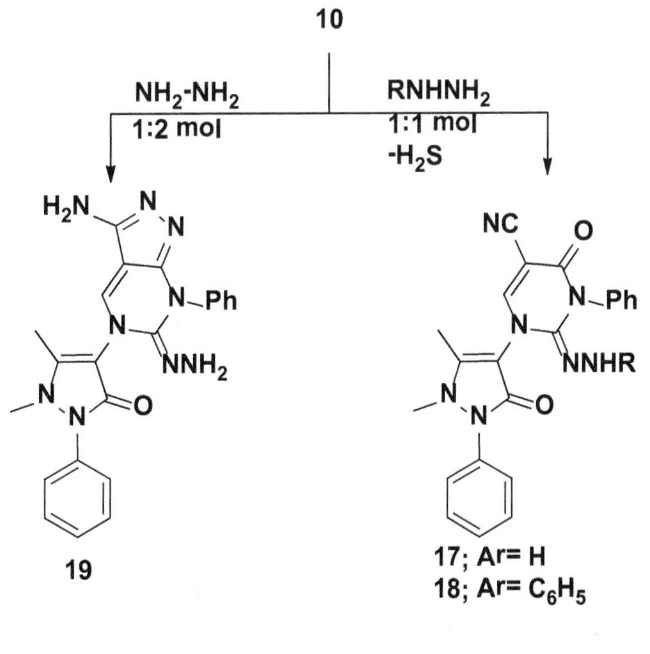

Scheme 4. Synthetic pathways for compounds **20**, **21**.

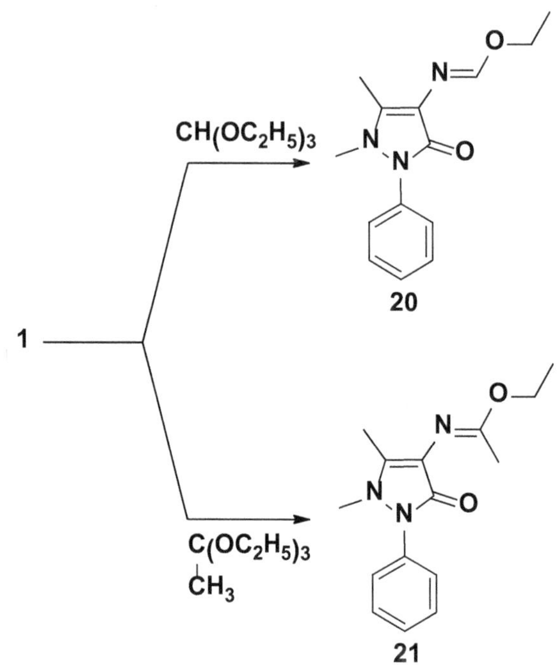

2.2. In-Vitro Anticancer Screening

Doxorubicin, the positive control used in this study, is an anticancer drug used to treat several cancer diseases including breast cancer. The relationship between surviving fraction and drug concentration was plotted; the response parameters calculated was IC_{50} value, which corresponds to the compound concentration causing 50% mortality in net cells (Table 1). The present work describes the synthesis of novel derivatives starting from 4-aminoantipyrine **1** by incorporating biologically active moieties, pyrazole, pyrrole, pyrimidine and pyrazolopyrimidine. From Table 1, we can observe that some of the tested compounds were found to be equipotent or even more potent than Doxorubicin on MCF7 cell line with IC_{50} values ranging from 30.68 to 70.65 µM compared to the reference drug (71.8 µM). The most potent compounds in this study were found to be those belonging to the pyrimidine derivatives of antipyrine especially the halogenated ones, where, the iodophenyl **14** (IC_{50} = 30.68 µM) and the bromophenyl **13** (IC_{50} = 43.41 µM) derivatives showed significant activities, also, the biscompound **16** (IC_{50} = 37.22 µM). In addition, pyrazole **5**, pyrimidines **17**, **18**, pyrazolopyrimidine **19** with IC_{50} values 60.72, 54.23, 44.99, and 44.49 µM exhibited a higher activity when compared with the Doxorubicin as positive control. The phenyl and 4-nitro phenyl derivatives **10** and **12** (IC_{50} = 72.04 and 70.65 µM) are nearly as active as Doxorubicin. On the other hand, reaction of one mole of hydrazine hydrate or phenyl hydrazine with compound **10** yielded the pyrimidine derivatives **17** and **18** with significant activities (IC_{50} = 54.23 and 44.99 µM), while, addition of two moles of hydrazine hydrate yielded the pyrazolopyrimidine **19** (IC_{50} = 44.49 µM) which is nearly as potent as compounds **17** and **18**. Moreover, the reaction of phenylhydrazine with compound **2** was also successful as it yielded the pyrazole derivative **5** which showed high activity (IC_{50} = 60.72 µM). All these compounds are more active than the reference drug. Considering the pyrrole derivatives **6**, **7** and **8**, they were found to exhibit lower activity compared to the reference drug (IC_{50} = 128.61, 104.11

and 85.12 μM, respectively). Compounds **2–4**, **9**, **11**, **15**, **20** and **21** are the least potent in this study with IC_{50} ranging from 109.58 to 173.83 μM.

Table 1. *In-vitro* anticancer screening of compounds **2–21** against human breast cell line (MCF7).

Compound No.	IC_{50} (μg/mL)	IC_{50} (μM)
2	48.2	173.83
3	38.0	116.56
4	34.9	111.50
5	23.5	60.72
6	40.9	128.61
7	38.0	104.11
8	28.6	85.12
9	38.9	109.58
10	29.9	72.04
11	NA	NA
12	32.5	70.65
13	21.4	43.41
14	16.6	30.68
15	NA	NA
16	33.2	37.22
17	22.4	54.23
18	22.0	44.99
19	19.0	44.49
20	35.8	138.22
21	NA	NA
Doxorubicin	39.0	71.8

NA: Compound having IC_{50} value > 100 μg/mL.

Generally, incorporation of pyrimidine ring yielded the most potent compounds and these results point to the possible use of pyrimidine derivatives of antipyrine for treatment of breast tumors.

3. Experimental Section

3.1. General

Reagents were obtained from commercial suppliers and were used without purification. Melting points were determined in open capillary tubes using Thermo system FP800 Mettler FP80 central processor supplied with FP81 MBC cell apparatus (Stuart Scientific, Redhill, UK), and were uncorrected. Elemental analyses (C, H, N) were performed on a Perkin-Elmer 2400 Instrument (Perkin-Elmer, Norwalk, CT, USA). All compounds were within ±0.4% of the theoretical values. Infrared (IR) spectra (KBr disc) were recorded on FT-IR spectrophotometer (Perkin Elmer, Norwalk, CT, USA) at the Research Center, College of Pharmacy, King Saud University, Saudi Arabia.^{1}H and ^{13}C NMR spectra were recorded on a Ultra Shield Plus 500 MHz (Bruker, Munich, Germany) spectrometer operating at 500 MHz for proton and 125 MHz for carbon, respectively. The chemical shift values are reported in δ (ppm) relative to the residual solvent peak, the coupling constants (*J*) are reported in Hertz (Hz).

3.2. Chemistry

3.2.1. 2-((1,5-Dimethyl-3-oxo-2-phenyl-2,3-dihydro-1*H*-pyrazol-4-ylamino)methylene)-malononitrile **2**

A mixture of 4-aminoantipyrine (0.01 mol), malononitrile (0.01 mol), triethylorthoformate (0.01 mol), and acetic acid (1 mL) in methanol (30 mL) was refluxed for 5 h, the reaction mixture was cooled, filtered, the filtered solid was crystallized from ethanol to give **2**. Yield%: 90, m.p. = 254.7 °C, IR, cm^{-1}: 3210 (NH), 3055 (CH arom.), 2941, 2818 (CH aliph.), 2200 (CN), 1658 (C=N). ^1H (DMSO-d_6, ppm): 2.2 [s, 3H, CH_3], 3.2 [s, 3H, N–CH_3], 7.3–7.9 [m, 5H, Ar–H], 8.1 [s, 1H, CH], 10.5 [s, 1H, NH, D_2O-exchangeable]. ^{13}C (DMSO-d_6, ppm): 10.3 (CH_3), 29.1 (N–CH_3), 50.3, 104.6, 114.1(2), 116.4(2), 117.2, 127.2(2), 129.1, 134.5, 160.1 (C=O), 165.5. Anal. Calcd. for $C_{15}H_{13}N_5O$ (279): C, 64.51; H, 4.69; N, 25.07. Found: C, 64.91; H, 4.80; N, 25.34.

3.2.2. (*Z*)-Ethyl-2-cyano-3-(1,5-dimethyl-3-oxo-2-phenyl-2,3-dihydro-1*H*-pyrazol-4-ylamino)acrylate **3**

A mixture of 4-aminoantipyrine (0.01 mol), ethylcyanoacetate (0.01 mol), triethylorthoformate (0.01 mol), and acetic acid (1 mL) in methanol (30 mL) was refluxed for 5 h, the reaction mixture was filtered, the filtered solid was crystallized from ethanol to give **3**. Yield%: 83, m.p. = 154.8 °C, IR, cm^{-1}: 3192 (NH), 3065 (CH arom.), 2965, 2841 (CH aliph.), 2214 (CN), 1710, 1658 (2C=O). ^1H (DMSO-d_6, ppm): 1.2 [t, 3H, CH_3, J = 7.9 Hz], 2.3 [s, 3H, CH_3], 3.2 [s, 3H, N–CH_3], 4.2 [q, 2H, CH_2, J = 8.1 Hz], 7.3–8.0 [m, 5H, Ar–H], 8.2 [d, 1H, CH, J = 7.12 Hz], 10.0 [d, 1H, NH, D_2O-exchangeable, J = 7.3 Hz]. ^{13}C (DMSO-d_6, ppm): 10.3, 14.3, 39.0, 60.2, 72.6, 109.7, 115.7(2), 116.0, 118,1, 129.0(2), 129.1, 134.3, 156.8, 161.0, 166.3. Anal. Calcd. for $C_{17}H_{18}N_4O_3$ (326): C, 62.57; H, 5.56; N, 17.17. Found: C, 62.90; H, 5.89; N, 17.25.

3.2.3. 3-((1,5-Dimethyl-3-oxo-2-phenyl-2,3-dihydro-1*H*-pyrazol-4-ylamino)methylene)-pentane-2,4-dione **4**

A mixture of 4-aminoantipyrine (0.01 mol), acetylacetone (0.01 mol), triethylorthoformate (0.01 mol), and acetic acid (1 mL) in methanol (30 mL) was refluxed for 5 h, the reaction mixture was filtered, the filtered solid was crystallized from ethanol to give **4**. Yield%: 90, m.p. = 201.8 °C, IR, cm^{-1}: 3209 (NH), 3100 (CH arom.), 2971, 2848 (CH aliph.), 1716, 1692, 1661 (3C=O), 1612 (C=N). ^1H (DMSO-d_6, ppm): 1.9 [s, 3H, CH_3], 2.1 [s, 6H, 2$COCH_3$], 3.0 [s, 3H, N–CH_3], 7.3–7.5 [m, 6H, Ar–H + CH], 9.0 [s, 1H, NH, D_2O-exchangeable]. ^{13}C (DMSO-d_6, ppm): 11.1, 22.4(2), 39.1, 104.4, 107.8(2), 108.4, 121.8, 128.8(2), 129.0, 135.0, 151.0, 161.8, 195.1(2). Anal. Calcd. for $C_{17}H_{19}N_3O_3$ (313): C, 65.16; H, 6.11; N, 13.41. Found: C, 65.87; H, 6.37; N, 13.21.

3.2.4. (*Z*)-4-((3-Amino-5-imino-1-phenyl-1*H*-pyrazol-4(5*H*)-ylidene)methylamino)-1,5-dimethyl-2-phenyl-1,2-dihydropyrazol-3-one **5**

Compound **2** (0.01 mol) was mixed with phenyl hydrazine (0.01 mol) in dioxane (20 mL) and refluxed for 5 h, the reaction mixture was cooled, poured onto ice water. The precipitated solid products were filtered and crystallized from methanol to give compound **5**. Yield%: 76, m.p. = 172.7 °C, IR, cm^{-1}: 3386, 3348, 3276 (NH, NH_2), 3026 (CH arom.), 2981, 2872 (CH aliph.), 1660 (C=O),

1595 (C=N). ^{1}H (DMSO-d_6, ppm): 2.2 [s, 3H, CH_3], 3.2 [s, 3H, N–CH_3], 7.2–7.9 [m, 10H, Ar–H], 8.3 [s, 1H, CH], 8.7 [s, 1H, NH, D_2O-exchangeable], 13.2 [s, 1H, NH-imino, D_2O-exchangeable]. ^{13}C (DMSO-d$_6$, ppm): 11.5, 39.5, 106.2, 108.0, 112.4(2), 116.1(2), 117.6, 124.1, 127.7(2), 128.9, 129.5(2), 137.9, 141.2, 148.4, 156.5, 163.1, 166.2. Anal. Calcd. for $C_{21}H_{21}N_7$ (387): C, 65.10; H, 5.46; N, 25.31. Found: C, 65.32; H, 5.09; N, 25.55.

3.2.5. 3-Amino-1-(1.5-dimethyl-3-oxo-2-phenyl-2,3-dihydro-1*H*-pyrazol-4-yl)-1*H*-pyrrole-2,4-dicarbonitrile **6**

Compound **2** (0.01 mol) was mixed with 2-chloroacetonitrile (0.01 mol) in dioxane (20 mL) containing 3 drops of triethylamine and refluxed for 5 h, the reaction mixture was cooled, poured onto ice water. The precipitated solid products were filtered and crystallized from methanol to give compound **6**. Yield%: 70, m.p. > 350 °C, IR, cm^{-1}: 3344, 3291 (NH_2), 3100 (CH arom.), 2966, 2881 (CH aliph.), 2200 (CN), 1699 (C=O). ^{1}H (DMSO-d_6, ppm): 1.6 [s, 3H, CH_3], 2.4 [s, 3H, N–CH_3], 6.5 [s, 2H, NH_2, D_2O-exchangeable], 7.0–8.0 [m, 6H, Ar–H + CH-pyrrole]. ^{13}C (DMSO-d_6, ppm): 13.9, 39.1, 101.2(2), 107.4, 110.4, 113.9(2), 116.2, 117.6(2), 119.1, 129.3(2), 138.1, 139.4, 161.2. Anal. Calcd. for $C_{17}H_{14}N_6O$ (318): C, 64.14; H, 4.43; N, 25.40. Found: C, 64.32; H, 4.67; N, 25.12.

3.2.6. Ethyl-3-amino-4-cyano-1-(1,5-dimethyl-3-oxo-2-phenyl-2,3-dihydro-1*H*-pyrazol-4-yl)-1*H*-pyrrole-2-carboxylate **7**

Compound **2** (0.01 mol) was mixed with ethyl bromoacetate (0.01 mol) in dioxane (20 mL) containing 3 drops of triethylamine and refluxed for 5 h, the reaction mixture was cooled, poured onto ice water. The precipitated solid products were filtered and crystallized from methanol to give compound **7**. Yield%: 89, m.p. = 143.4 °C, IR, cm^{-1}: 3411, 3396 (NH_2), 3100 (CH arom.), 2976, 2882 (CH aliph.), 2186 (CN), 1718, 1696 (2C=O). ^{1}H (DMSO-d_6, ppm): 1.2 [t, 3H, CH_3–ester], 2.0 [s, 3H, CH_3], 2.4 [s, 3H, N–CH_3], 4.1 [q, 2H, CH_2–ester], 7.3–8.0 [m, 7H, Ar–H + NH_2], 8.7 [s, 1H, CH–pyrrole]. ^{13}C (DMSO-d_6, ppm): 12.6, 13.4, 39.0, 59.8, 98.7, 112.0, 114.3(2), 115.6, 118.4, 122.7, 126.3, 129.1(2), 138.1, 139.6, 141.2, 160.0, 161.2. Anal. Calcd. for $C_{19}H_{19}N_5O_3$ (365): C, 62.46; H, 5.24; N, 19.17. Found: C, 62.79; H, 5.57; N, 19.34.

3.2.7. 3-Amino-4-cyano-1-(1,5-dimethyl-3-oxo-2-phenyl-2,3-dihydro-1*H*-pyrazol-4-yl)-1*H*-pyrrole-2-carboxamide **8**

Compound **2** (0.01 mol) was mixed with 2-chloroacetamide (0.01 mol) in dioxane (20 mL) containing 3 drops of triethylamine and refluxed for 5 h, the reaction mixture was cooled, poured onto ice water. The precipitated solid products were filtered and crystallized from methanol to give compound **8**. Yield%: 76, m.p. > 350 °C, IR, cm^{-1}: 3404, 3385, 3236 (NH_2), 3066 (CH arom.), 2961, 2836 (CH aliph.), 2196 (CN), 1700, 1680 (2C=O). ^{1}H (DMSO-d_6, ppm): 1.6 [s, 3H, CH_3], 2.3 [s, 3H, N–CH_3], 7.2–8.0 [m, 9H, Ar–H + $CONH_2$ + NH_2], 8.5 [s, 1H, CH–pyrrole]. ^{13}C (DMSO-d_6, ppm): 11.9, 39.1, 99.2, 111.8, 114.3(2), 115.6, 118.2, 124.4, 129.0(2), 131.8, 135.7, 138.2, 153.2, 162.4, 166.0. Anal. Calcd. for $C_{17}H_{16}N_6O_3$ (336): C, 60.71; H, 4.79; N, 24.99. Found: C, 60.99; H, 4.49; N, 24.70.

3.2.8. 4-((4,6-Diamino-2-thioxopyrimidin-5(2*H*)-ylidene)methylamino)-1,5-dimethyl-1,2-phenyl-1,2-dihydropyrazol-3-one **9**

A mixture of **2** (0.01 mol) and thiourea (0.01 mol) was refluxed for 5 h in ethanol containing sodium ethoxide (0.01 mol). The reaction mixture was cooled, poured onto ice water, acidified with dil. HCl, the precipitated solid product was filtered and crystallized from methanol to give **9**. Yield%: 90, m.p. = 219.6 °C, IR, cm^{-1}: 3410, 3362, 3350 (NH_2), 3054 (CH arom.), 2922, 2860 (CH aliph.), 1675 (C=O), 1624 (C=N), 1317 (C=S). ^1H (DMSO-d_6, ppm): 2.2 [s, 3H, CH_3], 3.1 [s, 3H, N–CH_3], 7.3 [s, 4H, $2NH_2$, D_2O-exchangeable], 7.5–7.9 [m, 5H, Ar–H], 9.4 [s, 1H, CH], 13.0 [s, 1H, NH, D_2O-exchangeable]. ^{13}C (DMSO-d_6, ppm): 10.3, 39.3, 84.2, 109.1, 116.4(2), 124.2, 127.2(2), 129.1, 134.4(2), 160.2, 170.8(2), 211.3 (C=S). Anal. Calcd. for $C_{16}H_{17}N_7OS$ (355): C, 54.07; H, 4.82; N, 27.59. Found: C, 54.34; H, 4.65; N, 27.25.

3.3. General Procedure for Preparation of Compounds **10–15**

A mixture of **2** (0.01 mol) and the appropriate aryl isothiocyanate (0.01 mol) was refluxed for 10 h in ethanol containing sodium ethoxide (0.01 mol). The reaction mixture was cooled, poured onto ice water, acidified with dil. HCl, the precipitated solid product was filtered and crystallized from methanol to give **10–15**, respectively.

3.3.1. 1-(1,5-Dimethyl-3-oxo-2-phenyl-2,3-dihydro-1*H*-pyrazol-4-yl)-4-oxo-3-phenyl-2-thioxo-1,2,3,4-tetrahydropyrimidine-5-carbonitrile **10**

Yield%: 81, m.p. = 132.9 °C, IR, cm^{-1}: 3100 (CH arom.), 2966, 2871 (CH aliph.), 2201 (CN), 1672, 1659 (2C=O), 1292 (C=S). ^1H (DMSO-d_6, ppm): 2.2 [s, 3H, CH_3], 3.2 [s, 3H, N–CH_3], 7.3 [s, 1H, CH–pyrimidine], 7.5–8.1 [m, 10H, Ar–H]. ^{13}C (DMSO-d_6, ppm): 14.4, 39.1, 104.6, 109.3, 114.1(2), 116.5, 118.1, 122.0(2), 126.3, 128.6(2), 129.1(2), 129.3, 134.5, 137.8, 139.1, 159.9, 160.5, 187.2 (C=S). Anal. Calcd. for $C_{22}H_{17}N_5O_2S$ (415): C, 63.60; H, 4.12; N, 16.86. Found: C, 63.34; H, 4.32; N, 16.60.

3.3.2. 1-(1,5-Dimethyl-3-oxo-2-phenyl-2,3-dihydro-1*H*-pyrazol-4-yl)-3-(4-methoxyphenyl)-4-oxo-2-thioxo-1,2,3,4-tetrahydropyrimidine-5-carbonitrile **11**

Yield%: 71, m.p. = 90.6 °C, IR, cm^{-1}: 3046 (CH arom.), 2991, 2875 (CH aliph.), 2208 (CN), 1684, 1654 (2C=O), 1257 (C=S). ^1H (DMSO-d_6, ppm): 2.4 [s, 3H, CH_3], 3.3 [s, 3H, N–CH_3], 3.7 [s, 3H, OCH_3], 6.8–7.5 [m, 10H, Ar–H + CH–pyrimidine]. ^{13}C (DMSO-d_6, ppm): 13.9, 39.1, 55.1, 95.2, 107.5, 113.5(2), 113.8(3), 123.3, 124.2(2), 124.9, 129.1(2), 130.8, 131.4, 143.6, 156.2, 156.6, 164.7, 188.0. Anal. Calcd. for $C_{23}H_{19}N_5O_3S$ (445): C, 62.01; H, 4.30; N, 15.72. Found: C, 62.34; H, 4.09; N, 15.51.

3.3.3. 1-(1,5-Dimethyl-3-oxo-2-phenyl-2,3-dihydro-1*H*-pyrazol-4-yl)-3-(4-nitrophenyl)-4-oxo-2-thioxo-1,2,3,4-tetrahydropyrimidine-5-carbonitrile **12**

Yield%: 79, m.p. = 190.9 °C, IR, cm^{-1}: 3076 (CH arom.), 2991, 2908 (CH aliph.), 2188 (CN), 1700, 1689 (2C=O), 1597, 1380 (NO_2), 1308 (C=S). ^1H (DMSO-d_6, ppm): 2.5 [s, 3H, CH_3], 3.3 [s, 3H,

N–CH_3], 7.8–8.2 [m, 10H, Ar–H + CH–pyrimidine]. ^{13}C (DMSO-d_6, ppm): 14.8, 39.3, 89.6, 108.2, 112.3(3), 117.5, 120.9, 124.5(2), 124.9(2), 126.3(2), 129.0, 137.4(2), 142.8, 144.0, 155.6, 162.4, 187.6 (C=S). Anal. Calcd. for $C_{22}H_{16}N_6O_4S$ (460): C, 57.38; H, 3.50; N, 18.25. Found: C, 57.69; H, 3.20; N, 18.56.

3.3.4. 3-(4-Bromophenyl)-1-(1,5-dimethyl-3-oxo-2-phenyl-2,3-dihydro-1*H*-pyrazol-4-yl)-4-oxo-2-thioxo-1,2,3,4-tetrahydropyrimidine-5-carbonitrile **13**

Yield%: 69, m.p. = 76.0 °C, IR, cm^{-1}: 3100 (CH arom.), 2986, 2861 (CH aliph.), 2218 (CN), 1684, 1653 (2C=O), 1216 (C=S). ^{1}H (DMSO-d_6, ppm): 2.2 [s, 3H, CH_3], 3.1 [s, 3H, N–CH_3], 7.0–7.6 [m, 10H, Ar–H + CH–pyrimidine]. ^{13}C (DMSO-d_6, ppm): 13.9, 39.5, 92.4, 104.6, 113.8(2), 114.1, 116.6, 119.9, 121.0(2), 127.2(2), 129.0, 132.6, 133.4(2), 137.7, 138.6, 159.9, 160.1, 186.6 (C=S). Anal. Calcd. for $C_{22}H_{16}BrN_5O_2S$ (493): C, 53.45; H, 3.26; N, 14.17. Found: C, 53.70; H, 3.11; N, 14.44.

3.3.5. 1-(1,5-Dimethyl-3-oxo-2-phenyl-2,3-dihydro-1*H*-pyrazol-4-yl)-3-(4-iodophenyl)-4-oxo-2-thioxo-1,2,3,4-tetrahydropyrimidine-5-carbonitrile **14**

Yield%: 90, m.p. = 114.1 °C, IR, cm^{-1}: 3092 (CH arom.), 2980, 2861 (CH aliph.), 2187 (CN), 1684, 1654 (2C=O), 1276 (C=S). ^{1}H (DMSO-d_6, ppm): 2.5 [s, 3H, CH_3], 3.1 [s, 3H, N–CH_3], 7.6–7.9 [m, 10H, Ar–H + CH–pyrimidine]. ^{13}C (DMSO-d_6, ppm): 13.9, 39.5, 88.8(2), 107.3, 114.6(2), 116.2, 120.2, 123.6(2), 129.0(3), 130.6, 137.2, 137.9(2), 139.1, 162.7, 166.1, 187.3. Anal. Calcd. for $C_{22}H_{16}N_5O_2S$ (541): C, 48.81; H, 2.98; N, 12.94. Found: C, 48.69; H, 2.69; N, 12.72.

3.3.6. 4-(5-Cyano-3-(1,5-dimethyl-3-oxo-2-phenyl-2,3-dihydro-1*H*-pyrazol-4-yl)-6-oxo-2-thioxo-2,3-tetrahydropyrimidin-1(6*H*)-yl)benzensulfonamide **15**

Yield%: 90, m.p. = 164.8 °C, IR, cm^{-1}: 3041 (CH arom.), 2934, 2881 (CH aliph.), 2217 (CN), 1714, 1662 (2C=O), 1296 (C=S). ^{1}H (DMSO-d_6, ppm): 2.2 [s, 3H, CH_3], 3.0 [s, 3H, N–CH_3], 7.3–8.0 [m, 11H, Ar–H + SO_2NH_2], 8.1 [s, 1H, CH–pyrimidine]. ^{13}C (DMSO-d_6, ppm): 13.9, 39.4, 96.2, 104.6, 114.2(2), 116.4, 117.2, 121.6(2), 125.1(2), 127.3(2), 129.1, 134.2, 134.5, 139.6, 140.9, 160.2, 160.5, 187.6 (C=S). Anal. Calcd. for $C_{22}H_{18}N_6O_4S_2$ (494): C, 53.43; H, 3.67; N, 16.99. Found: C, 53.69; H, 3.90; N, 16.34.

3.3.7. 3,3'-(4,4'-Sulfonylbis(4,1-phenylene))bis(1-(1,5-dimethyl-3-oxo-2-phenyl-2,3-dihydro-1*H*-pyrazol-4-yl)-4-oxo-2-thioxo-1,2,3,4-tetrahydropyrimidine-5-carbonitrile) **16**

A mixture of **2** (0.01 mol) and 1-(4-isothiocyanatophenylsulfonyl)-4-isothiocyanatobenzene (0.02 mol) was refluxed for 10 h in ethanol containing sodium ethoxide (0.01 mol). The reaction mixture was cooled, poured onto ice water, acidified with dil. HCl, the precipitated solid product was filtered and crystallized from methanol to give **16**. Yield%: 81, m.p. = 140.6 °C, IR, cm^{-1}: 3076 (CH arom.), 2981, 2861 (CH aliph.), 2219 (CN), 1661, 1643 (4C=O), 1322 (2C=S). ^{1}H (DMSO-d_6, ppm): 2.2 [s, 6H, 2CH_3], 3.1 [s, 6H, 2N–CH_3], 7.3–8.0 [m, 18H, Ar–H], 8.6 [s, 2H, 2CH–pyrimidine]. ^{13}C (DMSO-d_6, ppm): 13.8(2), 39.0(2), 92.6(2), 108.6(2), 113.5(4), 114.1(2), 118.4(2), 121.7(4),

127.0(4), 128.2(4), 129.1(2), 134.5(2), 136.2(2), 136.7(2), 142.4(2), 159.4(2), 160.2(2), 187.6(2). Anal. Calcd. for $C_{44}H_{32}N_{10}O_6S_3$ (892): C, 59.18; H, 3.61; N, 15.69. Found: C, 59.40; H, 3.80; N, 15.48.

3.4. General Procedure for Preparation of Compounds **17** *and* **18**

Compound **10** (0.01 mol) was mixed with either hydrazine hydrate or phenyl hydrazine (0.01 mol) in dioxane (20 mL) and refluxed for 5 h, the reaction mixture was cooled, poured onto ice water. The precipitated solid products were filtered and crystallized from methanol to give compounds **17** and **18**, respectively.

3.4.1. (*Z*)-1-(1,5-Dimethyl-3-oxo-2-phenyl-2,3-dihydro-1*H*-pyrazol-4-yl)-2-hydrazono-4-oxo-3-phenyl-1,2,3,4-tetrahydropyrimidine-5-carbonitrile **17**

Yield%: 68, m.p. = 78.0 °C, IR, cm^{-1}: 3213, 3191 (NH_2), 3047 (CH arom.), 2961, 2876 (CH aliph.), 2191 (CN). ^1H (DMSO-d_6, ppm): 2.5 [s, 3H, CH_3], 3.2 [s, 3H, N–CH_3], 4.5 [s, 2H, NH_2, D_2O-exchangeable], 7.1–7.5 [m, 11H, Ar–H + CH–pyrimidine]. ^{13}C (DMSO-d_6, ppm): 13.1, 39.0, 94.6, 106.2, 114.5(2), 116.7, 118.2, 120.6(2), 122.1, 127.6(2), 128.4(2), 129.7, 134.2, 137.7, 138.5, 156.2, 162.8, 168.9. Anal. Calcd. for $C_{22}H_{19}N_7O_2$ (413): C, 63.91; H, 4.63; N, 23.72. Found: C, 63.70; H, 4.91; N, 23.55.

3.4.2. (*Z*)-1-(1,5-Dimethyl-3-oxo-2-phenyl-2,3-dihydro-1*H*-pyrazol-4-yl)-4-oxo-3-phenyl-2-(2-phenylhydrazono)-1,2,3,4-tetrahydropyrimidine-5-carbonitrile **18**

Yield%: 65, m.p. = 90.6 °C, IR, cm^{-1}: 3381 (NH), 3074 (CH arom.), 2966, 2836 (CH aliph.), 2220 (CN), 1700, 1653 (2C=O). ^1H (DMSO-d_6, ppm): 2.4 [s, 3H, CH_3], 3.2 [s, 3H, N–CH_3], 7.0–8.0 [m, 15H, Ar–H], 8.4 [s, 1H, CH–pyrimidine], 9.5 [s, 1H, NH, D_2O-exchangeable]. ^{13}C (DMSO-d_6, ppm): 14.1, 39.6, 95.3, 108.3, 113.8(2), 114.6, 115.8, 116.4(2), 118.9, 119.5(2), 122.2, 128.6(2), 129.0(2), 129.6, 129.8(2), 130.2, 139.2, 141.5, 144.6, 153.5, 155.7, 165.6. Anal. Calcd. for $C_{28}H_{23}N_7O_2$ (489): C, 68.70; H, 4.74; N, 20.03. Found: C, 68.92; H, 4.99; N, 20.33.

3.4.3. (*Z*)-4-(3-Amino-6-hydrazono-7-phenyl-6,7-dihydropyrazolo[3,4-*d*]pyrimidin-5-yl)-1,5-dimethyl-2-phenyl-1,2-dihydropyrazol-3-one **19**

Compound **10** (0.01 mol) was mixed with hydrazine hydrate (0.02 mol) in dioxane (20 mL) and refluxed for 5 h, the reaction mixture was cooled, poured onto ice water. The precipitated solid products were filtered and crystallized from methanol to give compounds **19**. Yield%: 73, m.p. = 222.6 °C, IR, cm^{-1}: 3420, 3362 (NH_2), 3050 (CH arom.), 2971, 2861 (CH aliph.), 1654 (C=O), 1617 (C=N). ^1H (DMSO-d_6, ppm): 2.2 [s, 3H, CH_3], 3.2 [s, 3H, N–CH_3], 5.4 [s, 2H, N–NH_2, D_2O-exchangeable], 6.5 [s, 2H, NH_2, D_2O-exchangeable], 7.0–8.1 [m, 11H, Ar–H + CH–pyrimidine]. ^{13}C (DMSO-d_6, ppm): 11.4, 39.0, 97.6, 107.3, 112.6(2), 114.3(2), 116.7, 118.6, 123.7, 128.6(2), 129.1, 129.4(2), 134.1, 139.8, 155.7, 162.3, 166.0(2). Anal. Calcd. for $C_{22}H_{21}N_9O$ (427): C, 61.81; H, 4.95; N, 29.49. Found: C, 62.03; H, 5.12; N, 29.67.

3.5. General Procedure for Preparation of Compounds **20** *and* **21**

A solution of 4-aminoantipyrine **1** (0.001 mol) in either triethylorthoformate or triethylorthoacetate (0.001 mol) containing three drops of acetic anhydride was refluxed for 8 h, the reaction mixture was cooled and then poured onto cold water, the obtained solid was recrystallized from methanol to give compounds **20** and **21**, respectively.

3.5.1. (*E*)-Ethyl-*N*-1,5-dimethyl-3-oxo-2-phenyl-2,3-dihydro-1*H*-pyrazol-4-yl-formimidate **20**

Yield%: 90, m.p. = 196.9 °C, IR, cm^{-1}: 3078 (CH arom.), 2976, 2912 (CH aliph.), 1661 (C=O), 1612 (C=N). ^{1}H (DMSO-d_6, ppm): 1.0 [t, 3H, CH_3], 2.3 [s, 3H, CH_3], 3.1 [s, 3H, N–CH_3], 3.5 [q, 2H, CH_2], 7.2–7.5 [m, 5H, Ar–H], 8.1 [s, 1H, CH]. ^{13}C (DMSO-d_6, ppm): 11.3, 18.5, 39.3, 56.0, 106.3, 107.0(2), 120.0, 129.0(2), 135.1, 151.6, 160.1, 164.7. Anal. Calcd. for $C_{14}H_{17}N_3O_2$ (259): C, 64.85; H, 6.61; N, 16.34. Found: C, 64.66; H, 6.34; N, 16.67.

3.5.2. (*E*)-Ethyl-*N*-1,5-dimethyl-3-oxo-2-phenyl-2,3-dihydro-1*H*-pyrazol-4-yl-acetimidate **21**

Yield%: 88, m.p. = 81.6 °C, IR, cm^{-1}: 3086 (CH arom.), 2936, 2817 (CH aliph.), 1658 (C=O), 1598 (C=N). ^{1}H (DMSO-d_6, ppm): 1.2 [t, 3H, CH_3], 1.9 [s, 3H, N=C–CH_3], 2.1 [s, 3H, CH_3], 3.3 [s, 3H, N–CH_3], 4.1 [q, 2H, CH_2], 7.2–7.5 [m, 5H, Ar–H]. ^{13}C (DMSO-d_6, ppm): 10.1 (CH_3–pyrazole), 14.0 (CH_3–ethyl), 17.4 (N=C–CH_3), 39.1 (N–CH_3), 61.0 (CH_2–ethyl), 112.6, 118.7(2), 122.8, 128.9(2), 135.4, 146.1, 160.0, 164.0 (C=O). Anal. Calcd. for $C_{15}H_{19}N_3O_2$ (273): C, 65.91; H, 7.01; N, 15.37. Found: C, 66.13; H, 7.34; N, 15.48.

3.6. In-Vitro Anticancer Screening

The human tumor cell line (MCF7) was available from the National Cancer Institute, Cairo, Egypt. The antitumor activity of the newly synthesized compounds against the MCF7 cells was measured using the Sulforhodamine B (SRB) assay by the method of Skehan *et al.* (1990) [23,24]. The cell lines were grown in RPMI 1640 medium containing 10% fetal bovine serum and 2 mM L-glutamine. Cells were plated in 96-multi-well plates (10^4 cells/well) and were incubated at 37 °C, 5% CO_2 in a humidified atmosphere for 24 h to allow attachment prior to addition of compounds. The test compounds **3**–**14** were dissolved in DMSO and diluted with saline to the appropriate volume and maintained in RPMI 1640 medium. Different concentrations of the compounds under test were made: 5, 12.5, 25, 30 and 50 μM and were added to the cells. Triplicate wells were prepared for each individual dose. Cells were incubated with the compounds for 48 h at 37 °C, 5% CO_2. After 48 h, cells were fixed *in situ* by the gentle addition of 50 μL of cold 30% (*w*/*v*) trichloroacetic acid (TCA) (final concentration, 10%) and incubated for 60 min at 4 °C. The supernatant was discarded and the plates were washed five times with tap water and air dried. Sulforhodamine B (SRB) solution (50 μL) at 0.4% (*w*/*v*) in 1% acetic acid was added to each well and plates were incubated for 20 min at room temperature. After staining, unbounded dye was removed by four washes with 1% acetic acid, and attached stain was recovered with Tris-EDTA buffer. Color intensity was measured at wave length 564 nm in an ELISA reader (Gmbh, Viesbaden, Germany). The relation between surviving fraction and drug concentration was plotted to get the survival curve from each compound after the specified time. The concentration required for 50% inhibition of cell viability (IC_{50}) was calculated and compared with the reference drug doxorubicin and the results are given in Table 1.

4. Conclusions

The objective of the present study was to synthesize and investigate the anticancer activity of some novel pyrazole carrying a biologically active sulfonamide moieties. It was found that compounds **5**, **13**, **14**, and **16**–**19** showed promising anticancer activity, higher than that of doxorubicin as reference drug against human breast cancer cell line (MCF7), while compounds **10**, **12** are nearly as active as doxorubicin as positive control. Compound **8** exhibited a moderate activity and compounds **2**–**4**, **6**, **7**, **9**, and **20** showed a weak activity, while compounds **11**, **15** and **21** revealed no activity. Further investigations on different probable mechanisms of action and dose-response studies should be helpful in identifying the specific site(s) of action and optimum doses of the synthesized antipyrine derivatives. These investigations would be crucial in discovering more potent and more selective anti-breast cancer agents.

Acknowledgments

The authors would like to extend their sincere appreciation to the Deanship of Scientific Research at King Saud University (Riyadh, Saudi Arabia) for its funding of this research through the Research Group Project No. RGP-VPP-302.

Author Contributions

M.M.G. suggested the research idea, contributed in the experimental work and in writing the paper. M.G.E.-G. contributed in experimental work and in writing the paper. M.S.A. contributed in the experimental work, biological activity and in writing the paper.

References

1. Himly, M.; Jahn-Schmid, B.; Pittertschatscher, K.; Bohle, B.; Grubmayr, K.; Ferreira, F.; Ebner, H.; Ebner, C. Ig E-mediated immediate-type hypersensitivity to the pyrazolone drug propyphenazone. *J. Allergy Clin. Immunol.* **2003**, *111*, 882–888.
2. Gürsoy, A.; Demirayak, S.; Capan, G.; Erol, K.; Vural, K. Synthesis and preliminary evaluation of new 5-pyrazolinone derivatives as analgesic agents. *Eur. J. Med. Chem.* **2000**, *35*, 359–364.
3. Teng, Y.; Liu, R.; Li, C.; Zhang, H. Effect of 4-aminoantipyrine on oxidative stress induced by glutathione depletion in single human erythrocytes using a microfluidic device together with fluorescence imaging. *J. Hazard. Mater.* **2011**, *192*, 1766–1771.
4. Turan-Zitouni, G.; Sivaci, M.; Kiliç, F.S.; Erol, K. Synthesis of some triazolyl-antipyrine derivatives and investigation of analgesic activity. *Eur. J. Med. Chem.* **2001**, *36*, 685–689.

5. Lutsevich, A.N.; Bender, K.I.; Reshet'ko, O.V. The relationship between antipyrine kinetics, the seromucoid content and the xanthine oxidase activity in the plasma of rats with acute and chronic inflammation. *Eksp Klin. Farmakol.* **1995**, *58*, 51–55.
6. Bondock, S.; Rabie, R.; Etman, H.A.; Fadda, A.A. Synthesis and antimicrobial activity of some new heterocycles incorporating antipyrine moiety. *Eur. J. Med. Chem.* **2008**, *43*, 2122–2129.
7. Metwally, M.A.; Gouda, M.A.; Harmal, A.N.; Khalil, A.M. Synthesis, antitumor, cytotoxic and antioxidant evaluation of some new pyrazolotriazines attached to antipyrine moiety. *Eur. J. Med. Chem.* **2012**, *56*, 254–262.
8. Kakiuchi, Y.; Sasaki, N.; Satoh-Masuoka, M.; Murofushi, H.; Murakami-Murofushi, K. A novel pyrazolone, 4,4-dichloro-1-(2,4-dichlorophenyl)-3-methyl-5-pyrazolone, as a potent catalytic inhibitor of human telomerase q. *Biochem. Biophy. Res. Commun.* **2004**, *320*, 1351–1358.
9. Sigroha, S.; Narasimhan, B.; Kumar, P.; Khatkar, A.; Ramasamy, K.; Mani, V.; Mishra, R.K.; Abdul Majeed, A.B. Design, synthesis, antimicrobial, anticancer evaluation, and QSAR studies of 4-(substituted benzylidene-amino)-1,5-dimethyl-2-phenyl-1,2-dihydropyrazol-3-ones. *Med. Chem. Res.* **2012**, *21*, 3863–3875.
10. Chandrasekharan, N.V.; Dai, H.; Roos, K.L.T.; Evanson, N.K.; Tomsik, J.; Elton, T.S. COX-3, a cyclooxygenase-1 variant inhibited by acetaminophen and other analgesic/antipyretic drugs: Cloning, structure, and expression. *Proc. Natl. Acad. Sci. USA* **2002**, *99*, 13926–13931.
11. Levy, M. Hypersensitivity to pyrazolones. *Thorax* **2000**, *55*, 72–74.
12. Al-Haiza, M.A.; El-Assiery, S.A.; Sayed, G.H. Synthesis and potential antimicrobial activity of some new compounds containing the pyrazol-3-one moiety. *Acta Pharm.* **2001**, *51*, 251–261.
13. Lin, R.; Chiu, G.; Yu, Y. Design, synthesis, and evaluation of 3,4-disubstituted pyrazole analogues as anti-tumor CDK inhibitors. *Bioorg. Med. Chem. Lett.* **2007**, *17*, 4557–4581.
14. Aly, H.M.; El-Gazzar, M.G. Novel pyrazole derivatives as anticancer and radiosensitizing agents. *Arzneimittelforschung* **2012**, *62*, 105–112.
15. Ghorab, M.M.; Ragab, F.A.; Heiba, H.I.; Hanan, A.Y.; El-Gazzar, M.G. Synthesis of novel pyrazole and pyrimidine derivatives bearing sulfonamide moiety as antitumor and radiosensitizing agents. *Med. Chem. Res.* **2012**, *21*, 1376–1383.
16. Ghorab, M.M.;Heiba, H.I.; Hassan, A.A.; Abd El-Aziz, A.B.; El-Gazzar, M.G. Antimicrobial evaluation of novel pyrrole, pyrazole, pyrimidine and pyrrolo [2,3-*d*]-pyrimidine derivatives brearing sulfonamide moiety. *J. Am. Sci.* **2011**, *7*, 1064–1073.
17. Ghorab, M.M.; Ragab, F.A.; Heiba, H.I.; Youssef, H.A.; Galal, M. Synthesis of some new pyrazole and pyrimidine derivatives carrying a sulfonamide moiety of expected antitumor activity and study of the synergistic effect of gamma-irradiation. *Arzneimittelforschung* **2010**, *60*, 48–55.
18. Ghorab, M.M.; Alsaid, M.S.; Nissan, Y.M. Dapson in heterocyclic chemistry, part V: Synthesis, molecular docking and anticancer activity of some novel sulfonylbiscompounds carrying biologically active dihydropyridine, dihydroisoquinoline, 1,3-dithiolan, 1,3-dithian, acrylamide, pyrazole, pyrazolopyrimidine and benzochromenemoieties. *Chem. Pharm. Bull. (Tokyo)* **2012**, *60*, 1019–1028.
19. Mohareb, R.M.; Sherif, S.M.; Zohdi, H.F. Heterocyclic synthesis with enamines: Convenient synthesis of polyfunctionally substituted pyrazole, pyridine, pyrimidine and pyrazolo[3,4-*d*]pyrimidine derivatives. *J. Chin. Chem. Soc.* **1993**, *40*, 181–187.

20. Mohamed, A.M.; El-Sayed, W.A.; Alsharari, M.A.; Al-Qalawi, H.R.; Germoush, M.O. Anticancer activities of some newly synthesized pyrazole and pyrimidine derivatives. *Arch. Pharm. Res.* **2013**, *36*, 1055–1065.
21. Ghorab, M.M.; Ragab, F.A.; Heiba, H.I.; Youssef, H.A.; El-Gazzar, M.G. Synthesis of novel pyrrole and pyrrolo[2,3-*d*]pyrimidine derivatives bearing sulfonamide moiety for evaluation as anticancer and radiosensitizing agents. *Bioorg. Med. Chem. Lett.* **2010**, *20*, 6316–6320.
22. Al-Issa, S.A. Synthesis and anticancer activity of some fused pyrimidines and related heterocycles. *Saudi Pharm. J.* **2013**, *21*, 305–316.
23. Skehan, P.; Storeng, R.; Scudiero, D.; Monks, A.; McMahon, J.; Vistica, D.; Warren, J.T.; Bokesch, H.; Kenney, S.; Boyd, M.R. New colorimetric cytotoxicity assay for anticancer-drug screening. *J. Natl. Cancer Inst.* **1990**, *82*, 1107–1112.
24. Rubinstein, L.V.; Shoemaker, R.H.; Paull, K.D.; Simon, R.M.; Tosini, S.; Skehan, P.; Scudiero, D.A.; Monks, A.; Boyd, M.R. Comparison of *in vitro* anticancer-drug-screening data generated with a tetrazolium assay *vs.* a protein assay against a diverse panel of human tumor cell lines. *J. Natl. Cancer Inst.* **1990**, *82*, 1113–1118.

4

PseAAC-General: Fast Building Various Modes of General Form of Chou's Pseudo-Amino Acid Composition for Large-Scale Protein Datasets

Pufeng Du [1,2,3,*], **Shuwang Gu** [1,2] **and Yasen Jiao** [1,2]

[1] School of Computer Science and Technology, Tianjin University, Tianjin 300072, China; E-Mails: shuwanggu@gmail.com (S.G.); yasenjiao@gmail.com (Y.J.)

[2] Tianjin Key Laboratory of Cognitive Computing and Application, Tianjin University, Tianjin 300072, China

[3] Department of Computer Science, City University of Hong Kong, Kowloon, Hong Kong

* Author to whom correspondence should be addressed; E-Mail: pufengdu@gmail.com

---

Abstract: The general form pseudo-amino acid composition (PseAAC) has been widely used to represent protein sequences in predicting protein structural and functional attributes. We developed the program PseAAC-General to generate various different modes of Chou's general PseAAC, such as the gene ontology mode, the functional domain mode, and the sequential evolution mode. This program allows the users to define their own desired modes. In every mode, 544 physicochemical properties of the amino acids are available for choosing. The computing efficiency is at least 100 times that of existing programs, which makes it able to facilitate the extensive studies on proteins and peptides. The PseAAC-General is freely available via SourceForge. It runs on both Linux and Windows.

Keywords: general form; large-scale datasets; pseudo-amino acid composition

---

1. Introduction

Over the last few years, machine learning has been introduced to predict protein structures and functions. In these studies, one of the keys is to formulate the protein sequences with a mathematical form that can reflect the intrinsic correlation with their structures and functions. To be more specific, this mathematical form should keep representing a protein sequence with a discrete form yet without completely losing its sequence-order information. The pseudo-amino acid compositions (PseAAC), which was originally introduced to predict protein attributes [1], is a typical mathematical form in this regard.

Ever since its first appearance, the PseAAC formulation has been widely applied for studying various problems in protein science, such as predicting eukaryotes and prokaryotes protein subcellular locations [2–11], protein sub-subcellular locations [12–22], membrane protein subcellular locations [23–26], viral protein subcellular locations [27,28], protein structural classes [29–35], secondary structures [36], super-secondary structures [37], quaternary structural attributes [38,39], GPCR classes [40–42], enzyme families [43,44], membrane protein types [45–47], metalloproteinase families [48], risk types of human papillomavirus [49], cell-wall lytic enzymes [50], cyclic proteins [51], allergenic proteins [52], bioluminescent proteins [53], DNA-binding proteins [54], GABA(A) receptor proteins [55], bacterial virulent proteins [56], essential proteins [57], anti-cancer peptides [58], anti-bacterial peptides [59], protein-protein interactions [60], protein solubility [61], drug-target network [62], and many more [63–76]. Recently, it was applied to represent DNA sequences in identifying the recombination spot [77].

Many different types of information, such as gene ontology annotations, functional domain compositions, and sequential evolution information, have been integrated skillfully with the concept of PseAAC to represent protein samples in order to enhance the prediction quality of their attributes. In essence, the protein sample thus formulated were actually various modes of Chou's general form PseAAC, as clearly indicated by Equations 9–14 in a comprehensive review [78]. On the contrary, the Type I PseAAC [1] and Type II PseAAC [79] belong to Chou's special form PseAAC. The modes of Chou's special form PseAAC can be calculated by several programs, such as PseAAC server [80], PseAAC-Builder [81] and the propy package [82].

However, so far no publicly accessible program could calculate Chou's general PseAAC. The current PseAAC-General is a universal software platform for users to generate various modes of general form PseAAC, including several widely used modes, such as the gene ontology mode [3], functional domain mode [83], and sequential evolution mode [18]. It is anticipated that PseAAC-General will become a very useful tool in bioinformatics, computational proteomics, and system biology.

2. Results and Discussion

The current PseAAC-General can generate 13 different modes of general form PseAAC, including conventional amino acid composition, di-peptide composition, tri-peptide composition, Type I PseAAC, Type II PseAAC, the gene ontology mode, the functional domain mode, the sequential evolution mode, the normalized Moreau-Broto autocorrelation coefficients, the Moran autocorrelation coefficients, the Geary autocorrelation coefficients, the composition-transition-distribution (CTD) descriptors and the quasi-sequence order descriptors. In every mode, 544 types of physicochemical properties are available for choosing. Over 20,000 different descriptor values can be calculated.

We list several commonly used modes of general form PseAAC as well as some program features in PseAAC-General program in Table 1. Several modes are uniquely available in PseAAC-General, which include the gene ontology mode, the functional domain mode and the sequential evolution mode. These modes have been mentioned in existing programs [81,82]. However, no program implemented these modes.

Table 1. Comparison of program features.

Program Functions [a]	PseAAC-General	PseAAC-Builder	Propy	PseAAC Server
Physicochemical Properties	544	544	8	6
	Output Features			
Type I PseAAC [1]	Y	Y	Y	Y
Type II PseAAC [79]	Y	Y	Y	Y
Amino acid composition	Y	Y	Y	Y
di-Peptide composition	Y	Y	Y	Y
tri-Peptide composition	Y	N	Y	N
Normalized Moreau-Broto autocorrelation [84,85]	Y	N	Y	N
Moran autocorrelation [86]	Y	N	Y	N
Geary autocorrelation [87]	Y	N	Y	N
Composition-Transition-Distribution (CTD) [88]	Y	N	Y	N
Quasi-sequence order [89]	Y	N	Y	N
Gene ontology mode [83]	Y	N	N	N
Functional domain mode [83]	Y	N	N	N
Sequential evolution mode [18]	Y	N	N	N
Other functions				
User defined	Y	N	N	N
Online updates	Y	N	N	N
Graphical User Interface (GUI)	Y	Y	N	Y
Execution efficiency [b]	~17,000 seqs/s	~170 seqs/s	N.A.	~15 seqs/s

[a] The program functions that were compared. There are three groups of functions, including the physicochemical properties, the sequence features that can be generated and the other function properties of the software. Y = YES; N = NO; [b] the execution time for PseAAC-General and PseAAC-Builder was tested on a dataset containing over 510,000 sequences by the wall-clock time. The execution time for PseAAC-Server was tested on a dataset containing 500 sequences due to the limitation of the service and the internet connection conditions. The execution time for Propy was not tested due the limitation of testing environments. Seqs/s means sequences per second.

PseAAC-General provided two methods for the users to create their own desired modes. The first method is called the Binary Extension Module (BEM). The gene ontology mode and functional domain mode were actually implemented by this method. A set of tools was provided along with the PseAAC-General, so that the users can create their own BEM to represent all kinds of descriptive information, which includes but not limited to the gene ontology annotations and the functional domain compositions.

The other method is the Lua script module. Lua script language is a very simple programming language that has been considered in analyzing sequence annotations [90]. We provided a programming interface that allows the user to use Lua script to access the internal data structures and functions of PseAAC-General. Furthermore, the algorithm modules of PseAAC-General can be replaced by the user-defined Lua script modules. This provides the maximal flexibility for the user-defined mode. Actually, the sequential evolution mode was implemented in this way.

Because of these extension modules, the input to the PseAAC-General is not only the protein sequences. These extension modules should also be loaded if they are needed. We illustrate the data flow of PseAAC-General in Figure 1.

Figure 1. The data flow of pseudo-amino acid composition (PseAAC)-General. The input data is FASTA format sequences. The output data is general form PseAAC. The mode of the general form PseAAC is chosen by the users. For the modes, which are implemented by Binary Extension Modules or Lua script modules, the corresponding modules should be loaded as well.

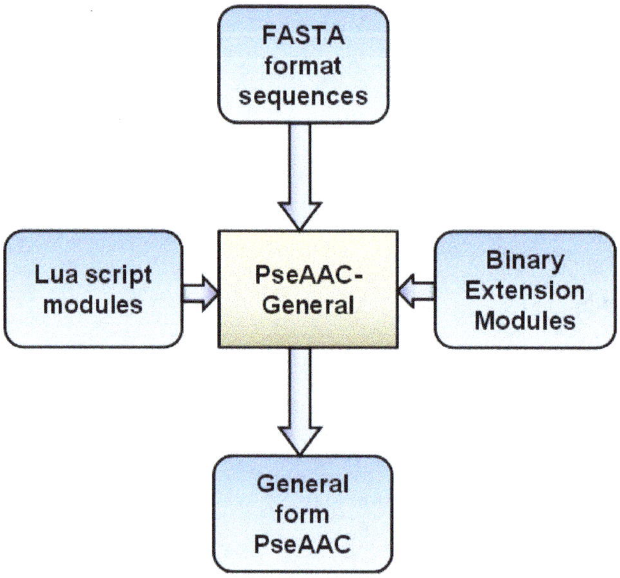

The usefulness of PseAAC-General is undisputed. In the early days of general form PseAAC, every study had to implement the PseAAC independently. This may bring a number of problems, including but not limited to inconsistent results, different computation efficiency and different basis in comparing predictive performance. PseAAC-General can serve as a standard program that saves time for all these studies. Furthermore, our program eliminates those unforeseen problems that were brought by the different implementations of PseAAC.

PseAAC-General is much faster than existing programs. We tested PseAAC-General by using it to calculate Type I PseAAC with default parameters. On the same machine that we tested PseAAC-Builder [81], it can process about 17,000 sequences per second. This is about 100 times faster than PseAAC-Builder. In other words, PseAAC-General can convert the entire Swiss-Prot database to Type I PseAAC within 30 s, while PseAAC-Builder needs about 40 min.

3. Implementations

PseAAC-General is released under GNU GPL (GNU General Public License). It can be integrated with other programs in the source code level. We have ported PseAAC-General to both Linux and Windows platforms. A GUI (Graphical User Interface) module was provided for both platforms. The users, who do not familiar with the command line, can use PseAAC-General through GUI. However, it should be noted that the most efficient way is the command line, which was designed to follow the GNU command line standard.

PseAAC-General was designed to be a stand-alone program running on the local machine without internet connection requirements. Therefore, we did not include the online sequence retrieving function within the program. On the other hand, the propy package has perfectly implemented the retrieving function. The best choice for the users is to let PseAAC-General work side by side with the propy package. For example, the users can use Propy to retrieve protein sequences and call PseAAC-General to calculate the PseAAC, as python environment has the built-in ability to call external programs, like PseAAC-General. In future versions of PseAAC-General, a similar function will be implemented. PseAAC-General and all its extension modules can be downloaded from its website [91]. To facilitate further studies, all source code of PseAAC-General, including the main program, GUI module and all extension modules, can be freely downloaded from the SourceForge website [92]. We also provided detailed documents within the software package, so that the users can learn not only how to use the existing modes, but also how to create their own modes by building their own extension modules. For the users' convenience to test their own modes, we provided four different testing dataset with different size. These testing datasets can also be downloaded from the website. Along with the testing datasets, we provided simple testing scripts to demonstrate the usage of PseAAC-General in a common case. The users can simply try the testing scripts to learn how to use the program.

Because the gene ontology mode and the functional domain mode should be upgraded along with the Swiss-Prot database, we deployed a cloud-computation based server in Amazon EC2 (Elastic Cloud 2, Amazon.com Inc., Seattle, WA, USA) to automatically upgrade the relevant extension modules on monthly basis.

4. Conclusions

As PseAAC-General is a very powerful and very flexible computation tool, we believe that PseAAC-General will facilitate all studies that apply the general form PseAAC, including those existing modes and those modes in development.

However, as a final reminder, we would like to remind the users to read the manual of PseAAC-General and those literatures describing the algorithm of general form PseAAC carefully before using it. Because of the powerful function and the flexibility of PseAAC-General, using it in your study without knowing the algorithms and technics behind the program and the source code could be very risky.

Acknowledgments

This work was supported by National Science Foundation of China (NSFC 61005041); Specialized Research Fund for the Doctoral Program of Higher Education (SRFDP 20100032120039); Tianjin Natural Science Foundation (No. 12JCQNJC02300); China Post-doctoral Science Foundation (2012T50240 and 2013M530114); HK Scholar Program (XJ2012033) and the Seed Foundation of Tianjin University (No. 60302006 and 60302024).

Author Contributions

P.D. designed the software, partially wrote the code and wrote the manuscript. S.G. and Y.J. partially wrote the code, carried out testing experiments and partially wrote the manuscript.

References

1. Chou, K.C. Prediction of protein cellular attributes using pseudo-amino acid composition. *Proteins* **2001**, *43*, 246–255.
2. Lee, K.; Chuang, H.-Y.; Beyer, A.; Sung, M.-K.; Huh, W.-K.; Lee, B.; Ideker, T. Protein networks markedly improve prediction of subcellular localization in multiple eukaryotic species. *Nucleic Acids Res.* **2008**, *36*, e136.
3. Chou, K.-C.; Shen, H.-B. Cell-PLoc: A package of web servers for predicting subcellular localization of proteins in various organisms. *Nat. Protoc.* **2008**, *3*, 153–162.
4. Huang, C.; Yuan, J. Using radial basis function on the general form of Chou's pseudo amino acid composition and PSSM to predict subcellular locations of proteins with both single and multiple sites. *BioSystems* **2013**, *113*, 50–57.
5. Jiang, X.; Wei, R.; Zhang, T.; Gu, Q. Using the concept of Chou's pseudo amino acid composition to predict apoptosis proteins subcellular location: An approach by approximate entropy. *Protein Pept. Lett.* **2008**, *15*, 392–396.
6. Lin, H.; Wang, H.; Ding, H.; Chen, Y.-L.; Li, Q.-Z. Prediction of subcellular localization of apoptosis protein using Chou's pseudo amino acid composition. *Acta Biotheor.* **2009**, *57*, 321–330.
7. Lin, J.; Wang, Y. Using a novel AdaBoost algorithm and Chou's Pseudo amino acid composition for predicting protein subcellular localization. *Protein Pept. Lett.* **2011**, *18*, 1219–1225.
8. Mei, S. Predicting plant protein subcellular multi-localization by Chou's PseAAC formulation based multi-label homolog knowledge transfer learning. *J. Theor. Biol.* **2012**, *310*, 80–87.
9. Pacharawongsakda, E.; Theeramunkong, T. Predict subcellular locations of singleplex and multiplex proteins by semi-supervised learning and dimension-reducing general mode of Chou's PseAAC. *NanoBioscience* **2013**, *12*, 311–320.
10. Wan, S.; Mak, M.-W.; Kung, S.-Y. GOASVM: A subcellular location predictor by incorporating term-frequency gene ontology into the general form of Chou's pseudo-amino acid composition. *J. Theor. Biol.* **2013**, *323*, 40–48.
11. Wang, X.; Li, G.-Z.; Lu, W.-C. Virus-ECC-mPLoc: A multi-label predictor for predicting the subcellular localization of virus proteins with both single and multiple sites based on a general

form of Chou's pseudo amino acid composition. *Protein Pept. Lett.* **2013**, *20*, 309–317.
12. Du, P.; Li, Y. Prediction of protein submitochondria locations by hybridizing pseudo-amino acid composition with various physicochemical features of segmented sequence. *BMC Bioinforma.* **2006**, *7*, 518.
13. Du, P.; Yu, Y. SubMito-PSPCP: Predicting protein submitochondrial locations by hybridizing positional specific physicochemical properties with pseudoamino acid compositions. *BioMed Res. Int.* **2013**, *2013*, 263829–263836.
14. Fan, G.-L.; Li, Q.-Z. Predicting protein submitochondria locations by combining different descriptors into the general form of Chou's pseudo amino acid composition. *Amino Acids* **2012**, *43*, 545–555.
15. Mei, S. Multi-kernel transfer learning based on Chou's PseAAC formulation for protein submitochondria localization. *J. Theor. Biol.* **2012**, *293*, 121–130.
16. Huang, C.; Yuan, J.-Q. Predicting protein subchloroplast locations with both single and multiple sites via three different modes of Chou's pseudo amino acid compositions. *J. Theor. Biol.* **2013**, *335*, 205–212.
17. Jiang, X.; Wei, R.; Zhao, Y.; Zhang, T. Using Chou's pseudo amino acid composition based on approximate entropy and an ensemble of AdaBoost classifiers to predict protein subnuclear location. *Amino Acids* **2008**, *34*, 669–675.
18. Shen, H.-B.; Chou, K.-C. Nuc-PLoc: A new web-server for predicting protein subnuclear localization by fusing PseAA composition and PsePSSM. *Protein Eng. Des. Sel.* **2007**, *20*, 561–567.
19. Li, F.-M.; Li, Q.-Z. Predicting protein subcellular location using Chou's pseudo amino acid composition and improved hybrid approach. *Protein Pept. Lett.* **2008**, *15*, 612–616.
20. Li, L.-Q.; Zhang, Y.; Zou, L.-Y.; Zhou, Y.; Zheng, X.-Q. Prediction of protein subcellular multi-localization based on the general form of Chou's pseudo amino acid composition. *Protein Pept. Lett.* **2012**, *19*, 375–387.
21. Nanni, L.; Lumini, A. Genetic programming for creating Chou's pseudo amino acid based features for submitochondria localization. *Amino Acids* **2008**, *34*, 653–660.
22. Zeng, Y.; Guo, Y.; Xiao, R.; Yang, L.; Yu, L.; Li, M. Using the augmented Chou's pseudo amino acid composition for predicting protein submitochondria locations based on auto covariance approach. *J. Theor. Biol.* **2009**, *259*, 366–372.
23. Pierleoni, A.; Martelli, P.L.; Casadio, R. MemLoci: Predicting subcellular localization of membrane proteins in eukaryotes. *Bioinformatics* **2011**, *27*, 1224–1230.
24. Du, P.; Tian, Y.; Yan, Y. Subcellular localization prediction for human internal and organelle membrane proteins with projected gene ontology scores. *J. Theor. Biol.* **2012**, *313*, 61–67.
25. Huang, C.; Yuan, J.-Q. A multilabel model based on Chou's pseudo-amino acid composition for identifying membrane proteins with both single and multiple functional types. *J. Membr. Biol.* **2013**, *246*, 327–334.
26. Zhang, S.-W.; Zhang, Y.-L.; Yang, H.-F.; Zhao, C.-H.; Pan, Q. Using the concept of Chou's pseudo amino acid composition to predict protein subcellular localization: An approach by incorporating evolutionary information and von Neumann entropies. *Amino Acids* **2008**, *34*, 565–572.

27. Cao, J.-Z.; Liu, W.-Q.; Gu, H. Predicting viral protein subcellular localization with Chou's pseudo amino acid composition and imbalance-weighted multi-label K-nearest neighbor algorithm. *Protein Pept. Lett.* **2012**, *19*, 1163–1169.
28. Shen, H.-B.; Chou, K.-C. Virus-mPLoc: A fusion classifier for viral protein subcellular location prediction by incorporating multiple sites. *J. Biomol. Struct. Dyn.* **2010**, *28*, 175–186.
29. Sahu, S.S.; Panda, G. A novel feature representation method based on Chou's pseudo amino acid composition for protein structural class prediction. *Comput. Biol. Chem.* **2010**, *34*, 320–327.
30. Chen, C.; Shen, Z.-B.; Zou, X.-Y. Dual-layer wavelet SVM for predicting protein structural class via the general form of Chou's pseudo amino acid composition. *Protein Pept. Lett.* **2012**, *19*, 422–429.
31. Kong, L.; Zhang, L.; Lv, J. Accurate prediction of protein structural classes by incorporating predicted secondary structure information into the general form of Chou's pseudo amino acid composition. *J. Theor. Biol.* **2013**, *344*, 12–18.
32. Li, Z.-C.; Zhou, X.-B.; Dai, Z.; Zou, X.-Y. Prediction of protein structural classes by Chou's pseudo amino acid composition: Approached using continuous wavelet transform and principal component analysis. *Amino Acids* **2009**, *37*, 415–425.
33. Liao, B.; Xiang, Q.; Li, D. Incorporating secondary features into the general form of Chou's PseAAC for predicting protein structural class. *Protein Pept. Lett.* **2012**, *19*, 1133–1138.
34. Liu, L.; Hu, X.-Z.; Liu, X.-X.; Wang, Y.; Li, S.-B. Predicting protein fold types by the general form of Chou's pseudo amino acid composition: Approached from optimal feature extractions. *Protein Pept. Lett.* **2012**, *19*, 439–449.
35. Qin, Y.-F.; Wang, C.-H.; Yu, X.-Q.; Zhu, J.; Liu, T.-G.; Zheng, X.-Q. Predicting protein structural class by incorporating patterns of over-represented k-mers into the general form of Chou's PseAAC. *Protein Pept. Lett.* **2012**, *19*, 388–397.
36. Chen, C.; Chen, L.; Zou, X.; Cai, P. Prediction of protein secondary structure content by using the concept of Chou's pseudo amino acid composition and support vector machine. *Protein Pept. Lett.* **2009**, *16*, 27–31.
37. Zou, D.; He, Z.; He, J.; Xia, Y. Supersecondary structure prediction using Chou's pseudo amino acid composition. *J. Comput. Chem.* **2011**, *32*, 271–278.
38. Sun, X.-Y.; Shi, S.-P.; Qiu, J.-D.; Suo, S.-B.; Huang, S.-Y.; Liang, R.-P. Identifying protein quaternary structural attributes by incorporating physicochemical properties into the general form of Chou's PseAAC via discrete wavelet transform. *Mol. Biosyst.* **2012**, *8*, 3178–3184.
39. Zhang, S.-W.; Chen, W.; Yang, F.; Pan, Q. Using Chou's pseudo amino acid composition to predict protein quaternary structure: A sequence-segmented PseAAC approach. *Amino Acids* **2008**, *35*, 591–598.
40. Gu, Q.; Ding, Y.S.; Zhang, T.L. Prediction of G-protein-coupled receptor classes in low homology using Chou's pseudo amino acid composition with approximate entropy and hydrophobicity patterns. *Protein Pept. Lett.* **2010**, *17*, 559–567.
41. Qiu, J.-D.; Huang, J.-H.; Liang, R.-P.; Lu, X.-Q. Prediction of G-protein-coupled receptor classes based on the concept of Chou's pseudo amino acid composition: An approach from discrete wavelet transform. *Anal. Biochem.* **2009**, *390*, 68–73.
42. Zia-Ur-Rehman; Khan, A. Identifying GPCRs and their types with Chou's pseudo amino acid

composition: An approach from multi-scale energy representation and position specific scoring matrix. *Protein Pept. Lett.* **2012**, *19*, 890–903.
43. Qiu, J.-D.; Huang, J.-H.; Shi, S.-P.; Liang, R.-P. Using the concept of Chou's pseudo amino acid composition to predict enzyme family classes: An approach with support vector machine based on discrete wavelet transform. *Protein Pept. Lett.* **2010**, *17*, 715–722.
44. Zhou, X.-B.; Chen, C.; Li, Z.-C.; Zou, X.-Y. Using Chou's amphiphilic pseudo-amino acid composition and support vector machine for prediction of enzyme subfamily classes. *J. Theor. Biol.* **2007**, *248*, 546–551.
45. Chen, Y.-K.; Li, K.-B. Predicting membrane protein types by incorporating protein topology, domains, signal peptides, and physicochemical properties into the general form of Chou's pseudo amino acid composition. *J. Theor. Biol.* **2013**, *318*, 1–12.
46. Han, G.-S.; Yu, Z.-G.; Anh, V. A two-stage SVM method to predict membrane protein types by incorporating amino acid classifications and physicochemical properties into a general form of Chou's PseAAC. *J. Theor. Biol.* **2013**, *344*, 31–39.
47. Hayat, M.; Khan, A. Discriminating outer membrane proteins with fuzzy K-nearest neighbor algorithms based on the general form of Chou's PseAAC. *Protein Pept. Lett.* **2012**, *19*, 411–421.
48. Mohammad Beigi, M.; Behjati, M.; Mohabatkar, H. Prediction of metalloproteinase family based on the concept of Chou's pseudo amino acid composition using a machine learning approach. *J. Struct. Funct. Genomics* **2011**, *12*, 191–197.
49. Esmaeili, M.; Mohabatkar, H.; Mohsenzadeh, S. Using the concept of Chou's pseudo amino acid composition for risk type prediction of human papillomaviruses. *J. Theor. Biol.* **2010**, *263*, 203–209.
50. Ding, H.; Luo, L.; Lin, H. Prediction of cell wall lytic enzymes using Chou's amphiphilic pseudo amino acid composition. *Protein Pept. Lett.* **2009**, *16*, 351–355.
51. Mohabatkar, H. Prediction of cyclin proteins using Chou's pseudo amino acid composition. *Protein Pept. Lett.* **2010**, *17*, 1207–1214.
52. Mohabatkar, H.; Mohammad Beigi, M.; Abdolahi, K.; Mohsenzadeh, S. Prediction of allergenic proteins by means of the concept of Chou's pseudo amino acid composition and a machine learning approach. *Med. Chem.* **2013**, *9*, 133–137.
53. Fan, G.-L.; Li, Q.-Z. Discriminating bioluminescent proteins by incorporating average chemical shift and evolutionary information into the general form of Chou's pseudo amino acid composition. *J. Theor. Biol.* **2013**, *334*, 45–51.
54. Fang, Y.; Guo, Y.; Feng, Y.; Li, M. Predicting DNA-binding proteins: Approached from Chou's pseudo amino acid composition and other specific sequence features. *Amino Acids* **2008**, *34*, 103–109.
55. Mohabatkar, H.; Mohammad Beigi, M.; Esmaeili, A. Prediction of GABAA receptor proteins using the concept of Chou's pseudo-amino acid composition and support vector machine. *J. Theor. Biol.* **2011**, *281*, 18–23.
56. Nanni, L.; Lumini, A.; Gupta, D.; Garg, A. Identifying bacterial virulent proteins by fusing a set of classifiers based on variants of Chou's pseudo amino acid composition and on evolutionary information. *IEEE/ACM Trans. Comput. Biol. Bioinforma.* **2012**, *9*, 467–475.
57. Sarangi, A.N.; Lohani, M.; Aggarwal, R. Prediction of essential proteins in prokaryotes by

incorporating various physico-chemical features into the general form of Chou's pseudo amino acid composition. *Protein Pept. Lett.* **2013**, *20*, 781–795.

58. Hajisharifi, Z.; Piryaiee, M.; Mohammad Beigi, M.; Behbahani, M.; Mohabatkar, H. Predicting anticancer peptides with Chou's pseudo amino acid composition and investigating their mutagenicity via Ames test. *J. Theor. Biol.* **2014**, *341*, 34–40.
59. Khosravian, M.; Faramarzi, F.K.; Beigi, M.M.; Behbahani, M.; Mohabatkar, H. Predicting antibacterial peptides by the concept of Chou's pseudo-amino acid composition and machine learning methods. *Protein Pept. Lett.* **2013**, *20*, 180–186.
60. Zhao, X.-W.; Ma, Z.-Q.; Yin, M.-H. Predicting protein–protein interactions by combing various sequence-derived features into the general form of Chou's pseudo amino acid composition. *Protein Pept. Lett.* **2012**, *19*, 492–500.
61. Niu, X.-H.; Hu, X.-H.; Shi, F.; Xia, J.-B. Predicting protein solubility by the general form of Chou's pseudo amino acid composition: Approached from chaos game representation and fractal dimension. *Protein Pept. Lett.* **2012**, *19*, 940–948.
62. Yu, H.; Chen, J.; Xu, X.; Li, Y.; Zhao, H.; Fang, Y.; Li, X.; Zhou, W.; Wang, W.; Wang, Y.A. Systematic prediction of multiple drug-target interactions from chemical, genomic, and pharmacological data. *PLoS One* **2012**, *7*, e37608.
63. Georgiou, D.N.; Karakasidis, T.E.; Nieto, J.J.; Torres, A. Use of fuzzy clustering technique and matrices to classify amino acids and its impact to Chou's pseudo amino acid composition. *J. Theor. Biol.* **2009**, *257*, 17–26.
64. Gupta, M.K.; Niyogi, R.; Misra, M. An alignment-free method to find similarity among protein sequences via the general form of Chou's pseudo amino acid composition. *SAR QSAR Environ. Res.* **2013**, *24*, 597–609.
65. Lin, H. The modified Mahalanobis discriminant for predicting outer membrane proteins by using Chou's pseudo amino acid composition. *J. Theor. Biol.* **2008**, *252*, 350–356.
66. Nanni, L.; Brahnam, S.; Lumini, A. Wavelet images and Chou's pseudo amino acid composition for protein classification. *Amino Acids* **2012**, *43*, 657–665.
67. Qiu, J.-D.; Suo, S.-B.; Sun, X.-Y.; Shi, S.-P.; Liang, R.-P. OligoPred: A web-server for predicting homo-oligomeric proteins by incorporating discrete wavelet transform into Chou's pseudo amino acid composition. *J. Mol. Graph. Model.* **2011**, *30*, 129–134.
68. Ren, L.-Y.; Zhang, Y.-S.; Gutman, I. Predicting the classification of transcription factors by incorporating their binding site properties into a novel mode of Chou's pseudo amino acid composition. *Protein Pept. Lett.* **2012**, *19*, 1170–1176.
69. Xiaohui, N.; Nana, L.; Jingbo, X.; Dingyan, C.; Yuehua, P.; Yang, X.; Weiquan, W.; Dongming, W.; Zengzhen, W. Using the concept of Chou's pseudo amino acid composition to predict protein solubility: An approach with entropies in information theory. *J. Theor. Biol.* **2013**, *332*, 211–217.
70. Xie, H.-L.; Fu, L.; Nie, X.-D. Using ensemble SVM to identify human GPCRs *N*-linked glycosylation sites based on the general form of Chou's PseAAC. *Protein Eng. Des. Sel.* **2013**, *26*, 735–742.
71. Yu, L.; Guo, Y.; Li, Y.; Li, G.; Li, M.; Luo, J.; Xiong, W.; Qin, W. SecretP: Identifying bacterial secreted proteins by fusing new features into Chou's pseudo-amino acid composition. *J. Theor. Biol.* **2010**, *267*, 1–6.

72. Zhang, G.-Y.; Fang, B.-S. Predicting the cofactors of oxidoreductases based on amino acid composition distribution and Chou's amphiphilic pseudo-amino acid composition. *J. Theor. Biol.* **2008**, *253*, 310–315.
73. Zhang, G.-Y.; Li, H.-C.; Gao, J.-Q.; Fang, B.-S. Predicting lipase types by improved Chou's pseudo-amino acid composition. *Protein Pept. Lett.* **2008**, *15*, 1132–1137.
74. Liu, B.; Wang, X.; Zou, Q.; Dong, Q.; Chen, Q. Protein remote homology detection by combining Chou's pseudo amino acid composition and profile-based protein representation. *Mol. Inform.* **2013**, *32*, 775–782.
75. Georgiou, D.N.; Karakasidis, T.E.; Nieto, J.J.; Torres, A. A study of entropy/clarity of genetic sequences using metric spaces and fuzzy sets. *J. Theor. Biol.* **2010**, *267*, 95–105.
76. Georgiou, T.N.; Karakasidis, T.E.; Megaritis, A.C. A short survey on genetic sequences, Chou's pseudo amino acid composition and its combination with fuzzy set theory. *Open Bioinforma. J.* **2013**, *7*, 41–48.
77. Chen, W.; Feng, P.-M.; Lin, H.; Chou, K.-C. iRSpot-PseDNC: Identify recombination spots with pseudo dinucleotide composition. *Nucleic Acids Res.* **2013**, *41*, e68.
78. Chou, K.-C. Some remarks on protein attribute prediction and pseudo amino acid composition. *J. Theor. Biol.* **2011**, *273*, 236–247.
79. Chou, K.-C. Using amphiphilic pseudo amino acid composition to predict enzyme subfamily classes. *Bioinformatics* **2005**, *21*, 10–19.
80. Shen, H.-B.; Chou, K.-C. PseAAC: A flexible web server for generating various kinds of protein pseudo amino acid composition. *Anal. Biochem.* **2008**, *373*, 386–388.
81. Du, P.; Wang, X.; Xu, C.; Gao, Y. PseAAC-Builder: A cross-platform stand-alone program for generating various special Chou's pseudo-amino acid compositions. *Anal. Biochem.* **2012**, *425*, 117–119.
82. Cao, D.-S.; Xu, Q.-S.; Liang, Y.-Z. Propy: A tool to generate various modes of Chou's PseAAC. *Bioinformatics* **2013**, *29*, 960–962.
83. Chou, K.-C.; Cai, Y.-D. Prediction of protein subcellular locations by GO-FunD-PseAA predictor. *Biochem. Biophys. Res. Commun.* **2004**, *320*, 1236–1239.
84. Feng, Z.P.; Zhang, C.T. Prediction of membrane protein types based on the hydrophobic index of amino acids. *J. Protein Chem.* **2000**, *19*, 269–275.
85. Lin, Z.; Pan, X.M. Accurate prediction of protein secondary structural content. *J. Protein Chem.* **2001**, *20*, 217–220.
86. Horne, D.S. Prediction of protein helix content from an autocorrelation analysis of sequence hydrophobicities. *Biopolymers* **1988**, *27*, 451–477.
87. Sokal, R.R.; Thomson, B.A. Population structure inferred by local spatial autocorrelation: An example from an Amerindian tribal population. *Am. J. Phys. Anthropol.* **2006**, *129*, 121–131.
88. Dubchak, I.; Muchnik, I.; Mayor, C.; Dralyuk, I.; Kim, S.H. Recognition of a protein fold in the context of the Structural Classification of Proteins (SCOP) classification. *Proteins* **1999**, *35*, 401–407.
89. Chou, K.-C. Prediction of protein subcellular locations by incorporating quasi-sequence-order effect. *Biochem. Biophys. Res. Commun.* **2000**, *27*, 477–483.

90. Steinbiss, S.; Gremme, G.; Schärfer, C.; Mader, M.; Kurtz, S. AnnotationSketch: A genome annotation drawing library. *Bioinformatics* **2009**, *25*, 533–534.
91. PseAAC-General. Available online: http://pseb.sf.net (accessed on 19 February 2014).
92. PseAAC-General SourceForge Site. Available online: http://sourceforge.net/projects/pseb/files (accessed on 19 February 2014).

5

iRSpot-TNCPseAAC: Identify Recombination Spots with Trinucleotide Composition and Pseudo Amino Acid Components

Wang-Ren Qiu [1], **Xuan Xiao** [1,2,4,*] **and Kuo-Chen Chou** [3,4]

[1] Computer Department, Jing-De-Zhen Ceramic Institute, Jingdezhen 333046, China; E-Mail: qiuone@163.com

[2] Information School, ZheJiang Textile & Fashion College, Ningbo 315211, China

[3] Center of Excellence in Genomic Medicine Research (CEGMR), King Abdulaziz University, Jeddah 21589, Saudi Arabia; E-Mail: kcchou@gordonlifescience.org

[4] Gordon Life Science Institute, Belmont, MA 02478, USA

* Author to whom correspondence should be addressed; E-Mail: xxiao@gordonlifescience.org or jdzxiaoxuan@163.com

---

Abstract: Meiosis and recombination are the two opposite aspects that coexist in a DNA system. As a driving force for evolution by generating natural genetic variations, meiotic recombination plays a very important role in the formation of eggs and sperm. Interestingly, the recombination does not occur randomly across a genome, but with higher probability in some genomic regions called "hotspots", while with lower probability in so-called "coldspots". With the ever-increasing amount of genome sequence data in the postgenomic era, computational methods for effectively identifying the hotspots and coldspots have become urgent as they can timely provide us with useful insights into the mechanism of meiotic recombination and the process of genome evolution as well. To meet the need, we developed a new predictor called "iRSpot-TNCPseAAC", in which a DNA sample was formulated by combining its trinucleotide composition (TNC) and the pseudo amino acid components (PseAAC) of the protein translated from the DNA sample according to its genetic codes. The former was used to incorporate its local or short-rage sequence order information; while the latter, its global and long-range one. Compared with the best existing predictor in this area, iRSpot-TNCPseAAC achieved higher rates in accuracy, Mathew's correlation coefficient, and sensitivity, indicating that the new predictor may become a useful tool for identifying the recombination hotspots and coldspots, or, at least, become a complementary tool to the existing methods. It has not escaped our notice that the aforementioned novel approach to incorporate the DNA sequence order information into a discrete model may also be used for many other genome analysis problems. The web-server for iRSpot-TNCPseAAC is available at http://www.jci-bioinfo.cn/iRSpot-TNCPseAAC. Furthermore, for the convenience of the vast majority of experimental scientists, a step-by-step guide is provided on how to use the current web server to obtain their desired result without the need to follow the complicated mathematical equations.

Keywords: genome; DNA; recombination spots; hotspots; coldspots; trinucleotide composition; pseudo amino acid composition; web-server; iRSpot-TNCPseAAC

1. Introduction

Meiosis and recombination are two indispensible aspects for cell reproduction and growth (Figure 1). The former is a special type of cell division by which the genome is divided in half to generate daughter cells for participating in sexual reproduction, while the latter is to produce single-strand ends that can invade the homologous chromosome [1].

Figure 1. An illustration to show the process of meiosis and recombination in a DNA system. Adapted from [2].

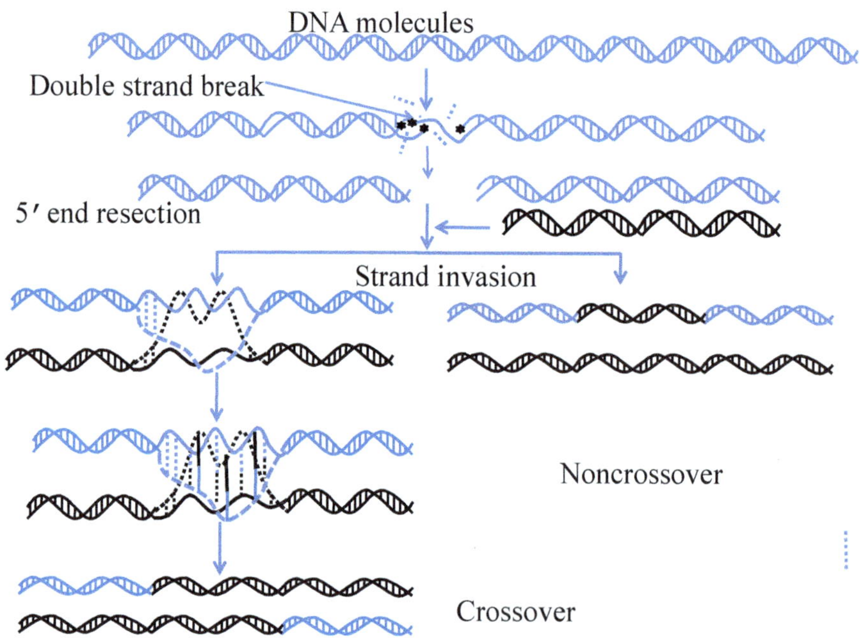

Recombination is initiated by double-strand breaks (or broken DNA ends); defecting in meiosis may lead to male infertility [3–5]. Meiotic recombination ensures accurate chromosome segregation during the first meiotic division and provides a mechanism to increase genetic heterogeneity among the meiotic products. Accordingly, identification of recombination spots may provide very useful information for in-depth understanding the reproduction and growth of cells.

In the past decades, a lot of global mapping studies have been performed to map double-strand break sites on chromosomes [6–13]. The following findings were observed through these studies for the meiotic recombination events. (i) They generally concentrate in 1:2.5 kilobase regions; (ii) They do not occur randomly across the entire genome but with a higher rate in some regions and lower in others; the former is a so-called "hotspot" while the latter, "coldspot"; (iii) They do not share a consensus sequence pattern.

With the rapid increasing number of genome sequences, it is important to address the following problem. Given a genome sequence, how can we predict which part of it is the hotspot for recombination, and which part is not?

Based on the nucleotide sequence contents, Liu *et al.* [14] proposed a computational method to deal with this problem. However, in their method no sequence-order effect whatsoever was taken into account, and, hence, its prediction power might be limited.

Actually, one of the most important, but also most difficult, problems in computational biology is how to formulate a biological sequence with a discrete model or a vector, yet still keep considerable sequence order information. This is as all the existing operation engines, such as covariance discriminant (CD) [15–20], neural network [21–23], support vector machine (SVM) [24–26], random forest [27,28], conditional random field [29], nearest neighbor (NN) [30,31], K-nearest neighbor (KNN) [32–34], OET-KNN (optimized evidence-theoretic k-nearest neighbors) [35–38], and Fuzzy K-nearest neighbor [39–43], can only handle vector, but not sequence, samples. However, a vector defined in a discrete model may completely lose all the sequence-order information.

To avoid completely losing the sequence-order information for proteins, the pseudo amino acid composition [44,45] or Chou's pseudo amino acid components (PseAAC) [46] was proposed. Ever since the concept of PseAAC was proposed in 2001 [44], it has penetrated into almost all the areas of computational proteomics, such as identifying cysteine S-nitrosylation sites in proteins [29], predicting bacterial virulent proteins [47], predicting antibacterial peptides [48], identifying bacterial secreted proteins [49], predicting supersecondary structure [50], predicting protein subcellular location [51–59], predicting membrane protein types [60,61], discriminating outer membrane proteins [62], identifying antibacterial peptides [48], identifying allergenic proteins [63], predicting metalloproteinase family [64], predicting protein structural class [65], identifying GPCRs (G protein-coupled receptors) and their types [66,67], identifying protein quaternary structural attributes [68,69], predicting protein submitochondria locations [70–73], identifying risk type of human papillomaviruses [74], identifying cyclin proteins [75], predicting GABA(A) receptor proteins [76], classifying amino acids [77], predicting the cofactors of oxidoreductases [78], predicting enzyme subfamily classes [79], detecting remote homologous proteins [80], analyzing genetic sequences [81], predicting anticancer peptides [82], among many others (see a long list of papers cited in the References section of [83]). Recently, the concept of PseAAC was further extended to represent the feature vectors of nucleotides [15], as well as other biological samples [84–86]. As it has been widely and increasingly used, recently two powerful soft-wares, called "PseAAC-Builder" [87] and "propy" [88], were established for generating various special Chou's pseudo-amino acid compositions, in addition to the web-server "PseAAC" [89], built in 2008.

Encouraged by the success of introducing PseAAC for proteins, recently, Chen *et al.* [25] proposed the pseudo dinucleotide composition or PseDNC to represent DNA sequences for identifying the recombination spots by counting some sequence effects, remarkably improving the prediction results in comparison with those by Liu *et al.* [14], without including any sequence information. However, in PseDNC, only the correlations of dinucleotides along a DNA sequence were considered, and, hence, some important sequence order effects might be missed.

The present study was initiated in an attempt to incorporate the long-range or global correlations of trinucleotides along a DNA sequences in hope to further improve the prediction quality in indentifying the recombination spots.

As demonstrated in a series of recent publications [24,42,90–92] and summarized in a comprehensive review [83], to establish a really useful statistical predictor for a biological system, one needs to consider the following procedures: (i) construct or select a valid benchmark dataset to train and test the predictor; (ii) formulate the biological samples with an effective mathematical expression that can truly reflect their intrinsic correlation with the target to be predicted; (iii) introduce or develop a powerful algorithm (or engine) to operate the prediction; (iv) properly perform cross-validation tests to objectively evaluate the anticipated accuracy of the predictor; and (v) establish a user-friendly web-server for the predictor that is accessible to the public. Below, let us elaborate how to deal with these procedures one-by-one.

2. Results and Discussion

2.1. Benchmark Dataset

The benchmark dataset S used in this study was taken from Liu *et al.* [14], which contains 490 recombination hotspots and 591 recombination coldspots, as can be formulated by:

$$S = S^{+} \cup S^{-} \tag{1}$$

where subset S^{+} and S^{-} are respectively for the hot and cold spots, while $\cup$ represents the symbol for "union" in the set theory. For reader's convenience, the 490 DNA sequences in S^{+} and 591 sequences in S^{-} are given in the Supplementary Information S1.

2.2. Formulate DNA Samples by Combining Trinucleotide Composition and Pseudo Amino Acid Components

Suppose a DNA sequence $\mathbf{D}$ with L nucleotides; *i.e.*,

$$\mathbf{D} = N_1 N_2 N_3 N_4 N_5 N_6 N_7 \cdots N_L \tag{2}$$

where

$$N_i \in \{\text{A (adenine)}, \quad \text{C (cytosine)} \quad \text{G (guanine)} \quad \text{T (thymine)}\} \tag{3}$$

denotes the i-th (i = 1, 2, …, L) nucleotide in the DNA sequence. If the feature vector of the DNA sequence is formulated by its mononucleotide composition (MNC), we have:

$$\begin{aligned}\mathbf{D} &= \begin{bmatrix} f(\text{A}) & f(\text{C}) & f(\text{G}) & f(\text{T}) \end{bmatrix}^{\mathbf{T}} \\ &= \begin{bmatrix} f_1^{(1)} & f_2^{(1)} & f_3^{(1)} & f_4^{(1)} \end{bmatrix}^{\mathbf{T}}\end{aligned} \tag{4}$$

where $f_1^{(1)} = f(\mathrm{A})$, $f_2^{(1)} = f(\mathrm{C})$, $f_3^{(1)} = f(\mathrm{G})$, and $f_4^{(1)} = f(\mathrm{T})$ are the normalized occurrence frequencies of adenine (A), cytosine (C), guanine (G), and thymine (T), respectively, in the DNA sequence; and the symbol **T** is the transpose operator. As we can see from Equation (4), all the sequence order information is missed if using MNC to represent a DNA sequence. If using the dinucleotide composition (DNC) to represent the DNA sequence, instead of the four components as shown in Equation (4), the corresponding feature vector will contain 4 × 4 = 16 components, as given below:

$$\begin{aligned}\mathbf{D} &= \begin{bmatrix} f(\mathrm{AA}) & f(\mathrm{AC}) & f(\mathrm{AG}) & f(\mathrm{AT}) & \cdots & f(\mathrm{TT}) \end{bmatrix}^{\mathbf{T}} \\ &= \begin{bmatrix} f_1^{(2)} & f_2^{(2)} & f_3^{(2)} & f_4^{(2)} & \cdots & f_{16}^{(2)} \end{bmatrix}^{\mathbf{T}}\end{aligned} \tag{5}$$

where $f_1^{(2)} = f(\mathrm{AA})$ is the normalized occurrence frequency of AA in the DNA sequence; $f_2^{(2)} = f(\mathrm{AC})$, that of AC; $f_3^{(2)} = f(\mathrm{AG})$, that of AG; and so forth. If represented by the trinucleotide composition (TNC), the corresponding feature vector will contain $4 \times 4 \times 4 = 4^3 = 64$ components, as given below:

$$\begin{aligned}\mathbf{D} &= \begin{bmatrix} f(\mathrm{AAA}) & f(\mathrm{AAC}) & f(\mathrm{AAG}) & f(\mathrm{AAT}) & \cdots & f(\mathrm{TTT}) \end{bmatrix}^{\mathbf{T}} \\ &= \begin{bmatrix} f_1^{(3)} & f_2^{(3)} & f_3^{(3)} & f_4^{(3)} & \cdots & f_{64}^{(3)} \end{bmatrix}^{\mathbf{T}}\end{aligned} \tag{6}$$

where $f_1^{(3)} = f(\mathrm{AAA})$ is the normalized occurrence frequency of AAA in the DNA sequence; $f_2^{(3)} = f(\mathrm{AAC})$, that of AAC; and so forth. Generally speaking, if a DNA sequence is represented by the K-tuple nucleotide composition, the corresponding vector D for the DNA sequence will contain 4^K components; *i.e.*,

$$\mathbf{D} = \begin{bmatrix} f_1^{(K)} & f_2^{(K)} & f_3^{(K)} & f_4^{(K)} & \cdots & f_{4^K}^{(K)} \end{bmatrix}^{\mathbf{T}} \tag{7}$$

As we can see from Equations (5–7), with increasing the tuple number, although the base sequence-order information within a local or very short range could be gradually included, none of the global or long-range sequence-order information would be reflected by the formulation.

Actually, in computational proteomics, we have also faced exactly the same situation; *i.e.*, although the dipeptide composition, tripeptide composition, and K-tuple peptide composition were used by many investigators to represent protein sequences by incorporating their local sequence order information [93–97], their global or long-range sequence order information still could not be reflected. As mentioned above, to deal with this kind of problems in proteomics, the concept of PseAAC [44,45] was introduced.

Stimulated by the PseAAC approach [44,45] in computational proteomics, below let us propose a novel feature vector to represent the DNA sequence (cf. Equation (2)) by combining its TNC (see Equation (2)) and the pseudo amino acid components of its translated protein chain.

As is well known, three nucleotides encode an amino acid (see Figure 2). Thus, according the conversion table from DNA codons to amino acids (Table 1), the DNA sequence in Equation (2) can be translated into a protein sequence expressed by:

$$\mathbf{P} = A_1 A_2 A_3 \cdots A_{L^*} \tag{8}$$

with

$$\begin{cases} A_i \in \{20 \text{ native amino acids}\} \\ L^* = \text{Int}\{L/3\} \end{cases} \tag{9}$$

where the symbol "Int" is an integer truncation operator meaning to take the integer part for the number in the brackets immediately after it.

Figure 2. A graph to show how a DNA codon of three nucleotides is converted to an amino acid. The characters in the first three rings from the center represent four bases in DNA, while those in the fourth ring represent the single-letter codes of the 20 native amino acids in protein. The symbol * means the "Stop" sign.

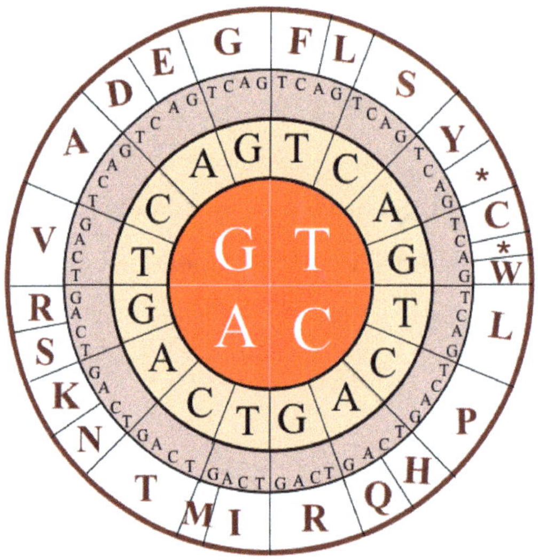

Table 1. The conversion code of the 64 trinucleotides in DNA to the 20 amino acids in protein.

Trinucleotide	Amino acid	Trinucleotide	Amino acid
AAA	Lys (K)	GAA	Glu (E)
AAC	Asn (N)	GAC	Asp (D)
AAG	Lys (K)	GAG	Glu (E)
AAT	Asn (N)	GAT	Asp (D)
ACA	Thr (T)	GCA	Ala (A)
ACC		GCC	
ACG		GCG	
ACT		GCT	
AGA	Arg (R)	GGA	Gly (G)
AGC	Ser (S)	GGC	
AGG	Arg (R)	GGG	
AGT	Ser (S)	GGT	

Table 1. *Cont.*

Trinucleotide	Amino acid	Trinucleotide	Amino acid
ATA	Ile (I)	GTA	Val (V)
ATC		GTC	
ATG	Met (M)	GTG	
ATT	Ile (I)	GTT	
CAA	Gln (Q)	TAA	Stop!
CAC	His (H)	TAC	Tyr (Y)
CAG	Gln (Q)	TAG	Stop!
CAT	His (H)	TAT	Tyr (Y)
CCA	Pro (P)	TCA	Ser (S)
CCC		TCC	
CCG		TCG	
CCT		TCT	
CGA	Arg (R)	TGA	Stop!
CGC		TGC	Cys (C)
CGG		TGG	Trp (W)
CGT		TGT	Cys (C)
CTA	Leu (L)	TTA	Leu (L)
CTC		TTC	Phe (F)
CTG		TTG	Leu (L)
CTT		TTT	Phe (F)

Now, according to the formulation of Chou's PseAAC approach [44,45], for the protein chain of Equation (8), we have:

$$\begin{cases} \theta_1 = \dfrac{1}{L^*-1}\sum_{i=1}^{L^*-1}\Theta(A_i\,,A_{i+1}) \\ \theta_2 = \dfrac{1}{L^*-2}\sum_{i=1}^{L^*-2}\Theta(A_i\,,A_{i+2}) \\ \theta_3 = \dfrac{1}{L^*-3}\sum_{i=1}^{L^*-3}\Theta(A_i\,,A_{i+3}) \\ \quad\vdots \\ \theta_\lambda = \dfrac{1}{L^*-\lambda}\sum_{i=1}^{L^*-1}\Theta(A_i\,,A_{i+\lambda}) \end{cases} \qquad (\lambda < L^*) \tag{10}$$

where θ_k $(k = 1,2,3,\cdots,\lambda)$ is called the k-th tier correlation factor that reflects the sequence order correlation between all the k-th most contiguous residues along a protein chain. In this study, the correlation function in Equation 10 is given by:

$$\Theta(A_i, A_j) = \frac{1}{6}\sum_{n=1}^{6}\left[H_n(A_j) - H_n(A_i)\right]^2 \tag{11}$$

where $H_n(A_j)$ $(n = 1, 2, \cdots, 6)$ is the six physicochemical properties of amino acid A_j ; they are, respectively, hydrophobicity, hydrophilicity, side-chain mass, pK1 (α-COOH), pK2 (NH3), and PI. Note that before substituting these physicochemical values into Equation (11), they were all subjected to a standard conversion as described by the following equation:

$$H_n(A_i) = \frac{H_n^0(A_i) - \langle H_n^0 \rangle}{\mathrm{SD}(H_n^0)} \tag{12}$$

where $H_n(A_i)$ $(n = 1, 2, \cdots, 6)$ is the n-th original physicochemical property value for the amino acid A_i as given in Table 2, the symbol < and > means taking the average of the quantity therein over 20 native amino acids, and SD means the corresponding standard deviation. Listed in Table 3 are the converted values obtained by Equation (12) that will have a zero mean value over the 20 native amino acids, and will remain unchanged if going through the same conversion procedure again.

Table 2. List of the original values of the six physical-chemical properties for each of the 20 native amino acids.

Amino acid	Hydro-phobicity [a] H_1^0	Hydro-philicity [b] H_2^0	Side-chain mass [c] H_3^0	pK1 [d] H_4^0	pK2 [e] H_5^0	PI [f] H_6^0
A	0.62	−0.5	15	2.35	9.87	6.11
C	0.29	−1.00	47	1.71	10.78	5.02
D	−0.90	3.00	59	1.88	9.60	2.98
E	−0.74	3.00	73	2.19	9.67	3.08
F	1.19	−2.50	91	2.58	9.24	5.91
G	0.48	0.00	1	2.34	9.60	6.06
H	−0.40	−0.50	82	1.78	8.97	7.64
I	1.38	−1.80	57	2.32	9.76	6.04
K	−1.50	3.00	73	2.20	8.90	9.47
L	1.06	−1.80	57	2.36	9.60	6.04
M	0.64	−1.30	75	2.28	9.21	5.74
N	−0.78	0.20	58	2.18	9.09	10.76
P	0.12	0.00	42	1.99	10.60	6.30
Q	−0.85	0.20	72	2.17	9.13	5.65
R	−2.53	3.00	101	2.18	9.09	10.76
S	−0.18	0.30	31	2.21	9.15	5.68
T	−0.05	−0.40	45	2.15	9.12	5.60
V	1.08	−1.50	43	2.29	9.74	6.02
W	0.81	−3.40	130	2.38	9.39	5.88
Y	0.26	−2.30	107	2.20	9.11	5.63

[a] Taken from [98]; [b] Taken from [99]; [c] Taken from any biochemistry text book; [d] Taken from [100] for C^{α}-COOH; [e] Taken from [100] for NH_3; [f] Taken from [101].

Table 3. The corresponding values obtained by the standard conversion of Equation12 on the original values in Table 2.

Amino acid	H_1	H_2	H_3	H_4	H_5	H_6
A	0.62	−0.15	−1.55	0.78	0.77	−0.10
C	0.29	−0.41	−0.52	−2.27	2.57	−0.64
D	−0.90	1.67	−0.13	−1.46	0.24	−1.65
E	−0.74	1.67	0.33	0.01	0.37	−1.61
F	1.19	−1.19	0.91	1.87	−0.48	−0.20
G	0.48	0.11	−2.00	0.73	0.24	−0.13
H	−0.40	−0.15	0.62	−1.94	−1.01	0.65
I	1.38	−0.82	−0.19	0.63	0.55	−0.14
K	−1.50	1.67	0.33	0.06	−1.15	1.56
L	1.06	−0.82	−0.19	0.82	0.24	−0.14
M	0.64	−0.56	0.39	0.44	−0.54	−0.29
N	−0.78	0.22	−0.16	−0.03	−0.77	2.20
P	0.12	0.11	−0.68	−0.94	2.21	−0.01
Q	−0.85	0.22	0.29	−0.08	−0.69	−0.33
R	−2.53	1.67	1.23	−0.03	−0.77	2.20
S	−0.18	0.27	−1.03	0.11	−0.65	−0.32
T	−0.05	−0.10	−0.58	−0.18	−0.71	−0.36
V	1.08	−0.67	−0.65	0.49	0.51	−0.15
W	0.81	−1.65	2.17	0.92	−0.18	−0.22
Y	0.26	−1.08	1.43	0.06	−0.73	−0.34

By combining the λ correlation factors with the 64 components in TNC (see Equation (6)), the DNA sequence is formulated by:

$$\mathbf{D}=\begin{bmatrix} d_1 & d_2 & \cdots & d_{64} & d_{64+1} & \cdots & d_{64+\lambda} \end{bmatrix}^{\mathrm{T}} \tag{13}$$

where:

$$d_u=\begin{cases} \dfrac{f_u^{(3)}}{\sum_{i=1}^{64} f_i^{(3)}+w\sum_{k=1}^{\lambda}\theta_k}, & (1\le u\le 64) \\ \dfrac{w\theta_{u-64}}{\sum_{i=1}^{64} f_i^{(3)}+w\sum_{k=1}^{\lambda}\theta_k}, & (64+1\le u\le 64+\lambda) \end{cases} \tag{14}$$

where w is the weight factor which is determined by optimizing the outcome as will be mentioned later. The rationale of using Equation (13) to represent the DNA sequence is that the local or short-range sequence order effect can be directly reflected via the occurrence frequencies of its 64 trinucleotides, while the global or long-range sequence order effect can be indirectly reflected via the λ pseudo amino acid components of its translated protein chain. As three nucleotides encode an amino acid, the above approach is both quite rational and natural.

2.3. Use Support Vector Machine as an Operation Engine

Support vector machine (SVM) has been widely to make classification prediction (see, e.g., [24,102–105]. The basic idea of SVM is to transform the input data into a high dimensional feature space and then determine the optimal separating hyperplane. A brief introduction about the formulation of SVM was given in [103,106]. Here, the DNA samples as formulated by Equation (13) were used as inputs for the SVM. Its software was downloaded from the LIBSVM package [107,108], which provided a simple interface. Due to this advantages, the users can easily perform classification prediction by properly selecting the built-in parameters C and γ . In order to maximize the performance of the SVM algorithm, the two parameters in the RBF kernel were preliminarily optimized through a grid search strategy in this study. To obtain the optimized parameters, the search function "SVMcgForClass" was downloaded from http://www.matlabsky.com.

The predictor obtained via the aforementioned procedures is called iRSpot-TNCPseAAC, where "i" means "identify", "RSpot" means "Recombination Spots", while TNCPseAAC means a combination of "Tri-Nucleotide Composition" and "Pseudo Amino Acid Components."

To objectively evaluate the quality of a new predictor, one should use proper metrics [109] and rigorous cross-validation [83] to test it. Below, let us address these problems.

2.4. Four Different Metrics for Measuring the Prediction Quality

In literature, the following metrics are often used for examining the performance quality of a predictor:

$$\begin{cases} Sn = \dfrac{TP}{TP+FN} \\ Sp = \dfrac{TN}{TN+FP} \\ Acc = \dfrac{TP+TN}{TP+TN+FP+FN} \\ MCC = \dfrac{(TP\times TN)-(FP\times FN)}{\sqrt{(TP+FP)(TP+FN)(TN+FP)(TN+FN)}} \end{cases} \tag{15}$$

where *TP* represents the number of the true positive; *TN*, the number of the true negative; *FP*, the number of the false positive; *FN*, the number of the false negative; *Sn*, the sensitivity; *Sp*, the specificity; Acc, the accuracy; MCC, the Mathew's correlation coefficient. To most biologists, however, the four metrics as formulated in Equation (15) are not quite intuitive and easier-to-understand, particularly for the Mathew's correlation coefficient. Here let us adopt the formulation proposed recently [25,29] based on the Chou's symbol and definition [110]; *i.e.*,

$$\begin{cases} Sn = 1-\dfrac{N_-^+}{N^+} \\ Sp = 1-\dfrac{N_+^-}{N^-} \\ Acc = 1-\dfrac{N_-^+ + N_+^-}{N^+ + N^-} \\ Mcc = \dfrac{1-\left(\dfrac{N_-^+ + N_+^-}{N^+ + N^-}\right)}{\sqrt{\left(1+\dfrac{N_+^- - N_-^+}{N^+}\right)\left(1+\dfrac{N_-^+ - N_+^-}{N^-}\right)}} \end{cases} \tag{16}$$

where N^+ is the total number of the hotspot samples investigated while N^+_- the number of the hotspot samples incorrectly predicted as coldspots; N^- the total number of the coldspot samples investigated while N^-_+ the number of the coldspot samples incorrectly predicted as the hotspots [111].

Now, it can be clearly seen from Equation (16) that when $N^+_- = 0$ meaning none of the hotspots was incorrectly predicted to be a coldspot, we have the sensitivity $Sn = 1$. When $N^+_- = N^+$ meaning that all the hotspots were incorrectly predicted to be the coldspots, we have the sensitivity $Sn = 0$. Likewise, when $N^-_+ = 0$ meaning none of the coldspots was incorrectly predicted to be the hotspot, we have the specificity $Sp = 1$; whereas $N^-_+ = N^-$ meaning all the coldspots were incorrectly predicted as the hotspots, we have the specificity $Sp = 0$. When $N^+_- = N^-_+ = 0$ meaning that none of hotspots in the positive dataset and none of the coldspots in the negative dataset was incorrectly predicted, we have the overall accuracy $Acc = 1$ and $MCC = 1$; when $N^+_- = N^+$ and $N^-_+ = N^-$ meaning that all the hotspots in the positive dataset and all the coldspots in the negative dataset were incorrectly predicted, we have the overall accuracy $Acc = 0$ and $MCC = -1$; whereas when $N^+_- = N^+/2$ and $N^-_+ = N^-/2$ we have $Acc = 0.5$ and $MCC = 0$ meaning no better than random guess. As we can see from the above discussion based on Equation (16), the meanings of sensitivity, specificity, overall accuracy, and Mathew's correlation coefficient have become much more intuitive and easier-to-understand.

It should be pointed out that the metrics as given in Equation (15) and Equation (16) are valid only for the single-label systems as in the current case. For the multi-label systems in which emergence has become increasingly frequent in cell's molecular systems [112–118] and biomedical systems [43,119], a completely different set of metrics as defined in [109] is needed.

2.5. Evaluate the Anticipated Success Rates by Jackknife Tests

The following three cross-validation methods are often used in statistical prediction to evaluate the anticipated accuracy of a predictor: independent dataset test, subsampling (*K*-fold cross-validation) test, and jackknife test [120]. However, as elucidated by a review article [83], among the three methods, the jackknife test is deemed the least arbitrary and most objective as it can always yield a unique outcome for a given benchmark dataset, and hence has been increasingly used and widely recognized by investigators to examine the accuracy of various predictor [48,60,63,65,69,76,121,122]. Accordingly, in this study we also used the results obtained by jackknife tests to optimizing the uncertain parameters and to compare with the other predictors in this area.

3. Experimental Section

The results obtained with iRSpot-TNCPseAAC on the benchmark dataset S of Supplementary Information S1 by the jackknife test are given in Table 4, where for facilitating comparison the corresponding results by the iRSpot-PseDNC [25] on the same benchmark dataset are also given.

Table 4. A comparison of iRSpot-TNCPseAAC with the best existing method.

Predictor	Test method	*Sn* (%)	*Sp* (%)	*Acc* (%)	MCC
iRSpot-PseDNC [a]	Jackknife	73.06	89.49	82.04	0.638
iRSpot-KNCPseAAC [b]	Jackknife	87.14	79.59	83.72	0.671

[a] From [25]; [b] This paper with $\lambda = 5$, $w = 1.1$, $C = 32$ and $\gamma = 0.5$ for the LIBSVM operation engine [107,108].

As we can clearly see from the table, the iRSpot-TNCPseAAC predictor is superior to iRSpot-PseDNC [25] in three of the four metrics as defined by Equation (16); *i.e.*, it can yield higher accuracy *Acc*, higher Mathew's correlation coefficient MCC, and higher sensitivity *Sn*. Therefore, it is anticipated that the new predictor will become a useful tool for identifying the recombination spots in DNA, or at the very least become a complementary tool to iRSpot-PseDNC, the best existing prediction method in this area.

4. Conclusions

The above fact has also proved that it is indeed a feasible and promising approach to extend the concept of pseudo amino acid composition [44,45,123] developed in computational proteomics to the area of computational genomics. As shown by Equation (13) and the related equations in defining its $64+\lambda$ components, each of the DNA samples investigated in this study was formulated by a combination of its trinucleotide composition (TNC) with the pseudo amino acid components (PseAAC) that were derived from the protein translated from the DNA sample according to its genetic codes. The former can better incorporate its local or short-rage sequence order information in comparison with the dinucleotide composition (DNC) used in iRSpot-PseDNC [25]; while the latter can incorporate its global or long-range sequence order effects in a more natural or logical manner. Accordingly, it is anticipated that the idea or approach by extending the Chou's pseudo amino acid composition [44,45,123] for protein sequences to the pseudo oligonucleotide composition for DNA or RNA sequences may also be used to deal with many other genome analysis problems.

5. Web Server and User Guide

To enhance the value of its practical applications, a web-server for the iRSpot-TNCPseAAC predictor was established. Moreover, for the convenience of the vast majority of experimental scientists, here a step-to-step guide is provided for how to use the web server to get the desired results without the need to follow the mathematic equations that were presented just for the integrity in developing the predictor.

Step 1. Open the web server at http://www.jci-bioinfo.cn/iRSpot-TNCPseAAC and you will see the top page of the predictor on your computer screen, as shown in Figure 3. Click on the Read Me button to see a brief introduction about the **iRSpot-TNCPseAAC** predictor and the caveat when using it.

Figure 3. A semi-screenshot for the top page of the web-server iRSpot-TNCPseAAC at http://www.jci-bioinfo.cn/iRSpot-TNCPseAAC.

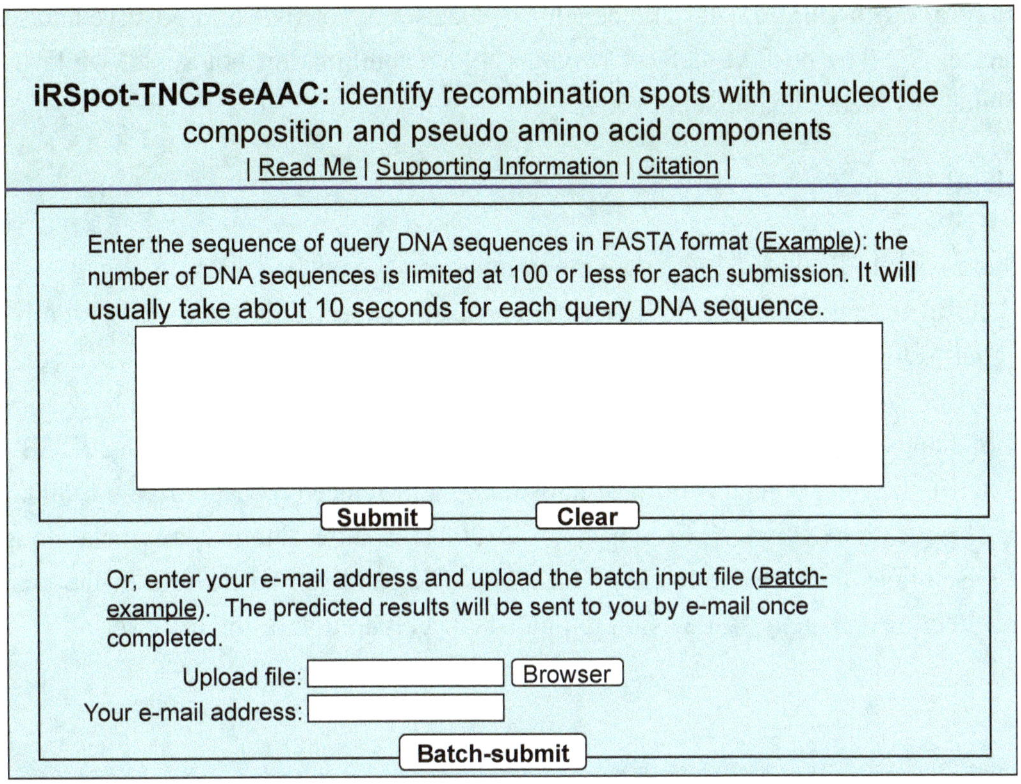

Step 2. Either type or copy/paste the query DNA sequences into the input box at the center of Figure 3. The input sequence should be in the FASTA format. For the examples of sequences in FASTA format, click the Example button right above the input box.

Step 3. Click on the Submit button to see the predicted result. For example, if you use the three query DNA sequences in the Example window as the input, after clicking the Submit button, you will see the following message shown on the screen of your computer: the outcome for the 1st query sample is "**recombination hotspot**"; the outcome for the 2nd query sample is "**recombination coldspot**". All these results are fully consistent with the experimental observations as summarized in the Supplementary Information S1. However, no result was given for the 3rd query sample as it contains some invalid characters as warned in the output screen. It takes about a few seconds for the above computation before the predicted result appears on your computer screen; the more number of query sequences and longer of each sequence, the more time it is usually needed.

Step 4. As shown on the lower panel of Figure 3, you may also choose the batch prediction by entering your e-mail address and your desired batch input file (in FASTA format) via the "**Browse**" button. To see the sample of batch input file, click on the button Batch-example. After clicking the button Batch-submit, you will see "Your batch job is under computation; once the results are available, you will be notified by e-mail."

Step 5. Click the Supporting Information button to download the benchmark dataset used to train and test the **iRSpot-TNCPseAAC** predictor.

Step 6. Click the Citation button to find the relevant papers that document the detailed development and algorithm of **iRSpot-TNCPseAAC**.

Supplementary Information

Supplementary Information S1. The benchmark dataset S consists of a positive dataset S^+ and a negative dataset S^-. The positive dataset contains 490 recombination hot spots, while the negative dataset contains 591 recombination cold spots.

Acknowledgments

The authors wish to thank the two anonymous reviewers for their constructive suggestions, which were very helpful for strengthening the presentation of this paper. This work was partially supported by the National Nature Science Foundation of China (No. 31260273, 61261027), the Jiangxi Provincial Foreign Scientific and Technological Cooperation Project (No.20120BDH80023), Natural Science Foundation of Jiangxi Province, China (No.20114BAB211013, 20122BAB211033, 20122BAB201044, 20122BAB2010), the Department of Education of JiangXi Province (GJJ12490), the LuoDi plan of the Department of Education of JiangXi Province(KJLD12083), and the JiangXi Provincial Foundation for Leaders of Disciplines in Science (20113BCB22008). The funders had no role in the design of this study, data collection and analysis, decision to publish, or preparation of the manuscript.

References

1. Hansen, L.; Kim, N.K.; Marino-Ramirez, L.; Landsman, D. Analysis of biological features associated with meiotic recombination hot and cold spots in *Saccharomyces cerevisiae*. *PLoS One* **2011**, *6*, e29711.
2. Keeney, S. Spo11 and the formation of DNA double-strand breaks in meiosis. *Genome Dyn. Stab.* **2008**, *2*, 81–123.
3. Ferguson, K.A.; Wong, E.C.; Chow, V.; Nigro, M.; Ma, S. Abnormal meiotic recombination in infertile men and its association with sperm aneuploidy. *Hum. Mol. Genet.* **2007**, *16*, 2870–2879.
4. Griffin, J.; Emery, B.R.; Christensen, G.L.; Carrell, D.T. Analysis of the meiotic recombination gene *REC8* for sequence variations in a population with severe male factor infertility. *Syst. Biol. Reprod. Med.* **2008**, *54*, 163–165.
5. Hann, M.C.; Lau, P.E.; Tempest, H.G. Meiotic recombination and male infertility: From basic science to clinical reality? *Asian J. Androl.* **2011**, *13*, 212–218.
6. Baudat, F.; Nicolas, A. Clustering of meiotic double-strand breaks on yeast chromosome III. *Proc. Natl. Acad. Sci. USA* **1997**, *94*, 5213–5218.
7. Klein, S.; Zenvirth, D.; Dror, V.; Barton, A.B.; Kaback, D.B.; Simchen, G. Patterns of meiotic double-strand breakage on native and artificial yeast chromosomes. *Chromosoma* **1996**, *105*, 276–284.
8. Zenvirth, D.; Arbel, T.; Sherman, A.; Goldway, M.; Klein, S.; Simchen, G. Multiple sites for double-strand breaks in whole meiotic chromosomes of Saccharomyces cerevisiae. *EMBO J.* **1992**, *11*, 3441–3447.
9. Petes, T.D. Meiotic recombination hot spots and cold spots. *Nat. Rev. Genet.* **2001**, *2*, 360–369.
10. Kohl, K.P.; Sekelsky, J. Meiotic and mitotic recombination in meiosis. *Genetics* **2013**, *194*, 327–334.

11. Lichten, M.; Goldman, A.S. Meiotic recombination hotspots. *Ann. Rev. Genet.* **1995**, *29*, 423–444.
12. Jeffreys, A.J.; Holloway, J.K.; Kauppi, L.; May, C.A.; Neumann, R.; Slingsby, M.T.; Webb, A.J. Meiotic recombination hot spots and human DNA diversity. *Philos. Trans. R. Soc. Lond. Ser. B* **2004**, *359*, 141–152.
13. Wahls, W.P. Meiotic recombination hotspots: Shaping the genome and insights into hypervariable minisatellite DNA change. *Curr. Top. Dev. Biol.* **1998**, *37*, 37–75.
14. Liu, G.; Liu, J.; Cui, X.; Cai, L. Sequence-dependent prediction of recombination hotspots in Saccharomyces cerevisiae. *J. Theor. Biol.* **2012**, *293*, 49–54.
15. Chen, W.; Lin, H.; Feng, P.M.; Ding, C.; Zuo, Y.C.; Chou, K.C. iNuc-PhysChem: A sequence-based predictor for identifying nucleosomes via physicochemical properties. *PLoS One* **2012**, *7*, e47843.
16. Chou, K.C. Prediction of G-protein-coupled receptor classes. *J. Proteome Res.* **2005**, *4*, 1413–1418.
17. Chou, K.C.; Elrod, D.W. Prediction of enzyme family classes. *J. Proteome Res.* **2003**, *2*, 183–190.
18. Wang, M.; Yang, J.; Xu, Z.J.; Chou, K.C. SLLE for predicting membrane protein types. *J. Theor. Biol.* **2005**, *232*, 7–15.
19. Xiao, X.; Wang, P.; Chou, K.C. Predicting protein structural classes with pseudo amino acid composition: An approach using geometric moments of cellular automaton image. *J. Theor. Biol.* **2008**, *254*, 691–696.
20. Chou, K.C. A novel approach to predicting protein structural classes in a (20–1)-D amino acid composition space. *Proteins: Struct. Funct. Genet* **1995**, *21*, 319–344.
21. Feng, K.Y.; Cai, Y.D.; Chou, K.C. Boosting classifier for predicting protein domain structural class. *Biochem. Biophys. Res. Commun.* **2005**, *334*, 213–217.
22. Cai, Y.D.; Chou, K.C. Artificial neural network for predicting alpha-turn types. *Anal. Biochem.* **1999**, *268*, 407–409.
23. Thompson, T.B.; Chou, K.C.; Zheng, C. Neural network prediction of the HIV-1 protease cleavage sites. *J. Theor. Biol.* **1995**, *177*, 369–379.
24. Feng, P.M.; Chen, W.; Lin, H.; Chou, K.C. iHSP-PseRAAAC: Identifying the heat shock protein families using pseudo reduced amino acid alphabet composition. *Anal. Biochem.* **2013**, *442*, 118–125.
25. Chen, W.; Feng, P.M.; Lin, H.; Chou, K.C. iRSpot-PseDNC: Identify recombination spots with pseudo dinucleotide composition. *Nucleic Acids Res.* **2013**, *41*, e69.
26. Xiao, X.; Wang, P.; Chou, K.C. iNR-PhysChem: A sequence-based predictor for identifying nuclear receptors and their subfamilies via physical-chemical property matrix. *PLoS One* **2012**, *7*, e30869.
27. Lin, W.Z.; Fang, J.A.; Xiao, X.; Chou, K.C. iDNA-Prot: Identification of DNA binding proteins using random forest with grey model. *PLoS One* **2011**, *6*, e24756.
28. Kandaswamy, K.K.; Chou, K.C.; Martinetz, T.; Moller, S.; Suganthan, P.N.; Sridharan, S.; Pugalenthi, G. AFP-Pred: A random forest approach for predicting antifreeze proteins from sequence-derived properties. *J. Theor. Biol.* **2011**, *270*, 56–62.
29. Xu, Y.; Ding, J.; Wu, L.Y.; Chou, K.C. iSNO-PseAAC: Predict cysteine *S*-nitrosylation sites in proteins by incorporating position specific amino acid propensity into pseudo amino acid composition. *PLoS One* **2013**, *8*, e55844.
30. Cai, Y.D.; Chou, K.C. Predicting subcellular localization of proteins in a hybridization space. *Bioinformatics* **2004**, *20*, 1151–1156.

31. Chou, K.C.; Cai, Y.D. Prediction of protease types in a hybridization space. *Biochem. Biophys. Res. Commun.* **2006**, *339*, 1015–1020.
32. Chou, K.C.; Shen, H.B. Predicting eukaryotic protein subcellular location by fusing optimized evidence-theoretic K-nearest neighbor classifiers. *J. Proteome Res.* **2006**, *5*, 1888–1897.
33. Chou, K.C.; Shen, H.B. Hum-PLoc: A novel ensemble classifier for predicting human protein subcellular localization. *Biochem. Biophys. Res. Commun.* **2006**, *347*, 150–157.
34. Chou, K.C.; Shen, H.B. Large-scale predictions of Gram-negative bacterial protein subcellular locations. *J. Proteome Res.* **2006**, *5*, 3420–3428.
35. Chou, K.C.; Shen, H.B. Euk-mPLoc: A fusion classifier for large-scale eukaryotic protein subcellular location prediction by incorporating multiple sites. *J. Proteome Res.* **2007**, *6*, 1728–1734.
36. Chou, K.C.; Shen, H.B. Signal-CF: A subsite-coupled and window-fusing approach for predicting signal peptides. *Biochem. Biophys. Res. Commun.* **2007**, *357*, 633–640.
37. Shen, H.B.; Chou, K.C. Using optimized evidence-theoretic K-nearest neighbor classifier and pseudo amino acid composition to predict membrane protein types. *Biochem. Biophys. Res. Commun.* **2005**, *334*, 288–292.
38. Shen, H.B.; Chou, K.C. A top-down approach to enhance the power of predicting human protein subcellular localization: Hum-mPLoc 2.0. *Anal. Biochem.* **2009**, *394*, 269–274.
39. Xiao, X.; Wang, P.; Chou, K.C. GPCR-2L: Predicting G protein-coupled receptors and their types by hybridizing two different modes of pseudo amino acid compositions. *Mol. Biosyst.* **2011**, *7*, 911–919.
40. Shen, H.B.; Yang, J.; Chou, K.C. Fuzzy KNN for predicting membrane protein types from pseudo amino acid composition. *J. Theor. Biol.* **2006**, *240*, 9–13.
41. Xiao, X.; Min, J.L.; Wang, P.; Chou, K.C. iGPCR-Drug: A web server for predicting interaction between GPCRs and drugs in cellular networking. *PLoS One* **2013**, *8*, e72234.
42. Xiao, X.; Min, J.L.; Wang, P.; Chou, K.C. iCDI-PseFpt: Identify the channel-drug interaction in cellular networking with PseAAC and molecular fingerprints. *J. Theor. Biol.* **2013**, *337C*, 71–79.
43. Xiao, X.; Wang, P.; Lin, W.Z.; Jia, J.H.; Chou, K.C. iAMP-2L: A two-level multi-label classifier for identifying antimicrobial peptides and their functional types. *Anal. Biochem.* **2013**, *436*, 168–177.
44. Chou, K.C. Prediction of protein cellular attributes using pseudo amino acid composition. *Proteins: Struct. Funct. Genet.* **2001**, *43*, 246–255.
45. Chou, K.C. Using amphiphilic pseudo amino acid composition to predict enzyme subfamily classes. *Bioinformatics* **2005**, *21*, 10–19.
46. Lin, S.X.; Lapointe, J. Theoretical and experimental biology in one—A symposium in honour of Professor Kuo-Chen Chou's 50th anniversary and Professor Richard Giegé's 40th anniversary of their scientific careers. *J. Biomed. Sci. Eng.* **2013**, *6*, 435–442.
47. Nanni, L.; Lumini, A.; Gupta, D.; Garg, A. Identifying bacterial virulent proteins by fusing a set of classifiers based on variants of Chou's pseudo amino acid composition and on evolutionary information. *IEEE/ACM Trans. Comput. Biol. Bioinform.* **2012**, *9*, 467–475.
48. Khosravian, M.; Faramarzi, F.K.; Beigi, M.M.; Behbahani, M.; Mohabatkar, H. Predicting antibacterial peptides by the concept of Chou's pseudo-amino acid composition and machine learning methods. *Protein Pept. Lett.* **2013**, *20*, 180–186.

49. Yu, L.; Guo, Y.; Li, Y.; Li, G.; Li, M.; Luo, J.; Xiong, W.; Qin, W. SecretP: Identifying bacterial secreted proteins by fusing new features into Chou's pseudo-amino acid composition. *J. Theor. Biol.* **2010**, *267*, 1–6.
50. Zou, D.; He, Z.; He, J.; Xia, Y. Supersecondary structure prediction using Chou's pseudo amino acid composition. *J. Comput. Chem.* **2011**, *32*, 271–278.
51. Zhang, S.W.; Zhang, Y.L.; Yang, H.F.; Zhao, C.H.; Pan, Q. Using the concept of Chou's pseudo amino acid composition to predict protein subcellular localization: An approach by incorporating evolutionary information and von Neumann entropies. *Amino Acids* **2008**, *34*, 565–572.
52. Kandaswamy, K.K.; Pugalenthi, G.; Moller, S.; Hartmann, E.; Kalies, K.U.; Suganthan, P.N.; Martinetz, T. Prediction of apoptosis protein locations with genetic algorithms and support vector machines through a new mode of pseudo amino acid composition. *Protein Pept. Lett.* **2010**, *17*, 1473–1479.
53. Mei, S. Predicting plant protein subcellular multi-localization by Chou's PseAAC formulation based multi-label homolog knowledge transfer learning. *J. Theor. Biol.* **2012**, *310*, 80–87.
54. Chang, T.H.; Wu, L.C.; Lee, T.Y.; Chen, S.P.; Huang, H.D.; Horng, J.T. EuLoc: A web-server for accurately predict protein subcellular localization in eukaryotes by incorporating various features of sequence segments into the general form of Chou's PseAAC. *J. Comput.-Aided Mol. Des.* **2013**, *27*, 91–103.
55. Fan, G.L.; Li, Q.Z. Predict mycobacterial proteins subcellular locations by incorporating pseudo-average chemical shift into the general form of Chou's pseudo amino acid composition. *J. Theor. Biol.* **2012**, *304*, 88–95.
56. Huang, C.; Yuan, J. Using radial basis function on the general form of Chou's pseudo amino acid composition and PSSM to predict subcellular locations of proteins with both single and multiple sites. *Biosystems* **2013**, *113*, 50–57.
57. Lin, H.; Wang, H.; Ding, H.; Chen, Y.L.; Li, Q.Z. Prediction of subcellular localization of apoptosis protein using Chou's pseudo amino acid composition. *Acta Biotheor.* **2009**, *57*, 321–330.
58. Wan, S.; Mak, M.W.; Kung, S.Y. GOASVM: A subcellular location predictor by incorporating term-frequency gene ontology into the general form of Chou's pseudo-amino acid composition. *J. Theor. Biol.* **2013**, *323*, 40–48.
59. Huang, C.; Yuan, J.Q. Predicting protein subchloroplast locations with both single and multiple sites via three different modes of Chou's pseudo amino acid compositions. *J. Theor. Biol.* **2013**, *335*, 205–212.
60. Chen, Y.K.; Li, K.B. Predicting membrane protein types by incorporating protein topology, domains, signal peptides, and physicochemical properties into the general form of Chou's pseudo amino acid composition. *J. Theor. Biol.* **2013**, *318*, 1–12.
61. Huang, C.; Yuan, J.Q. A Multilabel model based on Chou's pseudo-amino acid composition for identifying membrane proteins with both single and multiple functional types. *J. Membr. Biol.* **2013**, *246*, 327–334.
62. Hayat, M.; Khan, A. Discriminating outer membrane proteins with fuzzy K-nearest neighbor algorithms based on the general form of Chou's PseAAC. *Protein Pept. Lett.* **2012**, *19*, 411–421.
63. Mohabatkar, H.; Beigi, M.M.; Abdolahi, K.; Mohsenzadeh, S. Prediction of allergenic proteins by means of the concept of Chou's pseudo amino acid composition and a machine learning approach. *Med. Chem.* **2013**, *9*, 133–137.

64. Mohammad Beigi, M.; Behjati, M.; Mohabatkar, H. Prediction of metalloproteinase family based on the concept of Chou's pseudo amino acid composition using a machine learning approach. *J. Struct. Funct. Genomics* **2011**, *12*, 191–197.
65. Sahu, S.S.; Panda, G. A novel feature representation method based on Chou's pseudo amino acid composition for protein structural class prediction. *Comput. Biol. Chem.* **2010**, *34*, 320–327.
66. Zia Ur, R.; Khan, A. Identifying GPCRs and their types with Chou's pseudo amino acid composition: An approach from multi-scale energy representation and position specific scoring matrix. *Protein Pept. Lett.* **2012**, *19*, 890–903.
67. Xie, H.L.; Fu, L.; Nie, X.D. Using ensemble SVM to identify human GPCRs *N*-linked glycosylation sites based on the general form of Chou's PseAAC. *Protein Eng. Des. Sel.* **2013**, *26*, 735–742.
68. Zhang, S.W.; Chen, W.; Yang, F.; Pan, Q. Using Chou's pseudo amino acid composition to predict protein quaternary structure: A sequence-segmented PseAAC approach. *Amino Acids* **2008**, *35*, 591–598.
69. Sun, X.Y.; Shi, S.P.; Qiu, J.D.; Suo, S.B.; Huang, S.Y.; Liang, R.P. Identifying protein quaternary structural attributes by incorporating physicochemical properties into the general form of Chou's PseAAC via discrete wavelet transform. *Mol. BioSyst.* **2012**, *8*, 3178–3184.
70. Nanni, L.; Lumini, A. Genetic programming for creating Chou's pseudo amino acid based features for submitochondria localization. *Amino Acids* **2008**, *34*, 653–660.
71. Fan, G.L.; Li, Q.Z. Predicting protein submitochondria locations by combining different descriptors into the general form of Chou's pseudo amino acid composition. *Amino Acids* **2012**, *43*, 545–555.
72. Mei, S. Multi-kernel transfer learning based on Chou's PseAAC formulation for protein submitochondria localization. *J. Theor. Biol.* **2012**, *293*, 121–130.
73. Zeng, Y.H.; Guo, Y.Z.; Xiao, R.Q.; Yang, L.; Yu, L.Z.; Li, M.L. Using the augmented Chou's pseudo amino acid composition for predicting protein submitochondria locations based on auto covariance approach. *J. Theor. Biol.* **2009**, *259*, 366–372.
74. Esmaeili, M.; Mohabatkar, H.; Mohsenzadeh, S. Using the concept of Chou's pseudo amino acid composition for risk type prediction of human papillomaviruses. *J. Theor. Biol.* **2010**, *263*, 203–209.
75. Mohabatkar, H. Prediction of cyclin proteins using Chou's pseudo amino acid composition. *Protein Pept. Lett.* **2010**, *17*, 1207–1214.
76. Mohabatkar, H.; Mohammad Beigi, M.; Esmaeili, A. Prediction of GABA(A) receptor proteins using the concept of Chou's pseudo-amino acid composition and support vector machine. *J. Theor. Biol.* **2011**, *281*, 18–23.
77. Georgiou, D.N.; Karakasidis, T.E.; Nieto, J.J.; Torres, A. Use of fuzzy clustering technique and matrices to classify amino acids and its impact to Chou's pseudo amino acid composition. *J. Theor. Biol.* **2009**, *257*, 17–26.
78. Zhang, G.Y.; Fang, B.S. Predicting the cofactors of oxidoreductases based on amino acid composition distribution and Chou's amphiphilic pseudo amino acid composition. *J. Theor. Biol.* **2008**, *253*, 310–315.
79. Zhou, X.B.; Chen, C.; Li, Z.C.; Zou, X.Y. Using Chou's amphiphilic pseudo-amino acid composition and support vector machine for prediction of enzyme subfamily classes. *J. Theor. Biol.* **2007**, *248*, 546–551.

80. Liu, B.; Wang, X.; Zou, Q.; Dong, Q.; Chen, Q. Protein remote homology detection by combining Chou's pseudo amino acid composition and profile-based protein representation. *Mol. Informa.* **2013**, *32*, 775–782.
81. Georgiou, D.N.; Karakasidis, T.E.; Megaritis, A.C. A short survey on genetic sequences, Chou's pseudo amino acid composition and its combination with fuzzy set theory. *Open Bioinforma. J.* **2013**, *7*, 41–48.
82. Hajisharifi, Z.; Piryaiee, M.; Mohammad Beigi, M.; Behbahani, M.; Mohabatkar, H. Predicting anticancer peptides with Chou's pseudo amino acid composition and investigating their mutagenicity via Ames test. *J. Theor. Biol.* **2014**, *341*, 34–40.
83. Chou, K.C. Some remarks on protein attribute prediction and pseudo amino acid composition (50th Anniversary Year Review). *J. Theor. Biol.* **2011**, *273*, 236–247.
84. Li, B.Q.; Huang, T.; Liu, L.; Cai, Y.D.; Chou, K.C. Identification of colorectal cancer related genes with mRMR and shortest path in protein-protein interaction network. *PLoS One* **2012**, *7*, e33393.
85. Huang, T.; Wang, J.; Cai, Y.D.; Yu, H.; Chou, K.C. Hepatitis C virus network based classification of hepatocellular cirrhosis and carcinoma. *PLoS One* **2012**, *7*, e34460.
86. Jiang, Y.; Huang, T.; Lei, C.; Gao, Y.F.; Cai, Y.D.; Chou, K.C. Signal propagation in protein interaction network during colorectal cancer progression. *BioMed Res. Int.* **2013**, *2013*, 287019.
87. Du, P.; Wang, X.; Xu, C.; Gao, Y. PseAAC-Builder: A cross-platform stand-alone program for generating various special Chou's pseudo-amino acid compositions. *Anal. Biochem.* **2012**, *425*, 117–119.
88. Cao, D.S.; Xu, Q.S.; Liang, Y.Z. Propy: A tool to generate various modes of Chou's PseAAC. *Bioinformatics* **2013**, *29*, 960–962.
89. Shen, H.B.; Chou, K.C. PseAAC: A flexible web-server for generating various kinds of protein pseudo amino acid composition. *Anal. Biochem.* **2008**, *373*, 386–388.
90. Min, J.L.; Xiao, X.; Chou, K.C. iEzy-Drug: A web server for identifying the interaction between enzymes and drugs in cellular networking. *BioMed Res. Int.* **2013**, *2013*, 701317.
91. Xu, Y.; Shao, X.J.; Wu, L.Y.; Deng, N.Y.; Chou, K.C. iSNO-AAPair: Incorporating amino acid pairwise coupling into PseAAC for predicting cysteine S-nitrosylation sites in proteins. *PeerJ* **2013**, *1*, e171.
92. Liu, B.; Zhang, D.; Xu, R.; Xu, J.; Wang, X.; Chen, Q.; Dong, Q.; Chou, K.C. Combining evolutionary information extracted from frequency profiles with sequence-based kernels for protein remote homology detection. *Bioinformatics* **2013**, doi:10.1093/bioinformatics/btt709.
93. Lin, H.; Ding, H. Predicting ion channels and their types by the dipeptide mode of pseudo amino acid composition. *J. Theor. Biol.* **2011**, *269*, 64–69.
94. Liu, W.; Chou, K.C. Protein secondary structural content prediction. *Protein Eng.* **1999**, *12*, 1041–1050.
95. Lin, H.; Li, Q.Z. Using pseudo amino acid composition to predict protein structural class: Approached by incorporating 400 dipeptide components. *J. Comput. Chem.* **2007**, *28*, 1463–1466.
96. Chou, K.C. Using pair-coupled amino acid composition to predict protein secondary structure content. *J. Protein Chem.* **1999**, *18*, 473–480.
97. Lin, H.; Ding, C.; Yuan, L.F.; Chen, W.; Ding, H.; Li, Z.Q.; Guo, F.B.; Hung, J.; Rao, N.N.

Predicting subchloroplast locations of proteins based on the general form of Chou's pseudo amino acid composition: Approached from optimal tripeptide composition. *Int. J. Biomath.* **2013**, *6*, 1350003, doi:10.1142/S1793524513500034.

98. Tanford, C. Contribution of hydrophobic interactions to the stability of the globular conformation of proteins. *J. Am. Chem. Soc.* **1962**, *84*, 4240–4274.
99. Hopp, T.P.; Woods, K.R. Prediction of protein antigenic determinants from amino acid sequences. *Proc. Natl. Acad. Sci. USA* **1981**, *78*, 3824–3828.
100. Robert, C.W. *CRC Handbook of Chemistry and Physics*, 66th ed.; CRC Press: Boca Raton, FL, USA, 1985.
101. Dawson, R.M.C.; Elliott, D.C.; Elliott, W.H.; Jones, K.M. *Data for Biochemical Research*, 3rd ed.; Clarendon Press: Oxford, UK, 1986.
102. Chen, J.; Liu, H.; Yang, J.; Chou, K.C. Prediction of linear B-cell epitopes using amino acid pair antigenicity scale. *Amino Acids* **2007**, *33*, 423–428.
103. Chou, K.C.; Cai, Y.D. Using functional domain composition and support vector machines for prediction of protein subcellular location. *J. Biol. Chem.* **2002**, *277*, 45765–45769.
104. Lin, W.Z.; Fang, J.A.; Xiao, X.; Chou, K.C. Predicting secretory proteins of malaria parasite by incorporating sequence evolution information into pseudo amino acid composition via grey system model. *PLoS One* **2012**, *7*, e49040.
105. Wang, S.Q.; Yang, J.; Chou, K.C. Using stacked generalization to predict membrane protein types based on pseudo amino acid composition. *J. Theor. Biol.* **2006**, *242*, 941–946.
106. Cai, Y.D.; Zhou, G.P.; Chou, K.C. Support vector machines for predicting membrane protein types by using functional domain composition. *Biophys. J.* **2003**, *84*, 3257–3263.
107. Chang, C.-C.; Lin, C.-J. LIBSVM: A library for support vector machines. *ACM Trans. Intell. Syst. Technol.* **2011**, *2*, 1–27.
108. Cristianini, N.; Shawe-Taylor, J. *An Introduction to Support Vector Machines and Other Kernel-Based Learning Methods*; Cambridge University Press: Cambridge, UK, 2000; p. 189.
109. Chou, K.C. Some remarks on predicting multi-label attributes in molecular biosystems. *Mol. Biosyst.* **2013**, *9*, 1092–1100.
110. Chou, K.C. Using subsite coupling to predict signal peptides. *Protein Eng.* **2001**, *14*, 75–79.
111. Chou, K.C. Prediction of protein signal sequences and their cleavage sites. *Proteins: Struct. Funct. Genet.* **2001,** 42, 136–139.
112. Chou, K.C.; Wu, Z.C.; Xiao, X. iLoc-Euk: A multi-label classifier for predicting the subcellular localization of singleplex and multiplex eukaryotic proteins. *PLoS One* **2011**, *6*, e18258.
113. Wu, Z.C.; Xiao, X.; Chou, K.C. iLoc-Plant: A multi-label classifier for predicting the subcellular localization of plant proteins with both single and multiple sites. *Mol. BioSyst.* **2011**, *7*, 3287–3297.
114. Wu, Z.C.; Xiao, X.; Chou, K.C. iLoc-Gpos: A multi-layer classifier for predicting the subcellular localization of singleplex and multiplex gram-positive bacterial proteins. *Protein Pept. Lett.* **2012**, *19*, 4–14.
115. Xiao, X.; Wu, Z.C.; Chou, K.C. iLoc-Virus: A multi-label learning classifier for identifying the subcellular localization of virus proteins with both single and multiple sites. *J. Theor. Biol.* **2011**, *284*, 42–51.

116. Xiao, X.; Wu, Z.C.; Chou, K.C. A multi-label classifier for predicting the subcellular localization of gram-negative bacterial proteins with both single and multiple sites. *PLoS One* **2011**, *6*, e20592.
117. Chou, K.C.; Wu, Z.C.; Xiao, X. iLoc-Hum: Using accumulation-label scale to predict subcellular locations of human proteins with both single and multiple sites. *Mol. Biosyst.* **2012**, *8*, 629–641.
118. Lin, W.Z.; Fang, J.A.; Xiao, X.; Chou, K.C. iLoc-Animal: A multi-label learning classifier for predicting subcellular localization of animal proteins. *Mol. Biosyst.* **2013**, *9*, 634–644.
119. Chen, L.; Zeng, W.M.; Cai, Y.D.; Feng, K.Y.; Chou, K.C. Predicting Anatomical Therapeutic Chemical (ATC) classification of drugs by integrating chemical-chemical interactions and similarities. *PLoS One* **2012**, *7*, e35254.
120. Chou, K.C.; Zhang, C.T. Review: Prediction of protein structural classes. *Crit. Rev. Biochem. Mol. Biol.* **1995**, *30*, 275–349.
121. Fan, G.L.; Li, Q.Z. Discriminating bioluminescent proteins by incorporating average chemical shift and evolutionary information into the general form of Chou's pseudo amino acid composition. *J. Theor. Biol.* **2013**, *334*, 45–51.
122. Qiu, J.D.; Huang, J.H.; Liang, R.P.; Lu, X.Q. Prediction of G-protein-coupled receptor classes based on the concept of Chou's pseudo amino acid composition: an approach from discrete wavelet transform. *Anal. Biochem.* **2009**, *390*, 68–73.
123. Chou, K.C. Pseudo amino acid composition and its applications in bioinformatics, proteomics and system biology. *Curr. Proteomics* **2009**, *6*, 262–274.

6

Synthesis and Antioxidant Activity Evaluation of New Compounds from Hydrazinecarbothioamide and 1,2,4-Triazole Class Containing Diarylsulfone and 2,4-Difluorophenyl Moieties

Stefania-Felicia Barbuceanu [1,*], Diana Carolina Ilies [1,†], Gabriel Saramet [2,†], Valentina Uivarosi [3,†], Constantin Draghici [4,†] and Valeria Radulescu [1,†]

1 Organic Chemistry Department, Faculty of Pharmacy,
"Carol Davila" University of Medicine and Pharmacy, 6 Traian Vuia, 020956 Bucharest, Romania;
E-Mails: ilies_diana@hotmail.com (D.C.I.); valeria_radulescu@yahoo.com (V.R.)

2 Pharmaceutical Technology Department, Faculty of Pharmacy,
"Carol Davila" University of Medicine and Pharmacy, 6 Traian Vuia, 020956 Bucharest, Romania;
E-Mail: gsaramet@gmail.com

3 General and Inorganic Chemistry Department, Faculty of Pharmacy,
"Carol Davila" University of Medicine and Pharmacy, 6 Traian Vuia, 020956 Bucharest, Romania;
E-Mail: valentina_uivarosi@yahoo.com

4 "C.D. Nenitescu" Institute of Organic Chemistry, Romanian Academy, 202B Splaiul Independenţei, 060023 Bucharest, Romania; E-Mail: cst_drag@yahoo.com

† These authors contributed equally to this work.

* Author to whom correspondence should be addressed; E-Mail: sbarbuceanu@gmail.com or stefania.barbuceanu@umf.ro

---

Abstract: In the present investigation, new hydrazinecarbothioamides **4**–**6** were synthesized by reaction of 4-(4-X-phenylsulfonyl)benzoic acids hydrazides (X= H, Cl, Br) **1**–**3** with 2,4-difluorophenyl isothiocyanate and further these were treated with sodium hydroxide to obtain 1,2,4-triazole-3-thione derivatives **7**–**9**. The reaction of **7**–**9** with α-halogenated ketones, in basic media, afforded new S-alkylated derivatives **10**–**15**. The structures of the synthesized compounds have been established on the basis of ^{1}H-NMR, ^{13}C-NMR, IR, mass spectral studies and elemental analysis. The antioxidant activity of all compounds has been screened. Hydrazinecarbothioamides **4**–**6** showed excellent antioxidant activity and 1,2,4-triazole-3-thiones **7**–**9** showed good antioxidant activity using the DPPH method.

Keywords: hydrazinecarbothioamide; 1,2,4-triazole-3-thione; cyclization; alkylation; antioxidant activity, diarylsulfone, 2,4-difluorophenyl moiety

1. Introduction

Oxidation processes are intrinsic to the energy management of all living organisms and are therefore kept under strict control by several cellular mechanisms [1].

Free radicals are molecules, ions or atoms with unpaired electrons in their outermost shell of electrons [2]. These species, which are constantly formed in human body, can become toxic when generated in excess or in the presence of a deficiency in the naturally occurring antioxidant defenses. High levels of free radicals can cause damage to biomolecules such as lipids, proteins, enzymes and DNA in cells and tissues. This may result in many diseases such as: cancer, diabetes, cardiovascular and autoimmune diseases, and neurodegenerative disorders, aging, and other diseases through the violent reactivity of the free radicals [3–5].

Antioxidants are important compounds that reduce or neutralize the free radicals, thus protecting the cells from oxidative injury [6]. Therefore, considerable research has been directed towards the identification of new antioxidants to prevent radical-induced damage.

Over the years triazoles have become an important class of heterocyclic compounds in organic synthesis due to their various biological properties. It is well known that 1,2,4-triazole derivatives have therapeutic applications. Thus, there are various drugs incorporating in their structure the 1,2,4-triazole ring used as antifungal [7–9], antiviral [10] agents, aromatase inhibitors [11], *etc.* Among the 1,2,4-triazole derivatives, the mercapto- and the thione-substituted 1,2,4-triazole ring systems have been studied and so far a variety of biological properties have been reported for a large number of these compounds including antioxidant [12–14], antibacterial, antifungal [12,15–18], anticancer [17,19], hypolipidemic [20], anti-inflammatory [21] activity. Moreover, various S-alkylated 1,2,4-triazole-3-thiones showed antibacterial [22], antifungal [18,22], anti-inflammatory [23], and hypolipidemic [20] activities.

It has been reported that structural properties of triazoles, like moderate dipole character, hydrogen bonding capability, rigidity and stability under *in vivo* conditions are the main reasons for their superior pharmacological activities [24].

Many synthetic procedures exist for the synthesis of substituted 1,2,4-triazole-3-thiones. However, the development of simple, facile and efficient methodologies to get five-membered heterocycles is one of the major aspects in organic synthesis. Hydrazinecarbothioamides are valuable intermediates in a variety of synthetic transformations and useful as building blocks in the synthesis of biologically active heterocycles including synthesis of 1,2,4-triazole-thiones. In addition, hydrazinecarbothioamides derivatives exhibit various biological properties such as antioxidant [13,14,25,26], antibacterial [27], and antimycobacterial [28].

Moreover, sulfone derivatives provide examples of an important class of bioactive compounds with biological activities including antibacterial, and anti-HIV-1 [29,30].

On the other hand, incorporation of one or several fluorine atoms into an organic molecule can enhance their biological potency, bioavailability, metabolic stability and lipophilicity. Enhanced lipophilicity may lead to easier absorption and transportation of molecules within biological systems [31].

Considering these published data and as a sequel to our research on the design and synthesis of biologically active new heterocycles from the triazole class [32–35], it was thought worthwhile to synthesize the novel title compounds and to evaluate them for their antioxidant activity.

In this study, we present the design, synthesis, characterization and evaluation of the antioxidant activity of the new hydrazinecarbothioamides, 1,2,4-triazole-3-thiones and some S-alkylated 1,2,4-triazole derivatives incorporating in their molecule diarylsulfone and 2,4-difluorophenyl moieties.

2. Results and Discussion

2.1. Chemistry

The reaction sequences employed for synthesis of title compounds are showed in Scheme 1. In the present work, *2-(4-(4-X-phenylsulfonyl)benzoyl)-N-(2,4-difluorophenyl)hydrazinecarbo-thioamides* **4–6** were synthesized by reaction of *4-(4-X-phenylsulfonyl)benzoic acid hydrazides* **1–3** (X = H, Cl, Br) with 2,4-difluorophenyl isothiocyanate, in absolute ethanol, at reflux. The 4-(4-X-phenylsulfonyl)benzoic acid hydrazides precursors **1–3** were prepared starting from Friedel-Crafts reaction of benzene or halobenzene with *p*-tosyl chloride, according to a previously reported method [36,37]. The hydrazinecarbothioamides **4–6** were refluxed in 8% sodium hydroxide solution to obtain *5-(4-(4-X-phenylsulfonyl)phenyl)-4-(2,4-difluorophenyl)-2H-1,2,4-triazole-3(4H)-thiones* **7–9** in equilibrium with thiole tautomer. The treatment of 1,2,4-triazoles **7–9** with α-halogenated ketones (2-bromoacetophenone or 2-bromo-4′-fluoroacetophenone), in basic media, produced the new S-alkylated 1,2,4-triazoles namely *(2-(5-(4-(4-X-phenylsulfonyl)phenyl)-4-(2,4-difluorophenyl)-4H-1,2,4-triazol-3-ylthio)-1-(phenyl/4-fluorophenyl)ethanones* **10–15** and not *N*-alkylated derivatives.

The structures of all synthesized compounds **4–15** were proven by ^{1}H-NMR, ^{13}C-NMR, MS spectra and elemental analysis.

The IR spectra of hydrazinecarbothioamide derivatives **4–6** exhibit a new absorption band at 1243–1258 cm^{-1} corresponding to C=S stretching vibration which confirms the nucleophilic addition reaction of 4-(4-X-phenylsulfonyl)benzoic acid hydrazides **1–3** to 2,4-difluorophenyl isothiocyanate. Also, in the IR spectra of these compounds **4–6** was presented as a strong characteristic absorption band for carbonyl group at 1663–1682 cm^{-1}. The stretching bands corresponding to NH groups were observed in range 3150–3319 cm^{-1}. In the IR spectra of compounds **7–9** no absorption band was detected about 1663–1682 cm^{-1} indicating the absence of C=O group of hydrazinecarbothioamides **4–6** which is evidence for the conversion of these compounds to 1,2,4-triazoles. Compounds **7–9** can exist in two tautomeric forms, *5-(4-(4-X-phenylsulfonyl)phenyl)-4-(2,4-difluorophenyl)-4H-1,2,4-triazole-3-thioles* and *5-(4-(4-X-phenylsulfonyl)phenyl)-4-(2,4-difluorophenyl)-2H-1,2,4-triazole-3(4H)-thiones* **7–9**. The spectral analysis (IR, ^{1}H-NMR, ^{13}C-NMR) shows that these compounds exist in the latter tautomeric form. Thus, in the IR spectra, the νS-H vibration band (~2500–2600 cm^{-1}) was absent and the νC=S vibration band was observed in region 1247–1255 cm^{-1}. Also, the presence of the νNH absorption band in 3278–3414 cm^{-1} region is an additional proof for the thione tautomeric form [13,38,39]. The structure of compounds **10–12** and **13–15** obtained by alkylation of triazoles **7–9** with α-halogenated ketones was confirmed by the presence in their IR spectra of a new strong stretching band in a 1678–1703 cm^{-1} region characteristic to C=O group. Also, new bands appeared in 2920–2965 cm^{-1} region due to the presence of methylene group (νCH_2). The disappearance of C=S stretching band in IR spectra supported the S-alkylation leading to the formation of compounds **10–15**.

Scheme 1. Synthetic route of the title compounds.

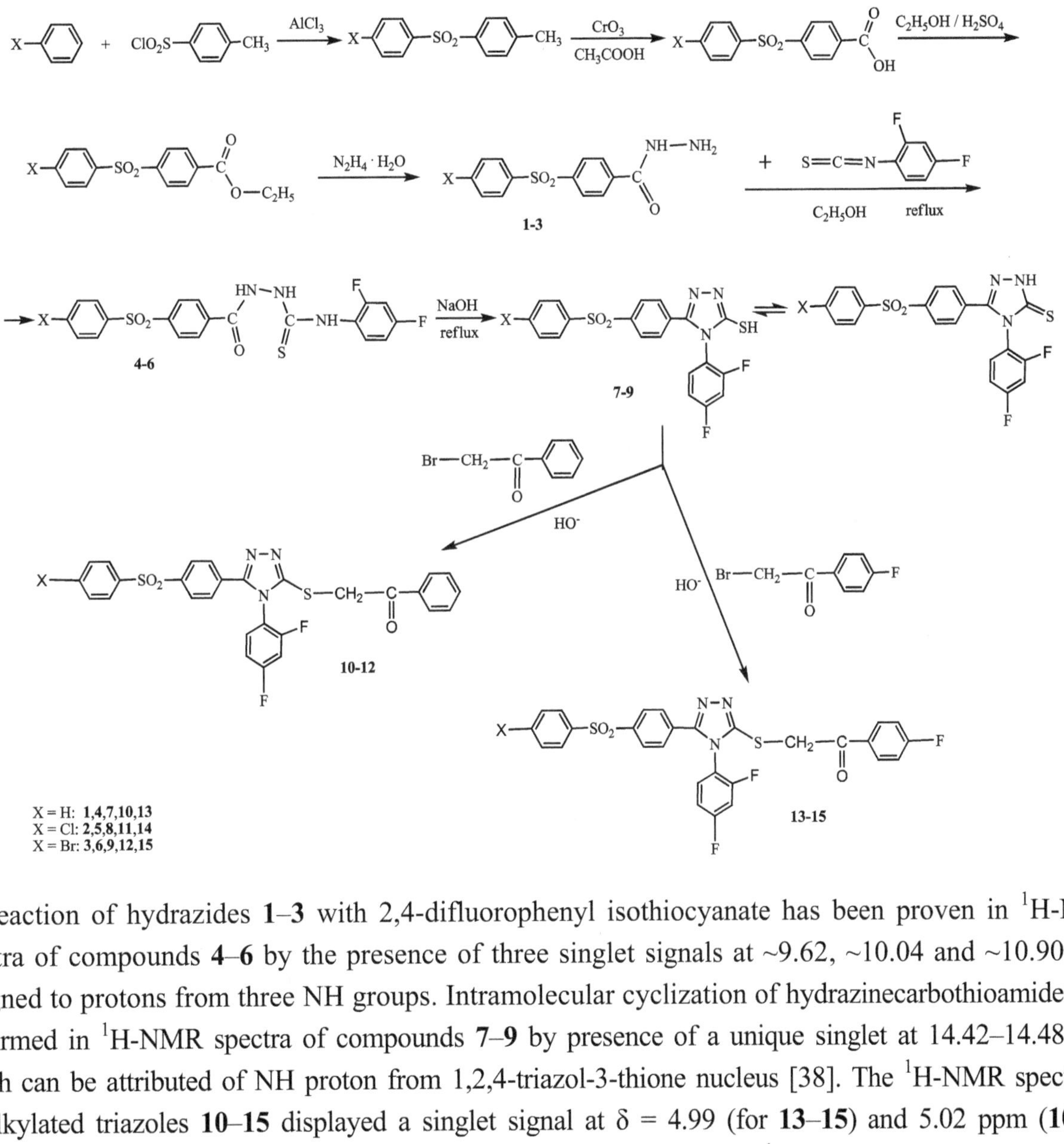

Reaction of hydrazides **1–3** with 2,4-difluorophenyl isothiocyanate has been proven in ^{1}H-NMR spectra of compounds **4–6** by the presence of three singlet signals at ~9.62, ~10.04 and ~10.90 ppm assigned to protons from three NH groups. Intramolecular cyclization of hydrazinecarbothioamides was confirmed in ^{1}H-NMR spectra of compounds **7–9** by presence of a unique singlet at 14.42–14.48 ppm which can be attributed of NH proton from 1,2,4-triazol-3-thione nucleus [38]. The ^{1}H-NMR spectra of all alkylated triazoles **10–15** displayed a singlet signal at δ = 4.99 (for **13–15**) and 5.02 ppm (**10–12**) assignable to S-CH_2 protons. The absence of the signal due to NH in ^{1}H-NMR spectra of compounds **10–15** and the presence of a new singlet for S-CH_2 confirmed that 1,2,4-triazole-3-thiones **7–9** were converted into alkylated derivatives (**10–15**) in the reaction with α-halogenated ketones.

The ^{13}C-NMR spectra of hydrazinecarbothioamides **4–6** showed two important signals characteristic of carbon atoms from C=O and C=S groups at δ 164.71–164.75 and 182.47 ppm, respectively [40]. In ^{13}C-NMR of compounds **7–9** the C-3 and C-5 heterocyclic carbon from triazole nucleus resonated at 169.52–169.54 and 149.01–149.03 ppm, respectively. The signal of the C-3 quaternary carbon atom at

~169 ppm is characteristic of C=S group [12,13,41–43] which indicates the presence of the thione tautomeric form in solution. The most significant proof of the alkylation of triazoles **7–9** with 2-bromoacetophenone or 2-bromo-4'-fluoroacetophenone was the presence in ^{13}C-NMR spectra of compounds **10–12** and **13–15** of two new signals at 191.42–192.73 and 40.33–40.46 ppm corresponding to C=O and S-CH_2 carbon atoms from a phenacyl/4-fluorophenacyl group. In addition, the formation of S-alkylated and not of *N*-alkylated products was confirmed by the absence of a C=S characteristic peak at ~169 ppm in ^{13}C-NMR spectra of **10–15**. The C-3 and C-5 heterocyclic carbons from these alkylated compounds resonate at 153.09–153.16 ppm (more shielded than the C-3 heterocyclic carbon from 1,2,4-triazoles **7–9**) and 153.01–153.09 ppm, respectively [12,43,44].

Moreover, the signals present in the NMR spectra corresponding to aromatic protons and carbons from 2,4-difluorophenyl-, 4-fluorophenyl- and 5-(4-(4-X-phenylsulfonyl)phenyl)-fragments prove the structure of the synthesized compounds. Further confirmations of the structure of the compounds were carried out by mass spectrometry and microanalysis (see experimental part).

2.2. Antioxidant Activity

The free radical scavenging activity of all compounds **4–15** was carried out in the presence of the stable free radical (1,1-diphenyl-2-picrylhydrazyl) DPPH using ascorbic acid (AA), *tert*-butyl-4-hydroxyanisole (BHA) and 2,6-bis(1,1-dimethylethyl)-4-methylphenol (BHT) antioxidant agents as positive control.

Although a number of methods are available for determination of the antioxidant activity, the DPPH method is very common, rapid and has been shown to be one of the most appropriate methods [12,45].

The DPPH solution has a deep purple color, with a strong absoption at 517 nm, and turns to yellow in the presence of antioxidants, which neutralizes the free radicals by pairing the DPPH odd electron with a hydrogen atom or by electron donation. Reduction of DPPH absorption at 517 nm represents the capacity of antioxidants to scavenge free radical [46].

The inhibitory effects of different concentrations of synthesized compounds on DPPH radical are presented in Tables 1 and 2. The antioxidant activity is expressed in terms of % inhibition and IC_{50} (effective concentration for scavenging 50% of the initial DPPH) value (μM).

Based on the experimental results, among all the compounds synthesized, hydrazinecarbothioamides **4–6** showed higher scavenging activity towards DPPH. These compounds have shown a strong inhibitory effect on DPPH radical at 250 μM concentration and inhibition rates were: 97.18% ± 1.42% (for **4**), 96.90% ± 1.39% (for **5**), 97.11% ± 1.12% (for **6**) better than the positive control AA (91.26% ± 0.49%) and BHA (89.30% ± 1.37%) and much stronger than BHT (23.05% ± 1.32%). These compounds **4–6** inhibited the DPPH activity with an IC_{50} = 39.39 μM (**4**), 39.79 μM (**5**) and 42.32 μM (**6**) which is better than the specific inhibitor BHA (IC_{50} = 51.62 μM) and AA (IC_{50} = 107.67 μM) and much stronger than BHT (423.37 μM).

The 1,2,4-triazole-3-thiones **7–9** obtained by cyclization of hydrazinecarbothioamides showed (at the same concentration, 250 μM) a good antioxidant activity (**7**: 67.70% ± 1.68%, **8**: 72.45% ± 1.42%, **9**: 58.52% ± 1.55%) but lower than AA (91.26% ± 0.49%) and BHA (89.30% ± 1.37%). However, triazoles had higher antioxidant activity than BHT. As deduced from the IC_{50} data, the triazole with the lowest anti-radical capacity were found to be derivative **9** (with 182.60 μM) followed by **7** (147.79 μM) and **8** was found to be slightly more active (133.80 μM) than its counterparts **7** and **9** (Table 1).

The S-alkylated 1,2,4-triazoles **10–15** showed weak inhibitory effect at 250 μM concentration, in the range of 7.73%–15.04% (Table 2). However, the presence of the third fluorine atom on phenyl radical linked to ketone groups determines a slight increase of antioxidant activity of compounds **13–15** compared with **10–12**. Because these compounds presented a weaker action even than BHT, IC_{50} was not calculated.

Table 1. Antioxidant activity of compounds **4–9** by DPPH method.

Compd.	Scavenging Effect (%)						IC_{50} (μM)
-	25 μM	50 μM	75 μM	100 μM	125 μM	250 μM	-
4	30.54 ± 1.32	64.37 ± 1.35	74.86 ± 1.40	85.39 ± 1.45	95.99 ± 1.50	97.18 ± 1.42	39.39
5	30.39 ± 1.18	63.58 ± 1.62	74.12 ± 1.34	84.69 ± 1.83	95.36 ± 1.87	96.90 ± 1.39	39.79
6	29.14 ± 1.53	59.28 ± 1.23	71.23 ± 1.32	83.23 ± 1.42	95.35 ± 1.18	97.11 ± 1.12	42.32
7	15.88 ± 1.03	24.74 ± 1.32	33.30 ± 1.67	37.93 ± 1.49	46.14 ± 1.45	67.70 ± 1.68	147.79
8	15.56 ± 0.95	24.36 ± 1.19	32.18 ± 1.48	40.58 ± 1.41	48.38 ± 1.54	72.45 ± 1.42	133.80
9	13.96 ± 0.97	22.99 ± 1.05	31.74 ± 1.56	38.63 ± 1.59	43.03 ± 1.63	58.52 ± 1.55	182.60
AA	0.70 ± 1.00	1.08 ± 0.84	17.48 ± 1.03	34.91 ± 0.69	84.12 ± 0.48	91.26 ± 0.49	107.67
BHA	23.27 ± 1.39	48.99 ± 1.42	64.77 ± 1.32	73.89 ± 1.59	81.74 ± 1.45	89.30 ± 1.37	51.62
BHT	-	-	-	-	-	23.05 ± 1.32	423.37

Table 2. Antioxidant activity of compounds **10–15** by DPPH method.

Compd.	Concentration (μM)	Scavenging Effect (%)
10	250	12.67 ± 0.82
11	250	8.24 ± 1.20
12	250	7.73 ± 0.96
13	250	13.23 ± 0.48
14	250	15.04 ± 0.43
15	250	12.73 ± 0.50
AA	250	91.26 ± 0.49
BHA	250	89.30 ± 1.37
BHT	250	23.05 ± 1.32

The higher antioxidant activity of hydrazinecarbothioamides **4–6** can be explained by the existence of the thiourea fragment [13] that determines stabilization of free radicals of nitrogen atoms (occurring due to the elimination of hydrogen atoms linked to these) by double conjugation, mainly with the thione group. The conjugation between free radicals of the nitrogen atom and π electrons of the aromatic ring represents an additional factor for increasing the stability of the radical structure. The probable mechanism for the reaction of compounds **4–6** with DPPH radical is presented in Scheme 2.

Scheme 2. The probable mechanism for the reaction of compounds **4**–**6** with DPPH radical

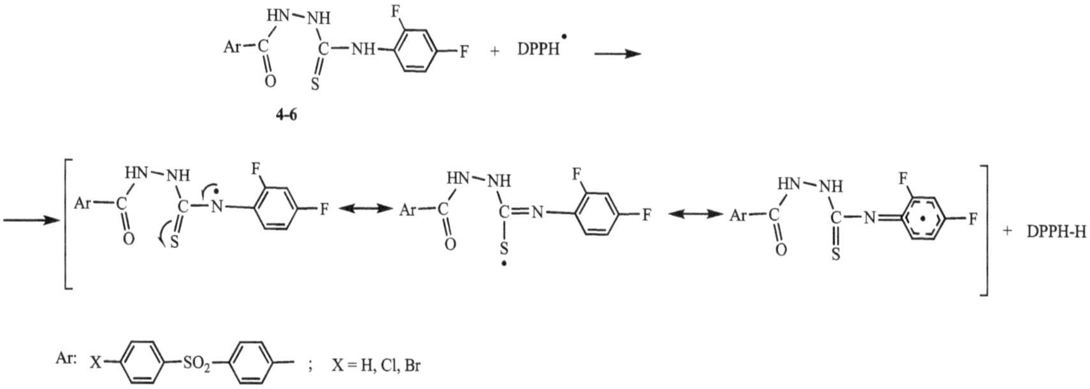

Heterocyclization to 1,2,4-triazole-3-thiones creates only the possibility to conjugate free radicals on the nitrogen atom N-2 with the thione group, which would explain the lower stability of this radical, probably responsible for a weaker antioxidant activity (Scheme 3).

Scheme 3. The probable mechanism for the reaction of compounds **7**–**9** with DPPH radical

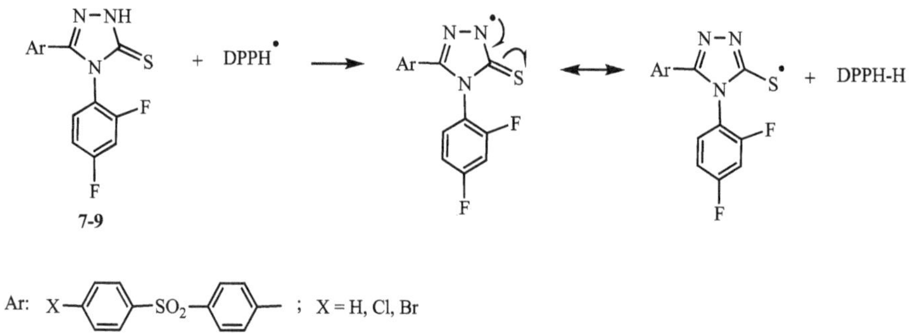

S-alkylation decreases almost entirely the possibilities of conjugation with thione group, causing the least stable radical structure and the weakest antioxidant activity, according to this interpretation.

The compounds tested displayed a considerable lipophilic character, with estimated mean logP values of 4.65 ± 0.71 (ADMET Predictor, Simulation Plus Inc., Lancaster, CA, USA). Based on the preliminary evaluation of biorelevant molecular descriptors and physico-chemical properties, it appears that the evaluated compounds are typical, low solubility—high permeability entities. Therefore, their bioavailability will dependent on the nature of the administration pathways. For oral route, the solubility in the hydrophilic gastro-intestinal fluids is probably the limiting step for absorption. The *in-vivo* distribution process may include binding and accumulation phenomenon in various organs, likely to be of interest for the antioxidant activity. Moreover, the high lipophilicity can limit the distribution to deeper skin layers or the systemic exposure, which is a considerable advantage for the safety profile. None of the compounds seems to present a high risk of low bioavailability, based on current mnemotic rules [47].

The lipophilicity, as estimate by logP values, was not directly correlated with the antioxidant activity (Supplementary data). Nevertheless, a rank order relationship seems apparent. The compounds showing higher scavenging activity towards DPPH (**4**–**6**) presented the lowest lipophilicity (except for triazole 7 which has lower antioxidant activity than hydrazinecarbothioamides **5** and **6** although it has lower lipophilicity than these derivatives).

3. Experimental

3.1. Chemistry

All reactants and solvents were obtained commercially with the highest purity and were used without further purification. Melting points were determined on a Boetius apparatus and are uncorrected. The IR spectra were recorded in KBr using a Vertex 70 Bruker spectrometer. Elemental analyses were performed on a ECS-40-10-Costeh micro-dosimeter (and are within ±0.4% of the theoretical values). The NMR spectra were recorded on a Varian Gemini 300 BB instrument operating at 300 MHz for a ^{1}H and 75 MHz for ^{13}C. Chemical shifts (δ, ppm) were assigned according to the internal standard signal of tetramethylsilane in DMSO-d_6 (δ = 0 ppm). Coupling constants, *J*, are expressed in hertz (Hz). Mass spectra were recorded on 1200 L/MS/MS triple quadrupole (Varian, Palo Alto, CA, USA) spectrometer. In case of compounds **4–9**, solutions of 2 μg/mL in methanol/ammonia (1/1, *v*/*v*) were directly injected into the electrospray interface (ESI), after a tenth dilution with methanol, at a flow rate of 20 μL/min. The instrument was operated in positive and negative ions mode. In case of compounds **10–15**, methanolic solutions of 0.1 μg/mL (with 0.1% ammonia) were directly infused into APCI (Atmospheric Pressure Chemical Ionization) source with a Prostar 240 SDM Pump (Varian). Parameters for APCI operation were set up as follows: air drying gas at 300 °C and 20 psi, nitrogen as nebulising gas at 40 psi, air as auxiliary gas at 20 psi, APCI torch at 300 °C, and corona discharge needle current at 10 μA. APCI generated only positive ions. Protonated molecular ions were fragmented by collision with argon at 1.5 mTorr.

3.1.1. General Procedure for the Preparation of 2-(4-(4-X-Phenylsulfonyl)benzoyl)-*N*-(2,4-difluorophenyl)hydrazinecarbothioamides **4–6**

Appropriate acid hydrazide **1–3** (5 mmol) in absolute ethanol (25 mL) and 2,4-difluorophenyl isothiocyanate (5 mmol) was heated under reflux for 10 h. The precipitate formed was cooled, filtered, washed with cold ethanol, dried and recrystallized from ethanol.

N-(2,4-Difluorophenyl)-2-(4-(phenylsulfonyl)benzoyl)hydrazinecarbothioamide **4**. Yield: 92.0%; m.p. 176–178 °C; IR (KBr, ν, cm^{-1}): 3267, 3169, 3150 (NH), 3067, 3001 (aromatic C-H), 1663 (C=O), 1539, 1510, 1483 (C=C), 1320, 1309, 1155 (SO_2), 1258 (C=S), 1144 (C-F); ^{1}H-NMR (DMSO-d_6, δ ppm): 10.89 (s, 1H; NH); 10.03 (s, 1H, NH); 9.61 (s, 1H, NH); 8.13 (d, 2H, *J* = 8.8 Hz, aromatic protons); 8.09 (d, 2H, *J* = 8.8 Hz; aromatic protons); 7.99 (dd, 2H, *J* = 7.4, 1.4 Hz, aromatic protons); 7.70 (tt, 1H, *J* = 7.4, 1.4 Hz, aromatic proton); 7.63 (t, 2H, *J* = 7.4 Hz, aromatic protons); 7.29 (m, 2H, aromatic protons); 7.07 (wt, 1H, *J* = 8.4 Hz, aromatic proton); ^{13}C-NMR (DMSO-d_6, δ ppm): 182.47 (C=S), 164.75 (C=O), 160.57 (dd, $J_{C\text{-}F}$ = 245.1; 11.2 Hz), 158.55 (dd, $J_{C\text{-}F}$ = 248.5; 13.7 Hz), 143.84,

140.64, 137.01, 134.12, 131.87 (d, J_{C-F} = 9.5 Hz), 129.95, 129.40, 127.57, 127.40, 123.81 (d, J_{C-F} = 12.9 Hz), 111.07 (d, J_{C-F} = 22.6 Hz), 104.28 (t, J_{C-F} = 25.5 Hz); (ESI-MS) *m/z*: 448 $[M + H]^+$, 319 (38) $[C_6H_5SO_2C_6H_4CONHNHCS]^+$, 277 (100, BP) $[C_6H_5SO_2C_6H_4CONHNH_2 + H]^+$, 245 (19) $[C_6H_5SO_2C_6H_4CO]^+$; (ESI-MS) *m/z*: 446 $[M - H]^-$, 426 (2) $[M - H\text{-}HF]^-$, 412 (11) $[M - H\text{-}H_2S]^-$, 275 (100, BP) $[C_6H_5SO_2C_6H_4CONHNH]^-$; Anal. calcd for $C_{20}H_{15}F_2N_3O_3S_2$ (447.48 g/mol): C, 53.68; H, 3.38; N, 9.39. Found: C, 53.61; H, 3.30; N, 9.28%.

2-(4-(4-Chlorophenylsulfonyl)benzoyl)-*N*-(2,4-difluorophenyl)hydrazinecarbothioamide **5**. Yield: 90%; m.p. 170–172 °C; IR (KBr, ν, cm^{-1}): 3290, 3160 (NH), 3090, 3010 (aromatic C-H), 1680 (C=O), 1531, 1478 (C=C), 1319, 1294, 1156 (SO_2), 1243 (C=S), 1145 (C-F), 761 (C-Cl); ^{1}H-NMR (DMSO-d_6, δ ppm): 10.90 (s, 1H, NH); 10.03 (s, 1H, NH); 9.61 (s, 1H, NH); 8.12 (d, 2H, *J* = 8.9 Hz, aromatic protons); 8.09 (d, 2H, *J* = 8.9 Hz, aromatic protons); 8.01 (d, 2H, *J* = 8.5 Hz, aromatic protons); 7.71 (d, 2H, *J* = 8.5 Hz, aromatic protons); 7.07 (wt, 1H, *J* = 8.4 Hz, aromatic protons); 7.29 (m, 2H, aromatic protons); ^{13}C-NMR (DMSO-d_6, δ ppm): 182.47 (C=S), 164.71 (C=O), 160.65 (dd, J_{C-F} = 246.0; 11.3 Hz), 157.80 (dd, J_{C-F} = 245.0; 13.7 Hz), 143.36, 139.45, 138.98, 137.20, 131.82 (d, J_{C-F} = 9.7 Hz), 130.11, 129.58, 129.47, 127.54, 123.72 (d, J_{C-F} = 19.9 Hz), 111.08 (d, J_{C-F} = 21.8 Hz), 104.28 (t, J_{C-F} = 25.5 Hz); (ESI-MS) *m/z*: 482 $[M + H]^+$, 484 $[M + H]^+$, 353 (31) $[^{35}ClC_6H_4SO_2C_6H_4CONHNHCS]^+$, 355 (58) $[^{37}ClC_6H_4SO_2C_6H_4CONHNHCS]^+$, 311 (100, BP) $[^{35}ClC_6H_4SO_2C_6H_4CONHNH_2 + H]^+$, 313 (100, BP) $[^{37}ClC_6H_4SO_2C_6H_4CONHNH_2 + H]^+$, 279 (5) $[^{35}ClC_6H_4SO_2C_6H_4CO]^+$, 281 (24) $[^{37}ClC_6H_4SO_2C_6H_4CO]^+$; (ESI-MS) *m/z*: 480 $[M - H]^-$, 482 $[M - H]^-$, 446 (9) $[^{35}ClM\text{-}H\text{-}H_2S]^-$, 448 (9) $[^{37}ClM\text{-}H\text{-}H_2S]^-$, 309 (100, BP) $[^{35}ClC_6H_4SO_2C_6H_4CONHNH]^-$, 311 (100, BP) $[^{37}ClC_6H_4SO_2C_6H_4CONHNH]^-$; Anal. calcd for $C_{20}H_{14}ClF_2N_3O_3S_2$ (481.92 g/mol): C, 49.84; H, 2.93; N, 8.72. Found: C, 49.75; H, 2.87; N, 8.60%.

2-(4-(4-Bromophenylsulfonyl)benzoyl)-*N*-(2,4-difluorophenyl)hydrazinecarbothioamide **6**. Yield: 88%; m.p. 175–177 °C; IR (KBr, ν, cm^{-1}): 3319, 3280 (NH), 3088, 3044, 3010 (aromatic C-H), 1682 (C=O), 1573, 1536, 1481 (C=C), 1321, 1293, 1157 (SO_2), 1245 (C=S), 1144 (C-F), 576 (C-Br); ^{1}H-NMR (DMSO-d_6, δ ppm): 10.90 (s, 1H, NH); 10.04 (s, 1H, NH); 9.62 (s, 1H, NH); 8.11 (d, 2H, *J* = 8.5 Hz, aromatic protons); 8.10 (d, 2H, *J* = 8.5 Hz, aromatic protons); 7.92 (d, 2H, *J* = 8.7 Hz; aromatic protons); 7.85 (d, 2H, *J* = 8.7 Hz, aromatic protons); 7.29 (m, 2H, aromatic protons); 7.07 (wt, 1H, *J* = 8.8 Hz, aromatic proton); ^{13}C-NMR (DMSO-d_6, δ ppm): 182.47 (C=S), 164.71 (C=O), 160.65 (dd, J_{C-F} = 243.0; 11.2 Hz), 157.40 (dd, J_{C-F} = 243.0; 13.2 Hz), 143.33, 139.86, 137.20, 133.05, 131.93 (d, J_{C-F} = 9.6 Hz), 129.60, 129.46, 128.46, 127.54, 123.70, 111.08 (d, J_{C-F} = 20.9 Hz), 104.28 (t, J_{C-F} = 25.2 Hz); (ESI-MS) *m/z*: 526 $[M + H]^+$, 528 $[M + H]^+$, 397 (40) $[^{79}BrC_6H_4SO_2C_6H_4CONHNHCS]^+$, 399 (33) $[^{81}BrC_6H_4SO_2C_6H_4CONHNHCS]^+$, 355 (100, BP) $[^{79}BrC_6H_4SO_2C_6H_4CONHNH_2 + H]^+$, 357 (100, BP) $[^{81}BrC_6H_4SO_2C_6H_4CONHNH_2 + H]^+$, 323 (1) $[^{79}BrC_6H_4SO_2C_6H_4CO]^+$, 325 (32) $[^{81}BrC_6H_4SO_2C_6H_4CO]^+$, 172 (5) $[2,4\text{-}diFC_6H_3NHCS]^+$, 130 (6) $[2,4\text{-}diFC_6H_3NH_2 + H]^+$; (ESI-MS) *m/z*: 524 $[M - H]^-$, 526 $[M - H]^-$, 504 (3) $[M - H\text{-}HF]^-$, 506 (4) $[M - H\text{-}HF]^-$, 490 (7) $[M - H\text{-}H_2S]^-$, 492 (11) $[M - H\text{-}H_2S]^-$, 353 (100, BP) $[^{79}BrC_6H_4SO_2C_6H_4CONHNH]^-$, 355 (100, BP) $[^{81}BrC_6H_4SO_2C_6H_4CONHNH]^-$; Anal. calcd for $C_{20}H_{14}BrF_2N_3O_3S_2$ (526.37 g/mol): C, 45.64; H, 2.68; N, 7.98. Found: C, 45.58; H, 2.60; N, 7.88%.

3.1.2. General Procedure for the Preparation of 5-(4-(4-X-Phenylsulfonyl)phenyl)-4-(2,4-difluorophenyl)-2H-1,2,4-triazole-3(4H)-thiones **7–9**

The corresponding hydrazinecarbothioamide **4–6** (3 mmol) was refluxed in aqueous sodium hydroxide solution (8%, 45 mL) for 5 h. The filtrate obtained by filtration of reaction mixture was cooled and acidified to pH~5 with hydrochloric acid (1%). The precipitated obtained was filtered, washed with water, dried and recristallized from $CHCl_3$/petroleum ether (1:2, *v*/*v*).

4-(2,4-Difluorophenyl)-5-(4-(phenylsulfonyl)phenyl)-2H-1,2,4-triazole-3(4H)-thione **7** Yield: 71%; m.p. 256–258 °C; IR (KBr, ν, cm^{-1}): 3414 (NH), 3065, 3015 (aromatic C-H), 1614, 1580, 1518, 1474 (C=N + C=C), 1338, 1290, 1160 (SO_2), 1247 (C=S), 1143 (C-F); ^{1}H-NMR (DMSO-d_6, δ ppm): 14.48 (s, 1H, NH); 8.00 (d, 2H, *J* = 8.6 Hz, aromatic protons); 7.95 (dd, 2H, *J* = 7.7, 1.5 Hz, aromatic protons); 7.73 (td, 1H, *J* = 8.7, 6.1 Hz, aromatic proton); 7.70 (t, 1H, *J* = 7.7, 1.5 Hz, aromatic proton); 7.61 (t, 2H, *J* = 7.7 Hz, aromatic protons); 7.58 (d, 2H, *J* = 8.6 Hz, aromatic protons); 7.54 (ddd, 1H, *J* = 10.2, 8.9, 2.7 Hz, aromatic protons); 7.31 (dddd, 1H, *J* = 9.8, 6.1, 2.7, 1.5 Hz, aromatic proton); ^{13}C-NMR (DMSO-d_6, δ ppm): 169.52 (C3-triazolic ring), 162.96 (dd, $J_{C\text{-}F}$ = 251.4; 11.4 Hz), 157.72 (dd, $J_{C\text{-}F}$ = 252.8; 13.5 Hz), 149.03 (C5-triazolic ring), 142.85, 140.24, 134.17, 132.75 (d, $J_{C\text{-}F}$ = 10.6, Hz), 129.93, 129.86, 128.80, 128.03, 127.62, 118.39 (d, $J_{C\text{-}F}$ = 12.7 Hz), 112.99 (d, $J_{C\text{-}F}$ = 22.9 Hz), 105.68 (t, $J_{C\text{-}F}$ = 23.8 Hz); (ESI-MS) *m*/*z*: 430 $[M + H]^+$; 356 (8) $[M + H\text{-}SCNNH_2]^+$; 289 (100, BP) $[M + H\text{-}C_6H_5SO_2]^+$; 172 (10.9) $[F_2C_6H_3NCS + H]^+$; 153 (62) $[FC_6H_4NCS]^+$; (ESI-MS) *m*/*z*: 428 $[M - H]^-$; 408 (15.4) $[M - H\text{-}HF]^-$; 388 (15.4) $[M - H\text{-}2HF]^-$; 267 (7,3) $[M - H\text{-}HF\text{-}C_6H_5SO_2]^-$; 141 (100, BP) $[C_6H_5SO_2]^-$; Anal. calcd for $C_{20}H_{13}F_2N_3O_2S_2$ (429.46 g/mol): C, 55.93; H, 3.05; N, 9.78. Found: C, 55.83; H, 2.98; N, 9.65%.

5-(4-(4-Chlorophenylsulfonyl)phenyl)-4-(2,4-difluorophenyl)-2H-1,2,4-triazole-3(4H)-thione **8** Yield: 73%; m.p. 245–247 °C; IR (KBr, ν, cm^{-1}): 3278 (NH), 3091, 3053 (aromatic C-H), 1614, 1580, 1518, 1468 (C=N + C=C), 1338, 1276, 1159 (SO_2), 1248 (C=S), 1144 (C-F), 768 (C-Cl); ^{1}H-NMR (DMSO-d_6, δ ppm): 14.42 (s, 1H, NH); 8.01 (d, 2H, *J* = 8.5 Hz, aromatic protons); 7.96 (d, 2H, *J* = 8.8 Hz, aromatic proton); 7.73 (td, 1H, *J* = 8.8, 6.0 Hz, aromatic proton); 7.68 (d, 2H, *J* = 8.8 Hz, aromatic protons); 7.59 (d, 2H, *J* = 8.5 Hz, aromatic protons); 7.53 (ddd, 1H, *J* = 10.2, 9.1, 2.7 Hz, aromatic protons); 7.31 (dddd, 1H, *J* = 9.8, 6.4, 2.7, 1.5 Hz, aromatic proton); ^{13}C-NMR (DMSO-d_6, δ ppm): 169.54 (C3-triazolic ring), 162.98 (dd, *J* = 250.8; 11.7 Hz), 149.01 (C5-triazolic ring), 157.27 (dd, $J_{C\text{-}F}$ = 253.1, 13.1 Hz), 142.39, 139.36, 139.04, 132.77 (d, $J_{C\text{-}F}$ = 10.5 Hz), 130.78, 130.11, 129.63, 128.86, 128.13, 118.40 (d, $J_{C\text{-}F}$ = 12.6 Hz), 113.01 (d, $J_{C\text{-}F}$ = 22.6 Hz), 105.70 (t, $J_{C\text{-}F}$ = 23.5 Hz); (ESI-MS) *m*/*z*: 464 $[M + H]^+$; *m*/*z*: 466 $[M + H]^+$; 289 (100, BP) $[M + H\text{-}ClC_6H_4SO_2]^+$; (ESI-MS) *m*/*z*: 462 $[M - H]^-$; *m*/*z*: 464 $[M - H]^-$; Anal. calcd for $C_{20}H_{12}ClF_2N_3O_2S_2$ (463.91 g/mol): C, 51.78; H, 2.61; N, 9.06. Found: C, 51.89; H, 2.47; N, 8.96%.

5-(4-(4-Bromophenylsulfonyl)phenyl)-4-(2,4-difluorophenyl)-2H-1,2,4-triazole-3(4H)-thione **9** Yield: 81%; m.p. 264–266 °C; IR (KBr, ν, cm^{-1}): 3414 (NH), 3095, 3073, 3028 (aromatic C-H), 1614, 1572, 1516, 1471 (C=N + C=C), 1330, 1272, 1169 (SO_2), 1255 (C=S), 1145 (C-F), 578 (C-Br); ^{1}H-NMR (DMSO-d_6, δ ppm): 14.43 (s, 1H, NH); 8.00 (d, 2H, *J* = 8.5 Hz, aromatic protons); 7.88 (d, 2H, *J* = 8.8 Hz, aromatic protons); 7.83 (d, 2H, *J* = 8.8 Hz, aromatic protons); 7.73 (td, 1H, *J* = 8.8, 6.1 Hz, aromatic protons); 7.59 (d, 2H, J = 8.5 Hz, aromatic protons); 7.54 (ddd, 1H, J = 10.2, 9.0, 2.9 Hz, aromatic proton); 7.31 (dddd, 1H, J = 9.7, 6.5, 2.9, 1.4 Hz, aromatic proton); ^{13}C-NMR (DMSO-d_6, δ ppm): 169.54 (C3-triazolic ring), 162.98 (dd, $J_{C\text{-}F}$ = 251.0, 11.5 Hz), 149.01 (C5-triazolic ring), 157.50 (dd, $J_{C\text{-}F}$ = 254.0; 13.4 Hz), 142.35, 139.49, 133.06, 132.78 (d, $J_{C\text{-}F}$ = 10.6, Hz), 130.08, 129.66, 128.88, 128.51, 128.14, 118.48 (d, $J_{C\text{-}F}$ = 12.6 Hz), 113.03 (d, $J_{C\text{-}F}$ = 22.9 Hz), 105.66 (t, $J_{C\text{-}F}$ = 23.5 Hz); (ESI-MS) *m/z*: 508 $[M + H]^+$; *m/z*: 510 $[M + H]^+$; 289 (100, BP) $[M + H\text{-}BrC_6H_4SO_2]^+$; 155 (24.8) $[^{79}BrC_6H_4]^+$; 157 (25.6) $[^{81}BrC_6H_4]^+$; 129 (63.2) $[F_2C_6H_3NH_2]^+$; Anal. calcd for $C_{20}H_{12}BrF_2N_3O_2S_2$ (508.36 g/mol): C, 47.25; H, 2.38; N, 8.27. Found: C, 47.13; H, 2.30; N, 8.13%.

3.1.3. General Procedure for the Preparation of 2-(5-(4-(4-X-Phenylsulfonyl)phenyl)-4-(2,4-difluorophenyl)-4H-1,2,4-triazol-3-ylthio)-1-(phenyl/4-fluorophenyl)ethanones **10–15**

To a solution of sodium ethoxide (23 mg of sodium in 10 mL of absolute ethanol) was added the corresponding triazole **7–9** (1 mmol). The reaction mixture was stirred at room temperature until a solution was obtained. To this solution was added the corresponding α-halogenated ketone (1 mmol) and stirring was continuated for 10 h. The reaction mixture was poured into ice water and the precipitate was filtered off, washed with water and recristallized from ethanol.

2-(4-(2,4-Difluorophenyl)-5-(4-(phenylsulfonyl)phenyl)-4H-1,2,4-triazol-3-ylthio)-1-phenylethanone **10** Yield: 70%; m.p. 176–178 °C; IR (KBr, ν, cm^{-1}): 3070, 3038 (aromatic C-H), 2965, 2922 (CH_2), 1685 (C=O), 1614, 1598, 1515 (C=N + C=C), 1312, 1291, 1161 (SO_2), 1146 (C-F); ^{1}H-NMR (DMSO-d_6, δ ppm): 8.03 (dd, 2H, J = 7.7, 1.3 Hz, aromatic protons); 8.00 (d, 2H, J = 8.6 Hz, aromatic protons); 7.97 (dd, 2H, J = 7.7, 1.4 Hz, aromatic proton); 7.87 (dt, 1H, J = 8.8, 5.8 Hz, aromatic proton); 7.71 (m, 1H, aromatic proton); 7.65 (t, 2H, J = 7.7 Hz, aromatic proton); 7.62 (d, 2H, J = 8.6 Hz, aromatic protons); 7.60 (m, 2H, aromatic protons); 7.56 (t, 2H, J = 7.7 Hz, aromatic protons); 7.40 (m, 1H, aromatic proton); 5.02 (s, 2H, S-CH_2-); ^{13}C-NMR (DMSO-d_6, δ ppm): 192.73 (C=O), 163.34 (dd, $J_{C\text{-}F}$ = 251.9; 11.7 Hz), 156.66 (dd, $J_{C\text{-}F}$ = 253.4; 13.8 Hz), 153.11 (C3-triazolic ring), 153.05 (C5-triazolic ring), 142.27, 140.36, 135.14, 134.07, 133.82, 131.59 (d, $J_{C\text{-}F}$ = 10.9 Hz), 130.66, 129.87, 128.83, 128.41, 128.30, 128.04, 127.54, 117.50 (d, $J_{C\text{-}F}$ = 12.0 Hz), 113.56 (d, $J_{C\text{-}F}$ = 25.2 Hz), 106.84 (t, $J_{C\text{-}F}$ = 23.2 Hz), 40.46 (S-CH_2-); (APCI-MS) *m/z*: 548 $[M + H]^+$; 514 (5.6) $[M + H\text{-}H_2S]^+$; 430 (15.3) $[M + H\text{-}C_6H_5COCH]^+$; 398 (98.8) $[M + H\text{-}C_6H_5COCHS]^+$; 105 (88.8) $[C_6H_5CO]^+$; 91 (100, BP) $[\text{tropylium}]^+$; Anal. calcd for $C_{28}H_{19}F_2N_3O_3S_2$ (547.60 g/mol): C, 61.41; H, 3.50; N, 7.67. Found: C, 61.23; H, 3.29; N, 7.48%.

2-(5-(4-(4-Chlorophenylsulfonyl)phenyl)-4-(2,4-difluorophenyl)-4H-1,2,4-triazol-3-ylthio)-1-phenylethanone **11** Yield: 84%; m.p. 191–193 °C; IR (KBr, ν, cm^{-1}): 3084, 3040 (aromatic C-H), 2959, 2921 (CH_2), 1678 (C=O), 1612, 1598, 1580, 1516 (C=N) + C=C), 1328, 1283, 1161 (SO_2), 1146 (C-F), 767 (C-Cl); ^{1}H-NMR (DMSO-d_6, δ ppm): 8.03 (dd, 2H, J = 7.7, 1.4 Hz, aromatic protons); 8.00 (d, 2H, J = 8.8 Hz, aromatic protons); 7.96 (d, 2H, J = 8.8 Hz, aromatic protons); 7.70 (d, 2H, J = 8.8 Hz, aromatic proton); 7.65 (m, 1H, aromatic proton); 7.63 (d, 2H, J = 8.8 Hz, aromatic protons); 7.61 (dt, 1H, J = 8.8, 6.0 Hz, aromatic proton); 7.56 (t, 2H, J = 7.7 Hz, aromatic protons); 7.40 (ddd, 1H, J = 10.2, 9.1, 2.8 Hz, aromatic proton); 7.24 (m, 1H, aromatic proton); 5.02 (s, 2H, S-CH_2-); ^{13}C-NMR (DMSO-d_6, δ ppm): 192.72 (C=O), 163.35 (dd, $J_{C\text{-}F}$ = 251.9, 11.7 Hz), 156.57 (dd, $J_{C\text{-}F}$ = 253.4, 13.5 Hz),

153.09 (C3-triazolic ring), 153.06 (C5-triazolic ring), 141.80, 139.22, 139.16, 135.14, 133.82, 131.59 (d, $J_{C\text{-}F}$ = 10.6 Hz), 130.86, 130.03, 129.55, 128.83, 128.41, 128.34, 128.13, 117.55 (d, $J_{C\text{-}F}$ = 9.2 Hz), 113.57 (d, $J_{C\text{-}F}$ = 20.4 Hz), 106.84 (t, $J_{C\text{-}F}$ = 23.5 Hz), 40.35 (S-CH_2-); (APCI-MS) *m/z*: 582 $[M + H]^+$; *m/z*: 584 $[M + H]^+$; 476 (67.2) $[M + H\text{-}C_6H_5CHO]^+$; 478 (82.3) $[M + H\text{-}C_6H_5CHO]^+$; 464 (28.5) $[M + H\text{-}C_6H_5COCH]^+$; 466 (30.2) $[M + H\text{-}C_6H_5COCH]^+$; 444 (40.1) $[M + H\text{-}C_6H_5COCH\text{-}HF]^+$; 446 (41.2) $[M + H\text{-}C_6H_5COCH\text{-}HF]^+$; 432 (28.4) $[M + H\text{-}C_6H_5COCHS]^+$; 434 (84.1) $[M + H\text{-}C_6H_5COCHS]^+$; 305 (5.7) $[M + H\text{-}C_6H_5COCHS\text{-}F_2C_6H_3NH_2]^+$; 307 (7.2) $[M + H\text{-}C_6H_5COCHS\text{-}F_2C_6H_3NH_2]^+$; 159 (23.4) $[^{35}ClC_6H_4SO]^+$; 161 (10.3) $[^{37}ClC_6H_4SO]^+$; 105 (100, BP) $[C_6H_5CO]^+$; 91 (95.2) $[\text{tropylium}]^+$; Anal. calcd for $C_{28}H_{18}ClF_2N_3O_3S_2$ (582.04 g/mol): C, 57.78; H, 3.12; N, 7.22. Found: C, 57.67; H, 3.04; N, 7.07%.

2-(5-(4-(4-Bromophenylsulfonyl)phenyl)-4-(2,4-difluorophenyl)-4H-1,2,4-triazol-3-ylthio)-1-phenylethanone **12** Yield: 82%; m.p. 213–215 °C; IR (KBr, ν, cm^{-1}): 3083, 3050 (aromatic C-H), 2960, 2922 (CH_2), 1703 (C=O), 1615, 1598, 1572, 1517 (C=N + C=C), 1321, 1282, 1160 (SO_2), 1142 (C-F), 580 (C-Br); ^{1}H-NMR (DMSO-d_6, δ ppm): 8.03 (dd, 2H, *J* = 7.7, 1.4 Hz, aromatic protons); 8.00 (d, 2H, *J* = 8.8 Hz, aromatic protons); 7.89 (d, 2H, *J* = 8.8 Hz, aromatic protons); 7.87 (dt, 1H, *J* = 8.8, 5.8 Hz, aromatic proton); 7.83 (d, 2H, *J* = 8.8 Hz, aromatic protons); 7.69 (tt, 1H, *J* = 7.7, 1.4 Hz, aromatic proton); 7.65 (m, 1H, aromatic proton); 7.63 (d, 2H, *J* = 8.8 Hz, aromatic protons); 7.56 (t, 2H, *J* = 7.7 Hz, aromatic protons); 7.39 (m, 1H, aromatic proton); 5.02 (s, 2H, S-CH_2-); ^{13}C-NMR (DMSO-d_6, δ ppm): 192.71 (C=O), 163.26 (dd, $J_{C\text{-}F}$ = 251.7, 11.7 Hz), 156.65 (dd, $J_{C\text{-}F}$ = 253.4, 13.5 Hz), 153.11 (C3-triazolic ring), 153.06 (C5-triazolic ring), 141.75, 139.57, 135.13, 133.80, 132.98, 131.59 (d, $J_{C\text{-}F}$ = 10.6 Hz), 130.86, 129.56, 129.30, 128.83, 128.41, 128.35, 128.13, 117.51 (d, $J_{C\text{-}F}$ = 12.9 Hz), 113.59 (d, $J_{C\text{-}F}$ = 22.3 Hz), 106.85 (t, $J_{C\text{-}F}$ = 23.5 Hz), 40.46 (S-CH_2-); (APCI-MS) *m/z*: 626 $[M + H]^+$; *m/z*: 628 $[M + H]^+$; 476 (31.9) $[M + H\text{-}C_6H_5COCHS]^+$; 478 (26.3) $[M + H\text{-}C_6H_5COCHS]^+$; 434 (12.7) $[M + H\text{-}C_6H_5COCH_2SNCNH]^+$; 436 (33.2) $[M + H\text{-}C_6H_5COCH_2SNCNH]^+$; 159 (23.4) $[^{79}BrC_6H_4SO]^+$; 161 (10.3) $[^{81}BrC_6H_4SO]^+$; 105(100, BP) $[C_6H_5CO]^+$; 91 (95.2) $[\text{tropylium}]^+$; Anal. calcd for $C_{28}H_{18}BrF_2N_3O_3S_2$ (626.49 g/mol): C, 53.68; H, 2.90; N, 6.71. Found: C, 53.54; H, 2.79; N, 6.62%.

2-(4-(2,4-Difluorophenyl)-5-(4-(phenylsulfonyl)phenyl)-4H-1,2,4-triazol-3-ylthio)-1-(4-fluorophenyl)ethanone **13** Yield: 72%; m.p. 152–154 °C; IR (KBr, ν, cm^{-1}): 3071, 3035 (aromatic C-H), 2960, 2922 (CH_2), 1682 (C=O), 1614, 1598, 1515 (C=N + C=C), 1313, 1281, 1161 (SO_2), 1145 (C-F); ^{1}H-NMR (DMSO-d_6, δ ppm): 8.11 (dd, 2H, *J* = 8.8, 5.5 Hz, aromatic protons), 7.99 (d, 2H, *J* = 8.5 Hz, aromatic protons); 7.95 (dd, 2H, *J* = 7.4, 1.5 Hz, aromatic protons); 7.86 (dt, 1H, *J* = 8.8, 5.8 Hz, aromatic proton); 7.71 (tt, 1H, *J* = 7.4, 1.5 Hz, aromatic protons); 7.65 (m, 1H aromatic proton); 7.63 (d, 2H, *J* = 8.5 Hz, aromatic protons); 7.62 (t, 2H, *J* = 7.4 Hz, aromatic protons); 7.39 (t, 2H, *J* = 8.8 Hz, aromatic protons); 7.30 (m, 1H, aromatic proton); 4.99 (s, 2H, S-CH_2-); ^{13}C-NMR (DMSO-d_6, δ ppm): 191.45 (C=O), 165.36 (d, $J_{C\text{-}F}$ = 252.8 Hz), 163.04 (dd, $J_{C\text{-}F}$ = 250.5; 11.7 Hz), 156.76 (dd, $J_{C\text{-}F}$ = 250.9; 13.2 Hz), 153.16 (C3-triazolic ring), 153.01 (C5-triazolic ring), 142.32, 140.38, 134.10, 131.95 (d, $J_{C\text{-}F}$ = 2.7 Hz), 131.60 (d, $J_{C\text{-}F}$ = 9.6 Hz), 131.55 (d, $J_{C\text{-}F}$ = 9.4 Hz), 130.67, 129.90, 128.34, 128.07, 127.57, 117.48 (d, $J_{C\text{-}F}$ = 9.8 Hz), 115.92 (d, $J_{C\text{-}F}$ = 21.9 Hz), 113.60 (d, $J_{C\text{-}F}$ = 22.7 Hz), 106.16 (dd, $J_{C\text{-}F}$ = 235.0, 27.3 Hz), 40.34 (S-CH_2-); (APCI-MS) *m/z*: 566 $[M + H]^+$; 428 (18.9) $[M + H\text{-}FC_6H_4COCH_3]^+$; 398 (35.3) $[M + H\text{-}FC_6H_4COCHS]^+$; 356 (16.8) $[M + H\text{-}FC_6H_4COCH_2SNCNH]^+$; 137 (26.5) $[FC_6H_4COCH_2]^+$;

123 (82.2) $[FC_6H_4CO]^+$; 109 (100, BP) $[FC_6H_4N]^+$; Anal. calcd for $C_{28}H_{18}F_3N_3O_3S_2$ (565.59 g/mol): C, 59.46; H, 3.21; N, 7.43. Found: C, 59.23; H, 3.07; N, 7.26%.

2-(5-(4-(4-Chlorophenylsulfonyl)phenyl)-4-(2,4-difluorophenyl)-4H-1,2,4-triazol-3-ylthio)-1-(4-fluorophenyl)ethanone **14** Yield: 85%; m.p. 226–228 °C; IR (KBr, ν, cm^{-1}): 3068, 3030 (aromatic C-H), 2965, 2920 (CH_2), 1682 (C=O), 1615, 1599, 1514 (C=N + C=C), 1322, 1282, 1158 (SO_2); 1145 (C-F), 768 (C-Cl); ^{1}H-NMR (DMSO-d_6, δ ppm): 8.11 (dd, 2H, J = 8.8, 5.5 Hz, aromatic protons), 8.00 (d, 2H, J = 8.5 Hz, aromatic protons), 7.97 (d, 2H, J = 8.7 Hz, aromatic protons); 7.86 (dt, 1H, J = 8.8, 5.8 Hz, aromatic proton); 7.69 (d, 2H, J = 8.7 Hz, aromatic protons); 7.65 (m, 1H, aromatic proton), 7.63 (d, 2H, J = 8.5 Hz, aromatic protons); 7.39 (t, 2H, J = 8.8 Hz, aromatic protons); 7.38 (m, 1H, aromatic proton); 4.99 (s, 2H, S-CH_2-); ^{13}C-NMR (DMSO-d_6, δ ppm): 191.42 (C=O), 165.34 (d, $J_{C\text{-}F}$ = 252.5 Hz), 163.18 (dd, $J_{C\text{-}F}$ = 250.4, 11.8 Hz), 156.72 (dd, $J_{C\text{-}F}$ = 250.8, 13.1 Hz), 153.09 (C3-triazolic ring), 153.04 (C5-triazolic ring), 141.81, 139.22, 139.16, 131.94 (d, $J_{C\text{-}F}$ = 2.7 Hz), 131.59 (d, $J_{C\text{-}F}$ = 9.7 Hz), 131.52 (d, $J_{C\text{-}F}$ = 9.7 Hz), 130.85, 130.05, 128.55, 128.36, 128.14, 117.64 (d, $J_{C\text{-}F}$ = 9.8 Hz), 115.89 (d, $J_{C\text{-}F}$ = 21.9 Hz), 113.57 (d, $J_{C\text{-}F}$ = 19.6 Hz), 106.20 (dd, $J_{C\text{-}F}$ = 235.0, 27.3 Hz), 40.33 (S-CH_2-); (APCI-MS) m/z: 600 $[M + H]^+$; m/z: 602 $[M + H]^+$; 123 (52.2) $[FC_6H_4CO]^+$; 123 (48.3) $[FC_6H_4CO]^+$; 109 (100, BP) $[FC_6H_4N]^+$; Anal. calcd for $C_{28}H_{17}ClF_3N_3O_3S_2$ (600.03 g/mol): C, 56.05; H, 2.86; N, 7.00. Found: C, 55.97; H, 2.76; N, 6.87%.

2-(5-(4-(4-Bromophenylsulfonyl)phenyl)-4-(2,4-difluorophenyl)-4H-1,2,4-triazol-3-ylthio)-1-(4-fluorophenyl)ethanone **15** Yield: 80%; m.p. 228–230 °C; IR (KBr, ν, cm^{-1}): 3080, 3067 (aromatic C-H), 2963, 2920 (CH_2), 1682 (C=O), 1612, 1598, 1574, 1515 (C=N + C=C), 1323, 1282, 1159 (SO_2), 1144 (C-F), 578 (C-Br); ^{1}H-NMR (DMSO-d_6, δ ppm): 8.11 (dd, 2H, J = 8.9, 5.4 Hz, aromatic protons), 8.00 (d, 2H, J = 8.5 Hz, aromatic protons), 7.89 (d, 2H, J = 8.8 Hz, aromatic protons); 7.86 (dt, 1H, J = 8.8, 5.8 Hz, aromatic proton); 7.64 (d, 2H, J = 8.5 Hz, aromatic protons); 7.83 (d, 2H, J = 8.8 Hz, aromatic protons); 7.60 (m, 1H, aromatic proton); 7.38 (t, 2H, J = 8.9 Hz, aromatic protons); 7.30 (m, 1H, aromatic proton); 4.99 (s, 2H, S-CH_2-); ^{13}C-NMR (DMSO-d_6, δ ppm): 191.42 (C=O), 165.34 (d, $J_{C\text{-}F}$ = 252.5 Hz), 163.36 (dd, $J_{C\text{-}F}$ = 250.2, 11.8 Hz), 156.64 (dd, $J_{C\text{-}F}$ = 252.0, 13.4 Hz), 153.10 (C3-triazolic ring), 153.05 (C5-triazolic ring), 141.78, 139.58, 132.99, 131.92 (d, $J_{C\text{-}F}$ = 2.6 Hz), 131.59 (d, $J_{C\text{-}F}$ = 9.6 Hz), 131.52 (d, $J_{C\text{-}F}$ = 2.7 Hz), 130.86, 129.57, 129.15, 128.36, 128.13, 117.52 (d, $J_{C\text{-}F}$ = 9.4 Hz), 115.89 (d, $J_{C\text{-}F}$ = 21.9 Hz), 113.57 (d, $J_{C\text{-}F}$ = 20.0 Hz), 106.20 (dd, $J_{C\text{-}F}$ = 235.0, 27.3 Hz), 40.33 (S-CH_2-); (APCI-MS) m/z: 644 $[M + H]^+$; m/z: 646 $[M + H]^+$; 476 (31.9) $[M + H\text{-}FC_6H_4COCHS]^+$; 478 (26.3) $[M + H\text{-}FC_6H_4COCHS]^+$; 137 (26.5) $[FC_6H_4COCH_2]^+$; 137 (37.2) $[FC_6H_4COCH_2]^+$; 123 (100, BP) $[FC_6H_4CO]^+$; 109 (43.1) $[FC_6H_4N]^+$; 109 (74.2) $[FC_6H_4N]^+$; Anal. calcd for $C_{28}H_{17}BrF_3N_3O_3S_2$ (644.48 g/mol): C, 52.18; H, 2.66; N, 6.52. Found: C, 52.07; H, 2.57; N, 6.36%.

3.2. Antioxidant Activity

The antioxidant activity of all the synthesized compounds was evaluated by DPPH method [14,38] with some modifications and compared with standards (AA, BHA and BHT).

The 400 μM solution of DPPH (2 mL) in ethanol was added to tested sample solutions (2 mL) of different concentrations (50, 100, 125, 200, 250 and 500 μM) in acetone - ethanol 4:96 *v*/*v*. The samples were kept in the dark at room temperature. After 30 min the absorbance values were measured at 517 nm and were converted into the percentage antioxidant activity (%) using the formula [48]:

$$\% = \{1 - [(A_{sample} - A_{sampleblank})/A_{control}] \times 100 \quad (1)$$

where $A_{control}$ was the absorbance of DPPH solution without sample, A_{sample} was the absorbance of sample solution with DPPH, $A_{sampleblank}$ was the absorbance of the sample solutions without the DPPH.

All analyses were undertaken on three replicates and the results averaged. The IC_{50} values were calculated by linear regression plots, where the abscissa represented the concentration of tested compound solution (50, 100, 125, 200, 250 and 500 μM) and the ordinate represented the average percent of antioxidant activity from three separate tests. The absorbance was measured on a SPECORD 40 Analytik Jena spectrophotometer.

4. Conclusions

New hydrazinecarbothioamides, 1,2,4-triazole-3-thiones and S-alkylated 1,2,4-triazole derivatives were synthesized and characterized by IR, ^{1}H-NMR, ^{13}C-NMR and mass spectral data. All the synthesized compounds **4**–**15** have been investigated for their antioxidant activity. Some of these compounds were found to be significant scavengers of free radicals. The hydrazinecarbothioamides **4**–**6** showed excellent antioxidant activity, more than the standards. 1,2,4-Triazole-3-thiones showed good antioxidant activity, but lower than the key intermediates from hydrazinecarbothioamide class, unlike S-alkylates derivatives that had very low action. These results obtained by preliminary screening of antioxidant activity suggested that the molecules from hydrazinecarbothioamide class might serve as interesting compounds for the development of new antioxidant agents by synthesis of some new derivatives with this structure.

Acknowledgments

This work was supported by University of Medicine and Pharmacy "Carol Davila" Bucharest, a project number 28492/30.10.2012.

Author Contributions

Stefania-Felicia Barbuceanu designed the research, performed the synthesis of the compounds, contributed to the analysis of the data and wrote the paper; Diana Carolina Ilies and Valeria Radulescu performed the antioxidant experiments; Gabriel Saramet and Valentina Uivarosi contributed to the synthesis of the compounds and to the interpretation of the data; Constantin Draghici performed NMR data experiments and contributed to the interpretation of the data.

References and Notes

1. Ślusarczyk, S.; Hajnos, M.; Skalicka-Woźniak, K.; Matkowski, A. Antioxidant activity of polyphenols from *Lycopus lucidus* Turcz. *Food Chem.* **2009**, *113*, 134–138.

2. Dakubo, G.D. *Mitochondrial Genetics and Cance*; Springer-Verlag Berlin Heidelberg: Berlin, Germany, 2010; doi:10.1007/978-3-642-11416-8.
3. Torreggiani, A.; Tamba, M. Free radical scavenging and metal chelating activity of some therapeutic heterocyclic agents. *Trends Heterocycl. Chem.* **2005**, *10*, 115–137.
4. Karalı, N.; Güzel, Ö.; Özsoy, N.; Özbey, S.; Salman, A. Synthesis of new spiroindolinones incorporating a benzothiazole moiety as antioxidant agents. *Eur. J. Med. Chem.* **2010**, *45*, 1068–1077.
5. Patil, V.P.; Markad, V.L.; Kodam, K.M.; Waghmode, S.B. Facile preparation of tetrahydro-5*H*-pyrido[1,2,3-*de*]-1,4-benzoxazines via reductive cyclization of 2-(8-quinolinyloxy)ethanones and their antioxidant activity. *Bioorg. Med. Chem. Lett.* **2013**, *23*, 6259–6263.
6. Azam, F. *Therapeutic Potential of Free Radical Scavengers in Neurological Disorders in Handbook of Free Radicals: Formation, Types and Effects*; Chapter 2; Kozyrev, D., Slutsky, V., Eds.; Nova Science Pub. Inc.: Hauppauge, NY, USA, 2010; pp. 57–97.
7. Groll, A.H.; Kolve, H. Antifungal agents: *In vitro* susceptibility testing, pharmacodynamics, and prospects for combination therapy. *Eur. J. Clin. Microbiol. Infect. Dis.* **2004**, *23*, 256–270.
8. Kathiravan, M.K.; Salake, A.B.; Chothe, A.S.; Dudhe, P.B.; Watode, R.P.; Mukta, M.S.; Gadhwe, S. The biology and chemistry of antifungal agents: A review. *Bioorg. Med. Chem.* **2012**, *20*, 5678–5698.
9. Thompson, G.R., III; Cadena, J.; Patterson, T.F. Overview of antifungal agents. *Clin. Chest Med.* **2009**, *30*, 203–215.
10. Balfour, H.H., Jr. Antiviral drugs. *N. Engl. J. Med.* **1999**, *340*, 1255–1268.
11. Murthy, N.; Rao, A.R.; Sastry, G.N. Aromatase inhibitors: A new paradigm in breast cancer treatment. *Curr. Med. Chem. Anticancer Agents* **2004**, *4*, 523–534.
12. Koparir, M.; Orek, C.; Parlak, A.E.; Söylemez, A.; Koparir, P.; Karatepe, M.; Dastan, S.D. Synthesis and biological activities of some novel aminomethyl derivatives of 4-substituted-5-(2-thienyl)-2,4-dihydro-3*H*-1,2,4-triazole-3-thiones. *Eur. J. Med. Chem.* **2013**, *63*, 340–346.
13. Yehye, W.A.; Rahman, N.A.; Alhadi, A.A.; Khaledi, H.; Ng, S.W.; Ariffin, A. Butylated hydroxytoluene analogs: Synthesis and evaluation of their multipotent antioxidant activities. *Molecules* **2012**, *17*, 7645–7665.
14. Kuş, C.; Ayhan-Kılcıgil, G.; Özbey, S.; Kaynak, F.B.; Kaya, M.; Çoban, T.; Can-Eke, B. Synthesis and antioxidant properties of novel *N*-methyl-1,3,4-thiadiazol-2-amine and 4-methyl-2*H*-1,2,4-triazole-3(4*H*)-thione derivatives of benzimidazole class. *Bioorg. Med. Chem.* **2008**, *16*, 4294–4303.
15. Zoumpoulakis, P.; Camoutsis, C.; Pairas, G.; Soković, M.; Glamočlija, J.; Potamitis, C.; Pitsas, A. Synthesis of novel sulfonamide-1,2,4-triazoles, 1,3,4-thiadiazoles and 1,3,4-oxadiazoles, as potential antibacterial and antifungal agents. Biological evaluation and conformational analysis studies. *Bioorg. Med. Chem.* **2012**, *20*, 1569–1583.
16. Eswaran, S.; Adhikari, A.V.; Shetty, N.S. Synthesis and antimicrobial activities of novel quinoline derivatives carrying 1,2,4-triazole moiety. *Eur. J. Med. Chem.* **2009**, *44*, 4637–4647.
17. Hassan, G.S.; El-Messery, S.M.; Al-Omary, F.A.M.; Al-Rashood, S.T.; Shabayek, M.I.; Abulfadl, Y.S.; Habib, E.-S.E.; El-Hallouty, S.M.; Fayad, W.; Mohamed, K.M.; *et al.* Nonclassical antifolates, part 4. 5-(2-Aminothiazol-4-yl)-4-phenyl-4H-1,2,4-triazole-3-thiols as a new class of DHFR inhibitors: Synthesis, biological evaluation and molecular modeling study. *Eur. J. Med. Chem.* **2013**, *66*, 135–145.

18. Turan-Zitouni, G.; Kaplancikli, Z.A.; Yildiz, M.T.; Chevallet, P.; Kaya, D. Synthesis and antimicrobial activity of 4-phenyl/cyclohexyl-5-(1-phenoxyethyl)-3-[N-(2-thiazolyl)acetamido]-thio-4H-1,2,4-triazole derivatives. *Eur. J. Med. Chem.* **2005**, *40*, 607–613.
19. Duran, A.; Dogan, H.N.; Rollas, S. Synthesis and preliminary anticancer activity of new 1,4-dihydro-3-(3-hydroxy-2-naphthyl)-4-substituted-5*H*-1,2,4-triazoline-5-thiones. *Farmaco* **2002**, *57*, 559–564.
20. Idrees, G.A.; Aly, O.M.; Abuo-Rahma, G.E.D.A.A.; Radwan, M.F. Design, synthesis and hypolipidemic activity of novel 2-(naphthalen-2-yloxy)propionic acid derivatives as desmethyl fibrate analogs. *Eur. J. Med. Chem.* **2009**, *44* ,3973–3980.
21. Özadalı, K.; Özkanlı, F.; Jain, S.; Rao, P.P.N.; Velázquez-Martínez, C.A. Synthesis and biological evaluation of isoxazolo[4,5-*d*]pyridazin-4-(5*H*)-one analogues as potent anti-inflammatory agents. *Bioorg. Med. Chem.* **2012**, *20*, 2912–2922.
22. Orek, C.; Koparir, P.; Koparir, M. *N*-cyclohexyl-2-[5-(4-pyridyl)-4-(p-tolyl)-4H-1,2,4-triazol-3-ylsulfanyl]-acetamide dihydrate: Synthesis, experimental, theoretical characterization and biological activities. *Spectrochim. Acta A* **2012**, *97*, 923–934.
23. Navidpour, L.; Shafaroodi, H.; Abdi, K.; Amini, M.; Ghahremani, M.H.; Dehpour, A.R.; Shafiee, A. Design, synthesis, and biological evaluation of substituted 3-alkylthio-4,5-diaryl-4*H*-1,2,4-triazoles as selective COX-2 inhibitors. *Bioorg. Med. Chem.* **2006**, *14*, 2507–2517.
24. Stefanska, J.; Szulczyk, D.; Koziol, A.E.; Miroslaw, B.; Kedzierska, E.; Fidecka, S.; Busonera, B.; Sanna, G.; Giliberti, G.; La Colla, P.; *et al.* Disubstituted thiourea derivatives and their activity on CNS: Synthesis and biological evaluation. *Eur. J. Med. Chem.* **2012**, *55*, 205–213.
25. Šarkanj, B.; Molnar, M.; Čačić, M.; Gille, L. 4-Methyl-7-hydroxycoumarin antifungal and antioxidant activity enhancement by substitution with thiosemicarbazide and thiazolidinone moieties. *Food Chem.* **2013**, *139*, 488–495.
26. Kuş, C.; Ayhan-KIlcIgil, G.; Eke, B.C.; Işcan, M. Synthesis and antioxidant properties of some novel benzimidazole derivatives on lipid peroxidation in the rat liver. *Arch. Pharm. Res.* **2004**, *27*, 156–163.
27. Shelke, S.; Mhaske, G.; Gadakh, S.; Gill, C. Green synthesis and biological evaluation of some novel azoles as antimicrobial agents. *Bioorg. Med. Chem. Lett.* **2010**, *20*, 7200–7204.
28. Sriram, D.; Yogeeswari, P.; Priya, D.Y. Antimycobacterial activity of novel *N*-(substituted)-2-isonicotinoylhydrazinocarbothioamide endowed with high activity towards isoniazid resistant tuberculosis. *Biomed. Pharmacother.* **2009**, *63*, 36–39.
29. Elslager, E.F.; Gavrilis, Z.B.; Phillips, A.A.; Worth, D.F. Repository drugs. IV., 4',4'''-Sulfonylbisacetanilide (acedapsone, DADDS) and related sulfanilylanilides with prolonged antimalarial and antileprotic action. *J. Med. Chem.* **1969**, *12*, 357–363.
30. McMahon, J.B.; Gulakowski, R.J.; Weislow, O.S.; Schultz, R.J.; Narayanan, V.L.; Clanton, D.J.; Pedemonte, R.; Wassmundt, F.W.; Buckheit, R.W., Jr.; Decker, W.D.; *et al.* Diarylsulfones, a new chemical class of nonnucleoside antiviral anhibitors of human immunodeficiency virus Type 1 Reverse Transcriptase. *Antimicrob. Agents Chemother.* **1993**, *37*, 754–760.
31. Saeed, A.; Shaheen, U.; Hameed, A.; Kazmi, F. Synthesis and antimicrobial activity of some novel 2-(substituted fluorobenzoylimino)-3-(substituted fluorophenyl)-4-methyl-1,3-thiazolines. *J. Fluorine Chem.* **2010**, *131*, 333–339.

32. Barbuceanu, S.-F.; Saramet, G.; Almajan, G.L.; Draghici, C.; Barbuceanu, F.; Bancescu, G. New heterocyclic compounds from 1,2,4-triazole and 1,3,4-thiadiazole class bearing diphenylsulfone moieties. Synthesis, characterization and antimicrobial activity evaluation. *Eur. J. Med. Chem.* **2012**, *49*, 417–423.
33. Barbuceanu, S.-F.; Bancescu, G.; Saramet, G.; Barbuceanu, F.; Draghici, C.; Radulescu, F.S.; Ionescu, A.; Negres, S. Synthesis and biological evaluation of some new N^1-[4-(4-Chlorophenylsulfonyl)benzoyl]-N^4-(aryl)-thiosemicarbazides and products of their cyclization. *Heteroat. Chem.* **2013**, *24*, 309–321.
34. Almajan, G.L.; Innocenti, A.; Puccetti, L.; Manole, G.; Barbuceanu, S.; Saramet, I.; Scozzafava, A.; Supuran, C.T. Carbonic anhydrase inhibitors. Inhibition of the cytosolic and tumor-associated carbonic anhydrase isozymes I, II, and IX with a series of 1,3,4-thiadiazole- and 1,2,4-triazole-thiols. *Bioorg. Med. Chem. Lett.* **2005**, *15*, 2347–2352.
35. Socea, L.-I.; Apostol, T.V.; Şaramet, G.; Bărbuceanu, Ş.-F.; Drăghici, C.; Dinu, M. Synthesis and root growth activity of some new acetylhydrazinecarbothioamides and 1,2,4-triazoles substituted with 5H-dibenzo[a,d]annulene moiety. *J. Serb. Chem. Soc.* **2012**, *77*, 1541–1549.
36. Şaramet, I.; Almăjan, G.-L.; Barbuceanu, Ş.; Drăghici, C.; Banciu, M.D. Synthesis of some substituted aroyl thiosemicarbazides, -mercaptotriazoles and -aminothiadiazoles. *Rev. Roum. Chim.* **2005**, *50*, 19–27.
37. Mavrodin, A.; Zotta, V.; Stoenescu, V.M.; Oteleanu, D. Sulfones. IV. New sulfone-hydrazide derivatives. *Pharm. Zentr. Deutsch.* **1956**, *95*, 353–361.
38. Khan, I.; Ali, S.; Hameed, S.; Rama, N.H.; Hussain, M.T.; Wadood, A.; Uddin, R.; Ul-Haq, Z.; Khan, A.; Ali, S.; *et al.* Synthesis, antioxidant activities and urease inhibition of some new 1,2,4-triazole and 1,3,4-thiadiazole derivatives. *Eur. J. Med. Chem.* **2010**, *45*, 5200–5207.
39. Kumar, H.; Javed, S.A.; Khan, S.A.; Amir, M. 1,3,4-Oxadiazole/thiadiazole and 1,2,4-triazole derivatives of biphenyl-4-yloxy acetic acid: Synthesis and preliminary evaluation of biological properties. *Eur. J. Med. Chem.* **2008**, *43*, 2688–2698.
40. Liesen, A.P.; de Aquino, T.M.; Carvalho, C.S.; Lima, V.T.; de Araújo, J.M.; de Lima, J.G.; de Faria, A.R.; de Melo, E.J.T.; Alves, A.J.; Alves, E.W.; *et al.* Synthesis and evaluation of anti-Toxoplasma gondii and antimicrobial activities of thiosemicarbazides, 4-thiazolidinones and 1,3,4-thiadiazoles. *Eur. J. Med. Chem.* **2010**, *45*, 3685–3691.
41. Akhtar, T.; Hameed, S.; Al-Masoudi, N.A.; Khan, K.M. Synthesis and anti-HIV activity of new chiral 1,2,4-triazoles and 1,3,4-thiadiazoles. *Heteroat. Chem.* **2007**, *18*, 316–322.
42. Salgın-Gökşen, U.; Gökhan-Kelekçi, N.; Göktaş, Ö.; Köysal, Y.; Kılıç, E.; Işık, Ş.; Aktay, G.; Özalp, M. 1-Acylthiosemicarbazides, 1,2,4-triazole-5(4*H*)-thiones, 1,3,4-thiadiazoles and hydrazones containing 5-methyl-2-benzoxazolinones: Synthesis, analgesic-anti-inflammatory and antimicrobial activities. *Bioorg. Med. Chem.* **2007**, *15*, 5738–5751.
43. Al-Deeb, O.A.; Al-Omar, M.A.; El-Brollosy, N.R.; Habib, E.E.; Ibrahim, T.M.; El-Emam, A.A. Synthesis, antimicrobial, and antiinflammatory activities of novel 2-[3-(1-adamantyl)-4-substituted-5-tioxo-1,2,4-triazolin-1-yl]acetic acids, 2-[3-(1-adamantyl)-4-substituted-5-tioxo-1,2,4-triazolin-1-yl]-propionic acids and related derivatives. *Arzneim.-Forsch./Drug Res.* **2006**, *56*, 40–47.
44. Saadeh, H.A.; Mosleh, I.M.; Al-Bakri, A.G.; Mubarak, M.S. Synthesis and antimicrobial activity

of new 1,2,4-triazole-3-thiol metronidazole derivatives. *Monatsh. Chem.* **2010**, *141*, 471–478.

45. Kumar, A.; Sharma, P.; Kumari, P.; Kalal, B.L. Exploration of antimicrobial and antioxidant potential of newly synthesized 2,3-disubstituted quinazoline-4(3H)-ones. *Bioorg. Med. Chem. Lett.* **2011**, *21*, 4353–4357
46. Zhou, B.; Li, B.; Yi, W.; Bu, X.; Ma, L. Synthesis, antioxidant, and antimicrobial evaluation of some 2-arylbenzimidazole derivatives. *Bioorg. Med. Chem. Lett.* **2013**, *23*, 3759–3763.
47. Lipinski, C.A.; Lombardo, F.; Dominy, B.W.; Feeney P.J. Experimental and computational approaches to estimate solubility and permeability in drug discovery and development settings. *Adv. Drug. Deliv. Rev.* **2001**, *46*, 3–26.
48. Duan, X.-J.; Zhang, W.-W.; Li, X.-M.; Wang, B.-G. Evaluation of antioxidant property of extract and fractions obtained from a red alga, Polysiphonia urceolata. *Food Chem.* **2006**, *95*, 37–43.

7

Inhibitory Effects of Palmultang on Inflammatory Mediator Production Related to Suppression of *NF-κB* and *MAPK* Pathways and Induction of *HO-1* Expression in Macrophages

You-Chang Oh †, **Yun Hee Jeong** †, **Won-Kyung Cho, Min-Jung Gu and Jin Yeul Ma** *

Korean Medicine (KM)-Based Herbal Drug Development Group, Korea Institute of Oriental Medicine, 461-24, Jeonmin-dong, Yuseong, Daejeon 305-811, Korea; E-Mails: ulivuli@kiom.re.kr (Y.-C.O.); runxi0333@kiom.re.kr (Y.H.J.); wkcho@kiom.re.kr (W.-K.C.); guminjung@kiom.re.kr (M.-J.G.)

† These authors contributed equally to this work.

* Author to whom correspondence should be addressed; E-Mail: jyma@kiom.re.kr

---

Abstract: Palmultang (PM) is an herbal decoction that has been used to treat anorexia, anemia, general prostration, and weakness due to chronic illness since medieval times in Korea, China, and Japan. The present study focused on the inhibitory effects of PM on the production of inflammatory factors and on the activation of mechanisms in murine macrophages. PM suppressed the expression of nitric oxide (*NO*), inflammatory cytokines and inflammatory proteins by inhibiting nuclear factor (*NF*)-*κB* and mitogen-activated protein kinase (*MAPK*) signaling pathways and by inducing heme oxygenase (*HO*)-*1* expression. Collectively, our results explain the anti-inflammatory effect and inhibitory mechanism of PM in macrophages stimulated with lipopolysaccharide (LPS).

Keywords: palmultang; inducible nitric oxide synthase; heme oxygenase-1; nuclear factor-kappaB; mitogen-activated protein kinase

---

1. Introduction

Palmultang (PM) is a traditional herbal medication that has been used since medieval times in East Asia. Currently, PM is usually prescribed as an herbal medicine for the treatment of various symptoms associated with body weakness. Previous studies demonstrated that PM was an effective treatment for endometriosis [1]. In addition, a recent study revealed that PM has a beneficial effect on reproductive function in female mice [2]. However, the effects of PM on inflammation and inflammatory mechanisms still remain unknown.

Macrophages play a key role in the regulation of inflammatory and immune responses [3,4]. Activation of macrophages is induced by LPS stimulation, and activated macrophages secrete inflammatory factors, such as *NO*, prostaglandin *(PG)E*$_2$ and inflammatory cytokines [5,6]. *NO* and *PGE*$_2$ are synthesized by inducible nitric oxide synthase (*iNOS*) and cyclooxygenase (*COX*)-*2*, respectively, and the expression of *iNOS* is closely related to the induction of *HO-1*. *HO-1* is a stress-inducible protein that catalyzes the oxidative degradation of heme; two other heme oxygenase isoforms, *HO-2* and *HO-3*, have also been identified [7]. Enhancing the production of *HO-1* reduces the expression of *iNOS* and the level of free radicals [8].

NF-κB plays an important role in the expression of inflammatory genes. When unstimulated, *NF-κB* is present in the cytoplasm attached to *IκBα*; *NF-κB* is released through degradation of *IκBα* when induced by LPS [9]. Activated *NF-κB* can be transferred from the cytoplasm to the nucleus, where it binds to promoters and induces the expression of various inflammatory genes [10,11]. *MAPK* signaling pathways play an important role in transmitting inflammatory signals [12] and comprise extracellular signal-regulated kinase (*ERK*), *p38*, and c-Jun NH_2-terminal kinase (*JNK*) pathways. *MAPK*s are activated by phosphorylation and induce activation of the *NF-κB* pathway and expression of the *iNOS* gene.

In the present study, we evaluated the suppressive effect of PM on inflammation induced by LPS in RAW 264.7 macrophages. Further, we researched whether the effects of PM on *NF-κB* and *MAPK* signaling pathways and on induction of *HO-1* explain the anti-inflammatory mechanism of PM.

2. Results and Discussion

2.1. PM Did not Show Cytotoxicity and Had Inhibitory Activity against NO and Inflammatory Cytokine Production in Macrophages

In the present study, we demonstrated anti-inflammatory activity of PM in murine macrophages stimulated with LPS. First, we investigated the cytotoxicity of PM in RAW 264.7 macrophages at concentrations of 10–1000 μg/mL. As shown in Figure 1A, PM did not show cytotoxicity at concentrations up to 1000 μg/mL, indicating that it is not toxic to macrophages. Based on this result, we did experiments using up to 1000 μg/mL concentrations of PM.

The overproduction of *NO* is associated with various inflammatory diseases [13,14], so we preferentially investigated the inhibitory effect of PM on the production of *NO* induced by LPS stimulation. As shown in Figure 1B, the positive control, dexamethasone, which is known to be an anti-inflammatory drug, exerted a strong inhibitory effect on *NO* production. In addition, we discovered that PM dose-dependently repressed *NO* secretion to a statistically significant degree. Notably, PM inhibited *NO* production by more than 70% at a concentration of 500 μg/mL.

Further, we examined the inhibitory effect of PM on the production of the pro-inflammatory cytokines tumor necrosis factor (*TNF*)-*α*, interleukin (*IL*)-*6* and *IL-1β*. Cytokine expression was analyzed by ELISA and RT-PCR. PM did not inhibit *TNF-α* secretion (Figure 1C) and did not suppress the expression of *TNF-α* mRNA (Figure 1F). By contrast, PM effectively inhibited both *IL-6* production and mRNA expression in a dose-dependent fashion (Figure 1D,F). Likewise, PM strongly suppressed *IL-1β* cytokine and mRNA production at high concentrations (Figure 1E,F).

Figure 1. (**A**) The cytotoxicity of PM in RAW 264.7 cells. And the suppressive effect of PM on (**B**) *NO* production and (**C–F**) *TNF-α*, *IL-6* and *IL-1β* expression induced by LPS stimulation in macrophages. RAW 264.7 cells were pretreated with PM for 30 min before incubation with LPS for (**A–E**) 24 h or (**F**) 6 h. (**A**) Cytotoxicity was determined using CCK; (**B**) The culture supernatant was analyzed for nitrite production; (**C–E**) Production of cytokines was measured by ELISA and (**F**) mRNA levels were analyzed by RT-PCR. RNA values were quantitated using the i-MAX™ Gel Image Analysis System (Core Bio, Seoul, Korea). As a control, cells were incubated with vehicle alone. * $p < 0.01$ and ** $p < 0.001$ were calculated via comparisons with the LPS-stimulation value.

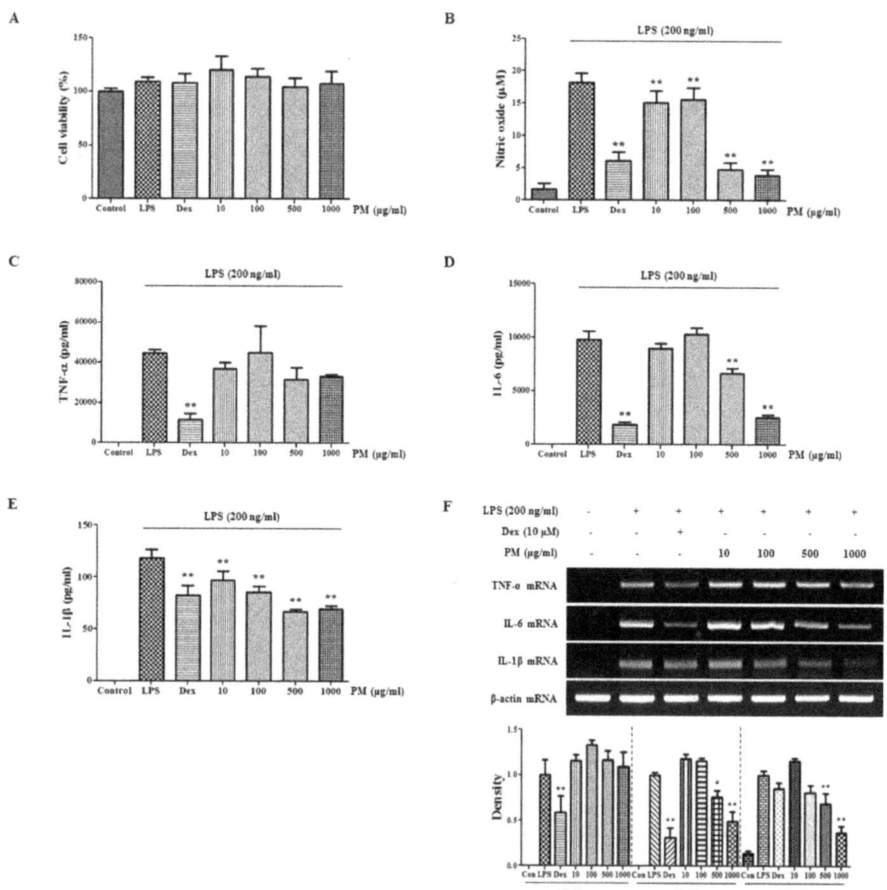

2.2. PM Strongly Suppresses Expression of iNOS but not COX-2 in LPS-Stimulated Macrophages and Induces HO-1 Induction

Because *COX-2* and *iNOS* are enzymes for *PGE₂* and *NO* synthesis, respectively, we further investigated the inhibitory effects of PM on *COX-2* and *iNOS* expression using Western blots and RT-PCR. As shown in Figure 2A, PM did not affect expression of *COX-2* at the protein or mRNA level. By contrast, PM showed a strong dose-dependent inhibitory effect on *iNOS* expression that was statistically significant (Figure 2B). The inhibitory effect of PM on *iNOS* production was believed to contribute to the suppression of *NO* secretion. These results indicate that PM has inhibitory activity against the production of pro-inflammatory mediators.

Figure 2. Inhibitory effect of PM on expression of (**A**) *COX-2* and (**B**) *iNOS*. And the inductive effect of PM on (**C**,**D**) *HO-1* in macrophages. Cells were treated with (**A**,**B**) LPS alone or LPS plus PM for 24 h and (**C**,**D**) with PM alone for the indicated time periods. Protein levels were determined by Western blot analysis, as described in the Materials and Methods, and quantitated using the Davinch-chemi™ CAS-400SM Chemiluminescence Imaging System (Core Bio, Seoul, Korea). Expression of mRNA was analyzed by RT-PCR. * $p < 0.01$ and ** $p < 0.001$ were calculated via comparisons with the (**A**,**B**) LPS-stimulation value or (**D**) vehicle alone.

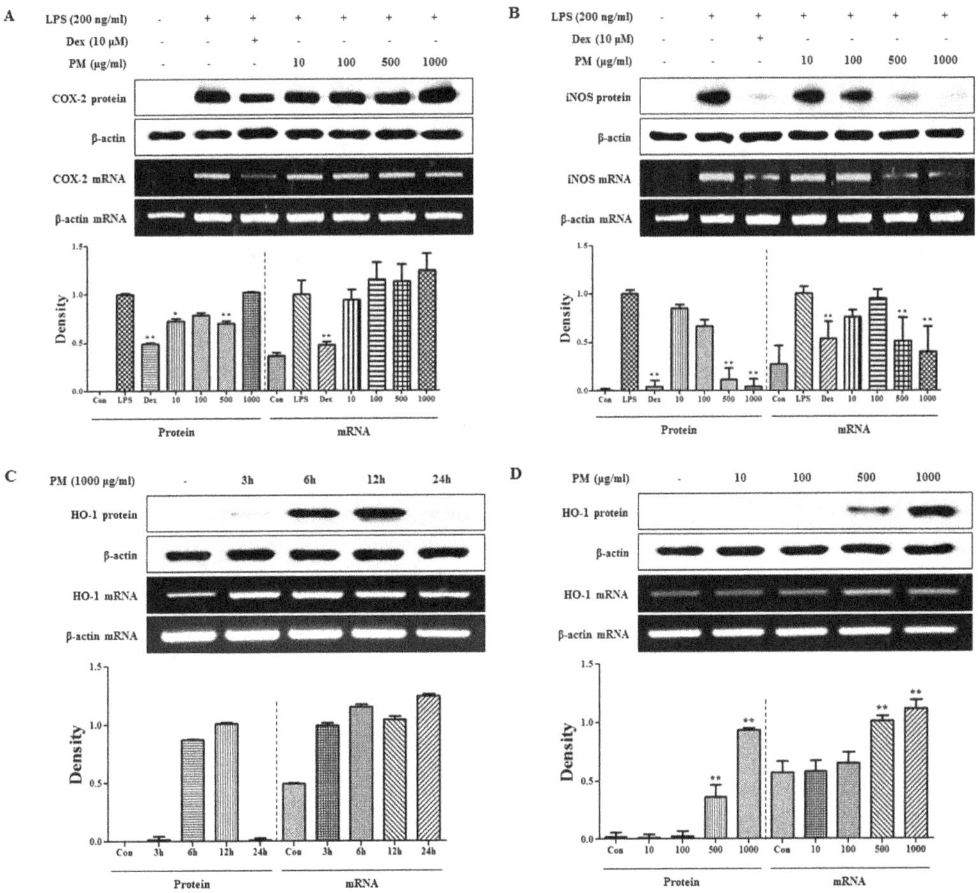

Increased *HO-1* induction has a direct effect on *iNOS* expression [8]. Therefore, we investigated whether the inhibitory effect of PM on *iNOS* expression was associated with increased *HO-1* production. We assessed *HO-1* induction in PM-treated macrophages using Western blot and RT-PCR analyses. First, we measured the induction of *HO-1* at 3–24 h after treatment with 1000 μg/mL PM. Protein and mRNA levels of *HO-1* were highest at 6 and 3 h, respectively (Figure 2C). Based on the results in Figure 2C, we investigated *HO-1* protein and mRNA expression at the indicated time points. PM induced *HO-1* expression at the protein and mRNA levels at concentrations of 500 and 1000 μg/mL in a dose-dependent manner (Figure 2D). These results suggest that pretreatment with PM inhibits *NO* and *iNOS* production by increasing *HO-1* induction.

2.3. *PM Inhibited NF-κB Pathway Activation via Blockade of IκBα Degradation in Macrophages upon LPS Stimulation*

We demonstrated a repressive effect of PM on secretion of the inflammatory cytokine *IL-6*. *NF-κB* is a key transcriptional factor associated with the cellular response to stimuli, such as LPS [15–17] and with the production of *NO*, *PGE_2*, inflammatory cytokines, and *iNOS* [18–20]. To investigate whether the inhibitory effect of PM on the expression of inflammatory mediators is associated with activity of the *NF-κB* pathway, we measured the effect of PM on *NF-κB* activation by analyzing translocation of p65 to the nucleus and the phosphorylation of *IκBα*. Western blot analysis showed that PM significantly repressed translocation of p65 to the nucleus at a concentration of 100 μg/mL or greater (Figure 3A). In addition, the phosphorylation level of *IκBα* was depressed dose-dependently after PM treatment (Figure 3B). Thus, PM inhibited the nuclear transcription of p65 by dose-dependently inhibiting *IκBα* degradation induced by LPS stimulation. These findings are consistent with previous studies showing that an *NF-κB* response drives the expression of the *iNOS* and *IL-6* genes [21–23].

Figure 3. Inhibitory effects of PM on (**A**) translocation of *NF-κB* to the nucleus and (**B**) phosphorylation of *IκBα*. Cells were treated with LPS alone or with LPS and PM for 30 min (*IκBα*) or 1 h (*NF-κB*). Proteins in the cytosol or nucleus were analyzed by Western blotting. $^{**}p < 0.001$ were calculated via comparisons with the LPS-stimulation value.

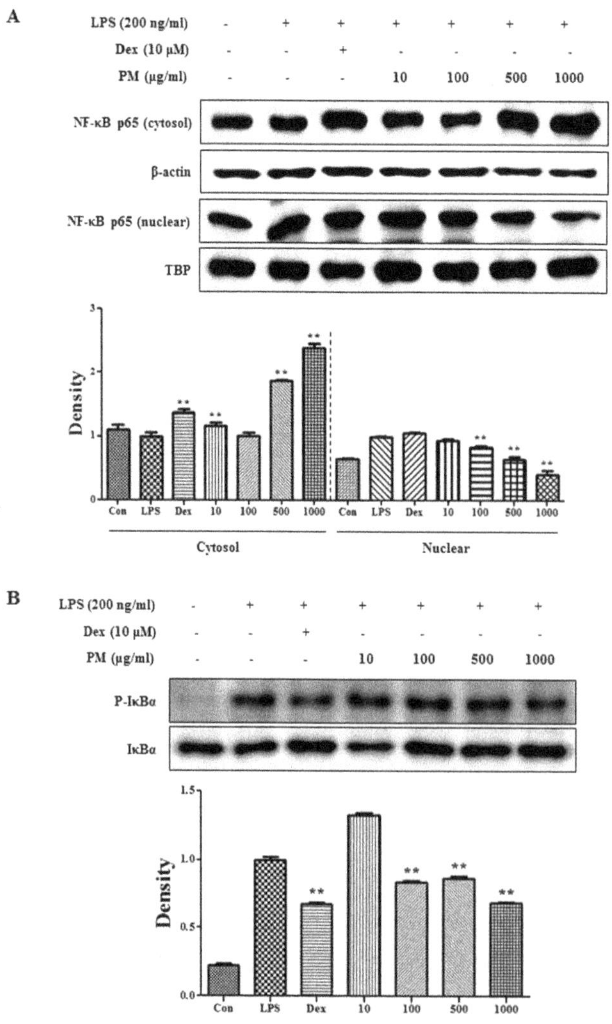

2.4. PM Suppressed LPS-Induced Phosphorylation of MAPKs in RAW 264.7 Cells

Because *MAPK*s activated by phosphorylation upon LPS stimulation are related to *iNOS* expression and *NF-κB* pathway activation in macrophages [24], we examined the inhibitory effect of PM on the phosphorylation of *MAPK*s. We assessed the phosphorylation levels of *MAPK*s, including *ERK 1/2*, *p38* and *JNK*. When RAW 264.7 cells were stimulated with LPS after pretreatment with PM, the levels of phosphorylated *ERK* and *JNK MAPK* were significantly decreased with no change in non-phosphorylated *MAPK* levels (Figure 4A,C). By contrast, PM showed only a slight inhibitory effect on *p38* phosphorylation (Figure 4B). These results indicate that the inhibitory effect of PM on the phosphorylation of *MAPK*s is directly related to inhibition of *NF-κB* activation and reduced production of inflammatory factors in RAW 264.7 cells.

Figure 4. Inhibitory effect of PM on the phosphorylation of (**A**) *ERK*; (**B**) *p38* and (**C**) *JNK MAPK* in macrophages. RAW 264.7 cells were treated with PM for 30 min and then incubated with LPS for 30 min. Cell lysates were analyzed by Western blotting using specific antibodies. ** $p < 0.001$ were calculated via comparisons with the LPS-stimulation value.

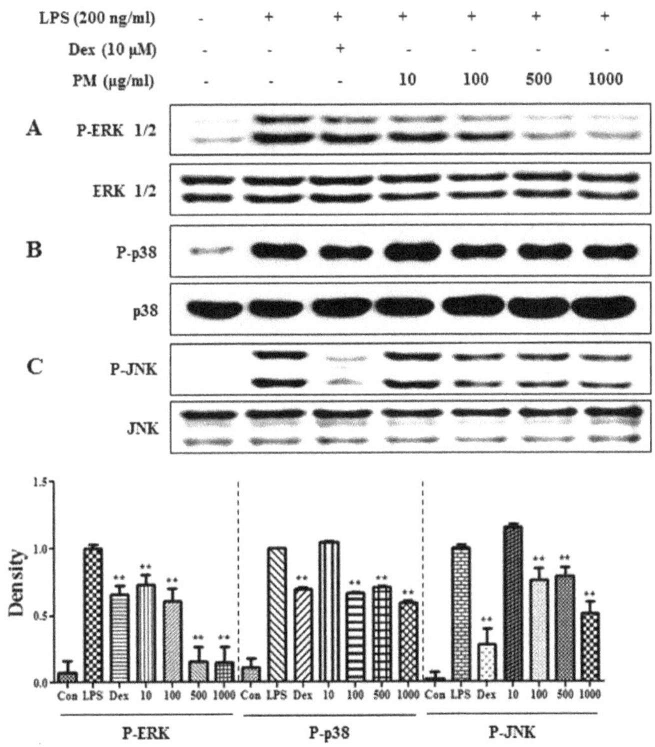

2.5. HPLC Analysis and Previous Reports on the Main Constituents of PM

HPLC-diode array detector (DAD) analysis conditions were successfully established for the separation of peaks in PM extracts. The retention times of eight peaks were as follows: 5-hydroxymethylfurfural (5-HMF), 10.30 min; paeoniflorin, 27.22 min; albiflorin, 30.28 min; ferulic acid, 35.20 min; nodakenin, 36.76 min; decursinol, 43.86 min; glycyrrhizin, 48.69 min; and decursin, 60.93 min. Figure 5 shows chromatograms of the reference components and of a 60% methanol extract of PM, with detection of eluents at 205 nm (for decursinol), 250 nm (for 5-HMF, albiflorin, ferulic acid, nodakenin, glycyrrhizin, and decursin), 330 nm (for paeoniflorin), with ultraviolet rays (UV) wavelengths selected according to the results of Figure 6. These compounds were identified by comparing the retention time and DAD spectra with those of authentic standard compounds. Peak purity checking and identification were conducted using a 190–400 nm UV scan with a DAD.

Figure 5. HPLC chromatograms of (A) a standard mixture and (B) PM at 250 nm. 1, 5-HMF, 10.30 min; 2, paeoniflorin, 27.22 min; 3, albiflorin, 30.28 min; 4, ferulic acid, 35.20 min; 5, nodakenin, 36.76 min; 6, decursinol, 43.86 min; 7, glycyrrhizin, 48.69 min; and 8, decursin, 60.93 min.

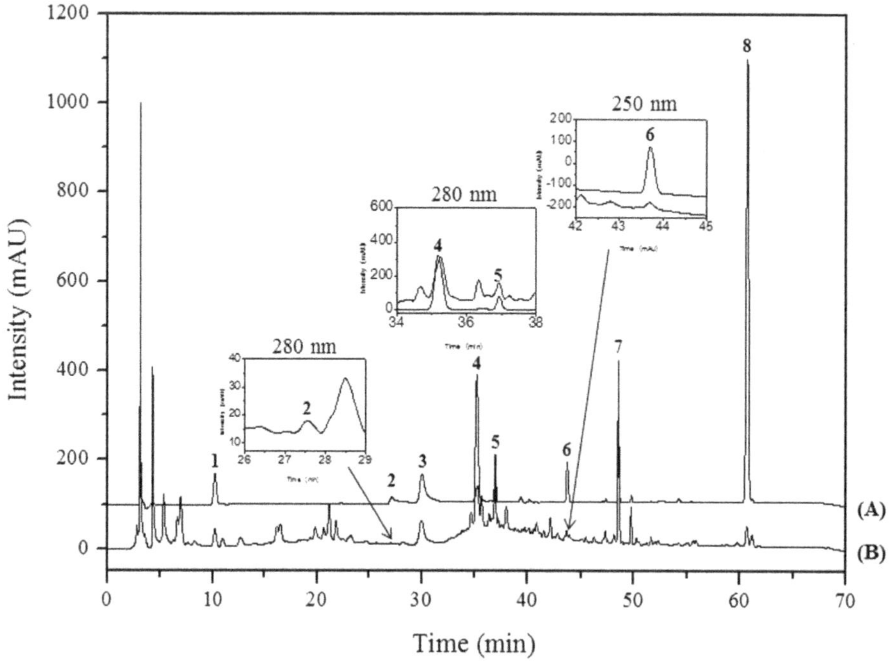

Figure 6. Chemical structures and HPLC DAD spectra of the main constituents of PM.

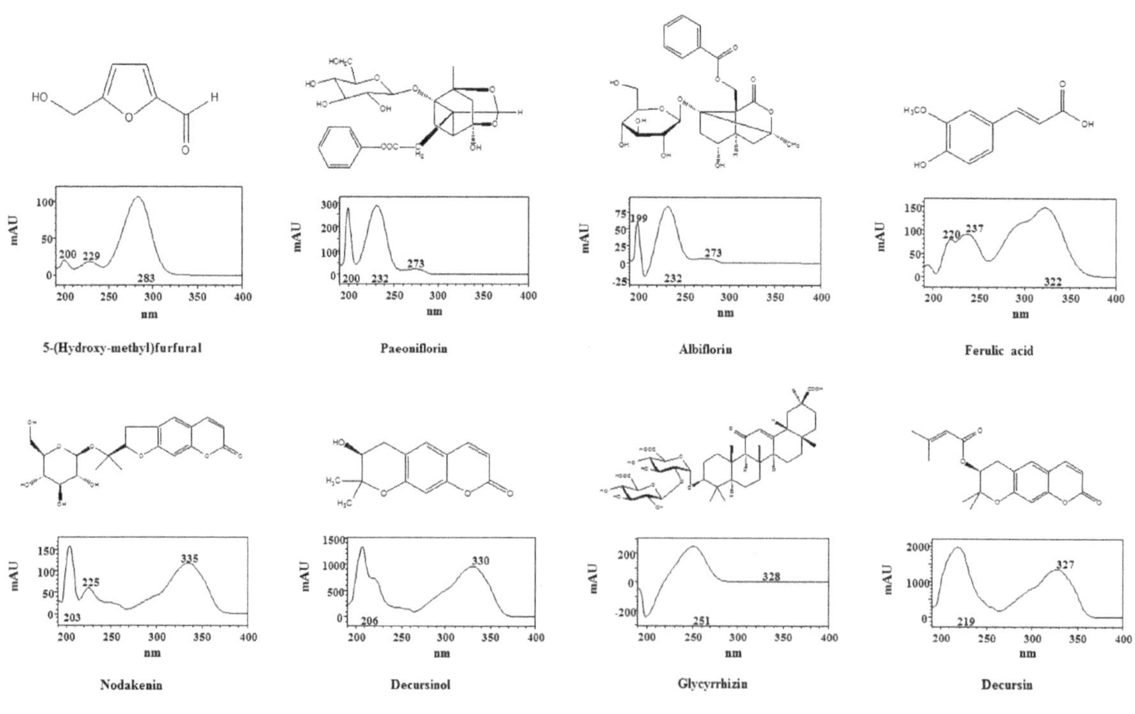

Calibration curves were obtained using standard solutions containing 1.25–10,000 μg/mL for 5-HMF, ferulic acid, nodakenin, decursinol, glycyrrhizin, and decursin, 20–20,000 μg/mL for peaoniflorin and albiflorin as marker components. Calibration curve showed good linearity ($r^2 > 0.9990$). The limits of detection (LOD) and limits of quantification (LOQ) were 0.16–0.50 μg/mL for 5-HMF, 0.22–0.68 μg/mL for ferulic acid, 0.13–0.40 μg/mL for nodakenin, 0.10–0.29 μg/mL for decursinol, 0.63–0.19 μg/mL for glycyrrhizin and 0.45–0.12 μg/mL for decursin, 48.17–16.05 μg/mL for peaoniflorin, 3.30–10.00 μg/mL for albiflorin (Table 1). The amounts of compounds 1–8 (5-HMF, peaoniflorin, albiflorin, ferulic acid, nodakenin, decursinol, glycyrrhizin, and decursin, respectively) were 11.09, 2.59, 2.30, 3.36, 8.23, 5.11, 0.36, and 1.17 mg/g, respectively. The analytical results for each component identified are summarized in Table 2.

Table 1. Linearity, correlation coefficient, limits of detection (LOD), and limits of quantification (LOQ) of the marker compound ($n = 3$).

Compound	Linear Range (μg/mL)	Regression Equation [a]	Correlation Coefficient (r^2)	LOD [b] (μg/mL)	LOQ [c] (μg/mL)
5-HMF	1.25–10,000	$y = 403917x - 87212$	0.9993	0.16	0.50
Ferulic acid	1.25–10,000	$y = 273782x + 89791$	0.9998	0.23	0.68
Nodakenin	1.25–10,000	$y = 239585x - 25958$	1.0000	0.13	0.40
Decursinol	1.25–10,000	$y = 598246x + 235041$	0.9996	0.10	0.29
Glycyrrhizin	1.25–10,000	$y = 43887x + 38994$	0.9991	0.63	0.19
Decursin	1.25–20,000	$y = 116410x + 1188529$	1.0000	0.45	0.12
Peaoniflorin	20–20,000	$y = 1871.8x + 16715$	0.9990	16.05	48.17
Albiflorin	20–20,000	$y = 8026.8x + 6805.9$	0.9993	3.33	10.00

[a] y = peak area (mAU) of the components, x = concentration (μg·mL^{-1}) of the components; [b] LOD = 3× signal-to-noise (*S*/*S*) ratio; [c] LOQ = 10× signal-to-noise (*S*/*S*) ratio.

Table 2. Content of the eight marker compounds of Palmultang ($n = 3$).

Compound	Content (mg/g)		
	Mean	SD	RSD (%)
5-HMF	11.09	0.35	3.11
Ferulic acid	2.59	0.00	0.15
Nodakenin	2.30	0.00	0.02
Decursinol	3.36	0.02	0.72
Glycyrrhizin	8.23	0.01	0.13
Decursin	5.11	0.00	0.01
Peaoniflorin	0.36	0.00	0.34
Albiflorin	1.17	0.03	2.41

A previous study reported that 5-HMF prevents *TNF-α*-induced monocytic cell adhesion to human umbilical vein endothelial cells (HUVECs) by suppression of vascular cell adhesion molecule-1 expression, reactive oxygen species generation and *NF-κB* activation [25]. Additionally, it was demonstrated that paeoniflorin suppresses *TNF-α*-induced chemokine production in human dermal microvascular endothelial cells by blocking *NF-κB* and *ERK* pathways [26]. Another recent study demonstrated that nodakenin exerts a suppressive effect on LPS-induced inflammatory responses in macrophages by inhibiting TNF receptor-associated factor 6 and *NF-κB* pathways, and it protects mice from lethal endotoxin shock [27]. A further recent study showed that glycyrrhizin inhibits *NO* and PGE_2 production in a bimodal fashion [28]. Another study demonstrated that decursin inhibits induction of inflammatory mediators by blocking *NF-κB* activation in macrophages [29]. These facts suggest that the anti-inflammatory activity of PM might be related to active components of PM, including 5-HMF, paeoniflorin, nodakenin, glycyrrhizin, and decursin.

3. Experimental Section

3.1. Materials and Reagents

Products related to cell culture (RPMI 1640, fetal bovine serum (FBS) and antibiotics) were purchased from Lonza (Basel, Switzerland). LPS and bovine serum albumin (BSA) were obtained from Sigma (St. Louis, MO, USA). The Cell-Counting Kit (CCK) was obtained from Dojindo Molecular Technologies, Inc. (Kumamoto, Japan). Various primary and secondary antibodies for Western blot analysis were purchased from Cell Signaling Technology, Inc. (Boston, MA, USA). Enzyme-linked immunosorbent assay (ELISA) antibody sets for cytokine detection were obtained from eBioscience (San Diego, CA, USA). An RNA extraction kit was purchased from iNtRON (Sungnam, Korea). DNA synthesizing kits and oligonucleotide primers were obtained from Bioneer (Daejeon, Korea). 5-(Hydroxy-methyl)furfural (5-HMF) and ferulic acid were purchased from Sigma (St. Louis, MO, USA). Paeoniflorin and glycyrrhizin were purchased from Tokyo Chemical Industry Co., Ltd. (Tokyo, Japan). Decursinol was purchased from Elcom Science (Seoul, Korea), nodakenin from Chem Faces (Wuhan, China), albiflorin from Wako (Osaka, Japan), and decursin from the Ministry of Food and Drug Safety (Osong, Korea). The purity of all representative standards was confirmed by high-performance liquid chromatography (HPLC) to be higher than 97%. HPLC grade solutions, acetonitrile and trifluoroacetic acid were purchased from J. T. Baker Inc. (Philipsburg, NJ, USA). Distilled water (DW) was filtered through a 0.45 μm membrane filter from ADVANTEC (Tokyo, Japan) before analysis.

3.2. Preparation of PM Extract

PM is composed of eight medicinal herbs listed in Table 3. All herbs were purchased from Yeongcheon Herbal Market (Yeongcheon, Korea). All voucher specimens were deposited in an herbal tank, placed in 19,200 mL of DW and then extracted by heating for 3 h at 115 °C and under high pressure (Gyeongseo Extractor Cosmos-600, Inchon, Korea). After extraction, the solution was filtered using standard testing sieves (150 μm) (Retsch, Haan, Germany), freeze-dried and kept in desiccators at 4 °C before use. The acquisition was 591 g and the yield was 30.8%. The freeze-dried extract powder was then dissolved in DW, centrifuged at 14,000 rpm for 10 min and supernatant was filtered (pore size, 0.2 μm) and kept at 4 °C prior to use.

Table 3. Herbal components and amount of Palmultang (PM) decoction.

Herbs	Amount of Herbs (g)
Ginseng Radix	240
Atractylodes Rhizome White	240
Poria	240
Glycyrrhizae Radix et Rhizoma	240
Angelica Gigas Root	240
Prepared Rehmannia Root	240
Peony Root	240
Cinidium Rhizome	240
Total weight	1920

3.3. Cell Culture and Drug Treatment

RAW 264.7 cells were obtained from the Korea Cell Line Bank (Seoul, Korea) and grown in complete RPMI 1640 medium. The cells were incubated in a humidified 5% CO_2 atmosphere at 37 °C. To stimulate the cells, the medium was replaced with fresh RPMI 1640 medium, and LPS (200 ng/mL) was added in the presence or absence of various concentrations of PM (10, 100, 500, and 1000 μg/mL) for the indicated time periods.

3.4. Cell Viability Assay

PM was added to the cells, which were incubated for 24 h at 37 °C in 5% CO_2. CCK solutions were added to each well, and the cells were incubated for an additional 1 h. The optical density was then read at 450 nm using an ELISA reader (Infinite M200, Tecan, Männedorf, Switzerland).

3.5. Determination of NO, TNF-α, IL-6 and IL-1β Cytokine Production

The cells were pretreated with PM and stimulated with LPS for 24 h. *NO* production was analyzed by measuring nitrite using Griess reagent (1% sulfanilamide, 0.1% naphthylethylenediamine dihydrochloride, 2.5% phosphoric acid) according to a previous study [30]. Secretion of the inflammatory cytokines *TNF-α, IL-6* and *IL-1β* was analyzed using a mouse ELISA antibody set (eBioscience, San Diego, CA, USA). The inhibitory effects of PM were determined at 570 and 450 nm for *NO* and cytokines, respectively, using an ELISA reader.

3.6. Preparation of Whole-Cell, Cytosolic and Nuclear Fractions and Western Blot Analysis

The expression of various proteins was analyzed by Western blot analysis according to standard procedures. Cells were stimulated with LPS with or without PM for the indicated time periods at 37 °C. After incubation, the cells were harvested and resuspended in radio immunoprecipitation assay (RIPA) lysis buffer (Millipore, Bedford, MA, USA) containing protease and phosphatase inhibitor cocktail (Roche, Basel, Switzerland) to obtain whole-cell lysates. Cytosolic and nuclear fractions were isolated using NE-PER Nuclear and Cytoplasmic Extraction Reagents (Thermo Scientific, Rockford, IL, USA) according to the procedure described by the manufacturer. After cell debris was removed by centrifugation, the concentration of protein was determined by Bradford's method, and equal amounts of protein were separated by sodium dodecyl sulfate-polyacrylamide gel electrophoresis (SDS-PAGE). The proteins were transferred onto a nitrocellulose membrane (Millipore, Bedford, MA, USA) and blocked with 3% BSA in Tris-buffered saline containing 0.1% Tween 20 (TBS-T). The membrane was then incubated with each primary antibody at 4 °C overnight, followed by incubation with HRP-conjugated secondary antibodies. The specific proteins were detected using SuperSignal West Femto Chemiluminescent Substrate (Thermo Scientific, Rockford, IL, USA).

3.7. RNA Extraction and Reverse Transcription-Polymerase Chain Reaction (RT-PCR)

Total RNA was isolated using an easy-BLUE™ RNA extraction kit (iNtRON, Daejeon, Korea) according to the procedure described by the manufacturer. cDNA was synthesized using AccuPower® CycleScript RT PreMix (Bioneer, Daejeon, Korea). The sequences of specific primers used for amplification by polymerase chain reaction are shown in Table 4. The following PCR conditions were applied for *TNF-α*, *IL-6*, *IL-1β*, *COX-2*, *iNOS*, *HO-1*, and β-actin: 35 cycles of denaturation at 94 °C for 30 s, annealing at the temperature indicated in Table 4 for 30 s, and extension at 72 °C for 30 s [30–34].

Table 4. Primer sequences and annealing temperatures used for RT-PCR analysis.

Target Gene	Primer Sequence	Annealing Temp
TNF-α	F: 5'-AGCACAGAAAGCATGATCCG-3' R: 5'-GTTTGCTACGACGTGGGCTA-3'	55 °C
IL-6	F: 5'-CATGTTCTCTGGGAAATCGTGG-3' R: 5'-AACGCACTAGGTTTGCCGAGTA-3'	58 °C
IL-1β	F: 5'-TGCAGAGTTCCCCAACTGGTACATC-3' R: 5'-GTGCTGCCTAATGTCCCCTTGAATC-3'	64 °C
COX-2	F: 5'-CACTCAGTTTGTTGAGTCATTC-3' R: 5'-GATTAGTACTGTAGGGTTAATG-3'	45 °C
iNOS	F: 5'-AGCCCAACAATACAAATGACCCTA-3' R: 5'-TTCCTGTTGTTTCTATTTCCTTTGT-3'	56 °C
HO-1	F: 5'-TGAAGGAGGCCACCAAGGAGG-3' R: 5'-AGAGGTCACCCAGGTAGCGGG-3'	62 °C
β-actin	F: 5'-ATGAAGATCCTGACCGAGCGT-3' R: 5'-AACGCAGCTCAGTAACAGTCCG-3'	58 °C

F, forward; R, reverse.

3.8. Preparation of Standard Solutions and Samples

An aqua 60% methanol standard stock solution containing compounds 5-HMF, ferulic acid, nodakenin, glycyrrhizin, decursinol, peaoniflorin, albiflorin, and decursin (each 1 mg/mL) were prepared and stored below −4 °C. Working standard solutions were prepared by serial dilution of stock solution with aqua 60% methanol. All calibration curves were obtains from assessement of peak areas of standards in the concentration ranges. A sample of 10 mg PM extract was prepared in 1 mL DW, extracted by ultra-sonication, and filtered through a 0.2 μm syringe membrane filter from Whatman Ltd. (Maidstone, UK) before injection into the HPLC system for analysis. Sample solutions were stored at −4 °C in a refrigerator before analysis.

3.9. General Experimental Procedures

Analytical HPLC data were obtained using an L-2130 pump, L-2200 auto-sampler, L-2300 column oven and L-2455 UV/VIS DAD. The output signal of the detector was recorded using EZChrom Elite software for the HPLC system (Hitachi, Tokyo, Japan). The OptimaPak C_{18} analytical HPLC column (4.6 × 250 mm, 5 μm; RS Tech Co., Daejeon, Korea) was used in this study.

3.10. Analytical Chromatographic Conditions

The mobile phase consisted of water containing (A) 0.1% trifluoroacetic acid and (B) acetonitrile with gradient elution at a flow rate of 1.0 mL/min. The sample injection volume was 20 μL, and the flow rate of the mobile phase was 1.0 mL/min (Table 5). The column temperature was maintained at 40 °C, and the wavelengths of the UV detector were set at 205, 250, and 330 nm.

Table 5. HPLC conditions used for the analysis of PM.

Item	Condition		
	Time (min)	Water (Containing 0.1% TFA)	Acetonitrile
Mobile phase	0	5	95
	5	5	95
	15	15	85
	25	15	85
	50	65	35
	60	65	35
Flow rate	1.0 mL/min		
Inject volume	20 μL		
Column	OptimaPak C_{18} (4.6 × 250 mm, 5 μm, RS tech Co., Daejeon, Korea)		
Column temperature	40 °C		
UV wavelength	205, 250 and 330 nm		

3.11. Statistical Analysis

The results are expressed as mean ± SE values. Statistical significance for each treated group compared with the negative control was determined using the Student's *t* test. Each experiment was repeated at least three times to yield comparable results. p values of <0.01 and <0.001 were considered significant.

4. Conclusions

In conclusion, PM shows significant inhibitory effects on the secretion of *NO* and expression of *IL-6*, *IL-1β* and *iNOS* in LPS-stimulated RAW 264.7 cells. These effects are due to inhibition of *NF-κB* activation through suppression of *IκBα* degradation and blockade of *MAPK* phosphorylation. Furthermore, the induction of *HO-1* by PM inhibits inflammatory factor production. These results show that PM could be developed as a new anti-inflammatory agent derived from natural products.

Acknowledgments

This work was supported by the grant K14050 awarded to Korea Institute of Oriental Medicine (KIOM) from Ministry of Education, Science and Technology (MEST), Korea.

References

1. Lee, M.J.; Lim, E.M.; Kwon, K.R. Effect of Paljin-tang on Surgically Induced Endometriosis in Rats. *J. Orient. Obstet. Gynecol.* **2006**, *19*, 83–94.
2. Joo, J.M.; Kim, D.C.; Back, S.H.; Kim, E.H. The Effect of Palmultang on the Ovarian Functions and Differential Gene Expression of Caspase-3, MAPK and MPG in Female Mice. *J. Orient. Obstet. Gynecol.* **2007**, *20*, 91–110.
3. Pierce, G.F. Macrophages: Important physiologic and pathologic sources of polypeptide growth factors. *Am. J. Respir. Cell Mol. Biol.* **1990**, *2*, 233–234.
4. Wadleigh, D.J.; Reddy, S.T.; Kopp, E.; Ghosh, S.; Herschman, H.R. Transcriptional activation of the cyclooxygenase-2 gene in endotoxin-treated RAW 264.7 macrophages. *J. Biol. Chem.* **2000**, *275*, 6259–6266.
5. Becker, S.; Mundandhara, S.; Devlin, R.B.; Madden, M. Regulation of cytokine production in human alveolar macrophages and airway epithelial cells in response to ambient air pollution particles: Further mechanistic studies. *Toxicol. Appl. Pharmacol.* **2005**, *207*, 269–275.
6. Kim, J.B.; Han, A.R.; Park, E.Y.; Kim, J.Y.; Cho, W.; Lee, J.; Seo, E.K.; Lee, K.T. Inhibition of LPS-induced iNOS, COX-2 and cytokines expression by poncirin through the NF-kappaB inactivation in RAW 264.7 macrophage cells. *Biol. Pharm. Bull.* **2007**, *30*, 2345–2351.
7. Pae, H.O.; Chung, H.T. Heme oxygenase-1: Its therapeutic roles in inflammatory diseases. *Immune Netw.* **2009**, *9*, 12–19.
8. Ashino, T.; Yamanaka, R.; Yamamoto, M.; Shimokawa, H.; Sekikawa, K.; Iwakura, Y.; Shioda, S.; Numazawa, S.; Yoshida, T. Negative feedback regulation of lipopolysaccharide-induced inducible nitric oxide synthase gene expression by heme oxygenase-1 induction in macrophages. *Mol. Immunol.* **2008**, *45*, 2106–2115.
9. De Martin, R.; Vanhove, B.; Cheng, Q.; Hofer, E.; Csizmadia, V.; Winkler, H.; Bach, F.H. Cytokine-inducible expression in endothelial cells of an I kappa B alpha-like gene is regulated by NF kappa B. *EMBO J.* **1993**, *12*, 2773–2779.
10. Pahl, H.L. Activators and target genes of Rel/NF-kappaB transcription factors. *Oncogene* **1999**, *18*, 6853–6866.
11. Baeuerle, P.A.; Baltimore, D. NF-kappa B: Ten years after. *Cell* **1996**, *87*, 13–20.
12. Robinson, M.J.; Cobb, M.H. Mitogen-activated protein kinase pathways. *Curr. Opin. Cell Biol.* **1997**, *9*, 180–186.
13. Guzik, T.J.; Korbut, R.; Adamek-Guzik, T. Nitric oxide and superoxide in inflammation and immune regulation. *J. Physiol. Pharmacol.* **2003**, *54*, 469–487.
14. Southan, G.J.; Szabo, C. Selective pharmacological inhibition of distinct nitric oxide synthase isoforms. *Biochem. Pharmacol.* **1996**, *51*, 383–394.
15. Brasier, A.R. The NF-kappaB regulatory network. *Cardiovasc. Toxicol.* **2006**, *6*, 111–130.

16. Gilmore, T.D. Introduction to NF-kappaB: Players, pathways, perspectives. *Oncogene* **2006**, *25*, 6680–6684.
17. Tian, B.; Brasier, A.R. Identification of a nuclear factor kappa B-dependent gene network. *Recent Prog. Horm. Res.* **2003**, *58*, 95–130.
18. Chen, F.; Kuhn, D.C.; Sun, S.C.; Gaydos, L.J.; Demers, L.M. Dependence and reversal of nitric oxide production on NF-kappa B in silica and lipopolysaccharide-induced macrophages. *Biochem. Biophys. Res. Commun.* **1995**, *214*, 839–846.
19. Roshak, A.K.; Jackson, J.R.; McGough, K.; Chabot-Fletcher, M.; Mochan, E.; Marshall, L.A. Manipulation of distinct NFkappaB proteins alters interleukin-1beta-induced human rheumatoid synovial fibroblast prostaglandin E2 formation. *J. Biol. Chem.* **1996**, *271*, 31496–31501.
20. Xie, W.; Merrill, J.R.; Bradshaw, W.S.; Simmons, D.L. Structural determination and promoter analysis of the chicken mitogen-inducible prostaglandin G/H synthase gene and genetic mapping of the murine homolog. *Arch. Biochem. Biophys.* **1993**, *300*, 247–252.
21. Ahn, K.S.; Noh, E.J.; Zhao, H.L.; Jung, S.H.; Kang, S.S.; Kim, Y.S. Inhibition of inducible nitric oxide synthase and cyclooxygenase II by Platycodon grandiflorum saponins via suppression of nuclear factor-kappaB activation in RAW 264.7 cells. *Life Sci.* **2005**, *76*, 2315–2328.
22. Barnes, P.J.; Karin, M. Nuclear factor-kappaB. A pivotal transcription factor in chronic inflammatory diseases. *N. Engl. J. Med.* **1997**, *336*, 1066–1071.
23. Kim, Y.M.; Lee, B.S.; Yi, K.Y.; Paik, S.G. Upstream NF-kappaB site is required for the maximal expression of mouse inducible nitric oxide synthase gene in interferon-gamma plus lipopolysaccharide induced RAW 264.7 macrophages. *Biochem. Pharmacol.* **1997**, *236*, 655–660.
24. Caivano, M. Role of MAP kinase cascades in inducing arginine transporters and nitric oxide synthetase in RAW 264.7 macrophages. *FEBS Lett.* **1999**, *429*, 249–253.
25. Kim, H.K.; Choi, Y.W.; Lee, E.N.; Park, J.K.; Kim, S.G.; Park, D.J.; Kim, B.S.; Lim, Y.T.; Yoon, S. 5-Hydroxymethylfurfural from black garlic extract prevents TNFα-induced monocytic cell adhesion to HUVECs by suppression of vascular cell adhesion molecule-1 expression, reactive oxygen species generation and NF-κB activation. *Phytother. Res.* **2011**, *25*, 965–974.
26. Chen, T.; Guo, Z.P.; Jiao, X.Y.; Jia, R.Z.; Zhang, Y.H.; Li, J.Y.; Huang, X.L.; Liu, H.J. Peoniflorin suppresses tumor necrosis factor-α induced chemokine production in human dermal microvascular endothelial cells by blocking nuclear factor-κB and ERK pathway. *Arch. Dermatol. Res.* **2011**, *303*, 351–360.
27. Rim, H.K.; Cho, W.; Sung, S.H.; Lee, K.T. Nodakenin suppresses lipopolysaccharide-induced inflammatory responses in macrophage cells by inhibiting tumor necrosis factor receptor-associated factor 6 and nuclear factor-κB pathways and protects mice from lethal endotoxin shock. *J. Pharmacol. Exp. Ther.* **2012**, *342*, 654–664.
28. Kato, T.; Horie, N.; Hashimoto, K.; Satoh, K.; Shimoyama, T.; Kaneko, T.; Kusama, K.; Sakagami, H. Bimodal effect of glycyrrhizin on macrophage nitric oxide and prostaglandin E2 production. *In Vivo* **2008**, *22*, 583–586.
29. Kim, J.H.; Jeong, J.H.; Jeon, S.T.; Kim, H.; Ock, J.; Suk, K.; Kim, S.I.; Song, K.S.; Lee, W.H. Decursin inhibits induction of inflammatory mediators by blocking nuclear factor-kappaB activation in macrophages. *Mol. Pharmacol.* **2006**, *69*, 1783–1790.
30. Choi, H.J.; Kang, O.H.; Park, P.S.; Chae, H.S.; Oh, Y.C.; Lee, Y.S.; Choi, J.G.; Lee, G.H.;

Kweon, O.H.; Kwon, D.Y. Mume Fructus water extract inhibits pro-inflammatory mediators in lipopolysaccharide-stimulated macrophages. *J. Med. Food* **2007**, *10*, 460–466.

31. Jo, H.Y.; Kim, Y.; Nam, S.Y.; Lee, B.J.; Kim, Y.B.; Yun, Y.W.; Ahn, B. The inhibitory effect of quercitrin gallate on iNOS expression induced by lipopolysaccharide in Balb/c mice. *J. Vet. Sci.* **2008**, *9*, 267–272.
32. Kim, H.Y.; Kim, J.K.; Choi, J.H.; Jung, J.Y.; Oh, W.Y.; Kim, D.C.; Lee, H.S.; Kim, Y.S.; Kang, S.S.; Lee, S.H.; *et al.* Hepatoprotective effect of pinoresinol on carbon tetrachloride-induced hepatic damage in mice. *J. Pharmacol. Sci.* **2010**, *112*, 105–112.
33. Srisook, K.; Palachot, M.; Mongkol, N.; Srisook, E.; Sarapusit, S. Anti-inflammatory effect of ethyl acetate extract from Cissus quadrangularis Linn may be involved with induction of heme oxygenase-1 and suppression of NF-κB activation. *J. Ethnopharmacol.* **2011**, *133*, 1008–1014.
34. Kwon, D.J.; Ju, S.M.; Youn, G.S.; Choi, S.Y.; Park, J. Suppression of iNOS and COX-2 expression by flavokawain A via blockade of NF-κB and AP-1 activation in RAW 264.7 macrophages. *Food Chem. Toxicol.* **2013**, *58*, 479–486.

8

The Discovery of Potentially Selective Human Neuronal Nitric Oxide Synthase (nNOS) Inhibitors: A Combination of Pharmacophore Modelling, CoMFA, Virtual Screening and Molecular Docking Studies

Guanhong Xu [1], Yue Chen [1], Kun Shen [1], Xiuzhen Wang [1,3], Fei Li [1,*] and Yan He [2,*]

[1] School of Pharmacy, Nanjing Medical University, Nanjing 210029, China;
E-Mails: xgh@njmu.edu.cn (G.X.); yuechen0311@126.com (Y.C.); mokingsk@sina.com (K.S.); showshow828@163.com (X.W.)

[2] Department of Internal Neurology, Nanjing Children's Hospital Affiliated to Nanjing Medical University, Nanjing 210008, China

[3] School of Pharmacy, China Pharmaceutical University, Nanjing 210009, China

* Authors to whom correspondence should be addressed;
E-Mails: kldlf@njmu.edu.cn (F.L.); kldhy2002@163.com (Y.H.)

Abstract: Neuronal nitric oxide synthase (nNOS) plays an important role in neurotransmission and smooth muscle relaxation. Selective inhibition of nNOS over its other isozymes is highly desirable for the treatment of neurodegenerative diseases to avoid undesirable effects. In this study, we present a workflow for the identification and prioritization of compounds as potentially selective human nNOS inhibitors. Three-dimensional pharmacophore models were constructed based on a set of known nNOS inhibitors. The pharmacophore models were evaluated by Pareto surface and CoMFA (Comparative Molecular Field Analysis) analyses. The best pharmacophore model, which included 7 pharmacophore features, was used as a search query in the SPECS database (SPECS®, Delft, The Netherlands). The hit compounds were further filtered by scoring and docking. Ten hits were identified as potential selective nNOS inhibitors.

Keywords: neuronal nitric oxide synthase; inhibitors; pharmacophore; virtual screening; docking

1. Introduction

Nitric oxide (NO) is one of the most studied biological signaling molecules and is produced by catalysis from nitric oxide synthase (NOS), which converts L-arginine to L-citrulline, and produces this tiny, short-lived molecule. To date, there are three distinct isoforms of NOS: neuronal NOS (nNOS), endothelial NOS (eNOS) and inducible NOS (iNOS). nNOS and eNOS are constitutively expressed and depend on increases in external calcium and binding of a calcium/calmodulin complex for activation. nNOS and eNOS play an important role in neurotransmission and smooth muscle relaxation, respectively, and iNOS is expressed during bacterial infection, tumor cell cytolysis and inflammation [1–3].

As an inorganic reactive free radical gas, NO is believed to be involved in a number of physiological processes such as inflammation, neurotransmission, blood pressure regulation, platelet aggregation and pain [4–6]. However, overproduction of NO has been implicated in numerous disease states [7]. In particular, excess NO in the central nervous system from nNOS activity can lead to many neurological disease states including neurodegeneration during Alzheimer's and Parkinson's diseases [8], altered spinal transmission of neuropathic pain [9,10], and progression of migraine and chronic tension-type headaches [11]. Consequently, an inhibitor of nNOS has the potential to be therapeutic in these diseases; however, the functions of eNOS in blood pressure regulation and iNOS in immune responses must be preserved, and the selective inhibition of nNOS has been the challenge of many researchers in the past decade [12–15].

Recently, several categories of selective inhibitors of nNOS have been designed and developed for the treatment of central nervous system (CNS) disorders [3,15–22]. Some showed significant efficacy in the rat Chung model of neuropathic pain [22] and in a rodent model of dural inflammation relevant to migraine pain [22]. X-ray structures of nNOS co-crystallized with various ligands [23–25] provided insights into the essential structural elements and motifs central to its catalytic mechanism and mode of binding. These findings provide useful information about the interaction between the ligands and the residues near the binding site and can be utilized to design even more selective and potent drug-like NOS inhibitors.

Virtual screening based on a pharmacophore model as a 3D search query has been successfully employed as an efficient alternative to high throughput screening approaches for the development of new compounds with the desired biological properties [26]. Pharmacophore modeling can be used to analyze the common functional groups responsible for specific drug receptor interactions or as a prelude to three dimensional quantitative structure activity relationship (3D-QSAR) analyses that are aligned accordingly with a set of known active compounds in 3D space. 3D-QSAR has been successfully applied in drug discovery and design. As a popular QSAR method, Comparative Molecular Field Analysis (CoMFA) [27] studies incorporate 3D information of the ligands by searching for the sites on molecules that are capable of being modified into more specific ligands. As a useful methodology for studying interaction mechanisms, receptor based molecular docking analysis can be used as a complementary tool to prioritize the hits from the pharmacophore-based virtual screening [28].

In the present study, a 3D pharmacophore model for nNOS inhibitors was assembled and the generated model was used as a search query in the SPECS database containing 197,000 compounds. The virtual screening approach, in combination with pharmacophore modeling and molecular docking can be used to identify and design novel nNOS inhibitors with high selectivity. These molecules may be potential lead compounds for future drug development.

2. Results and Discussion

2.1. Pharmacophore Results

Twenty pharmacophore models were generated using SYBYL X 1.3 (Tripos Associates Inc., St. Louis, MO, USA). Table 1 lists the parameters of each model. Specificity is a logarithmic indicator of the expected discrimination for each query and is based on the number of features it contains, their allotment across partial match constraints, and the degree to which the features are separated in space. Strong models should have a high Specificity value. Generally, the Specificity value should be at least 5 in a pharmacophore model used as the query for a UNITY flex search [29]. For this study, MODEL 012, MODEL 019, and MODEL 003 had the high Specificity values of 5.138, 5.128 and 4.8580, respectively. These models yielded reasonable pharmacophore models. The N_HITS column shows the actual number of ligands hit by the model query, with the majority of the models matching at least 5 ligands. The value in the FEATS column indicates the total number of features possessed by each model. All of the models had six or more features except for MODEL 011. The retained models had a PARETO rank value of 0, indicating that a single model is not superior to any other. The HBOND term is a measure of the overall pharmacophoric similarity among the ligand conformers. The STERIC term is a measure of the overall steric similarity among the ligand conformers; this term is basically the same as the HBOND term. The ENERGY term indicates the total energy (using the Tripos force field) of all molecules in the training set.

Table 1. Parameters of the pharmacophore model [a].

No.	SPECIFICITY	N_HITS	FEATS	PARETO	ENERGY	STERICS	HBOND
MOEDL_001	4.180	4	6	0	15.60	666.7	173.3
MOEDL_002	3.881	8	7	0	15.44	703.1	161.8
MOEDL_003	4.858	6	8	0	18.53	750.4	155.1
MOEDL_004	4.108	6	6	0	18.62	712.0	166.6
MOEDL_005	3.823	9	7	0	20.15	852.7	162.7
MOEDL_006	3.735	6	7	0	17.54	714.7	160.5
MOEDL_007	3.902	9	7	0	58.38	705.2	179.2
MOEDL_008	4.051	6	6	0	19.3	784.6	171.4
MOEDL_009	4.036	3	6	0	40.81	845.3	159.5
MOEDL_010	3.393	5	9	0	35.12	612.2	178.2
MOEDL_011	3.158	6	5	0	22.40	635.3	178.9

Table 1. *Cont.*

No.	SPECIFICITY	N_HITS	FEATS	PARETO	ENERGY	STERICS	HBOND
MOEDL_012 [b]	**5.138**	**5**	**7**	**0**	**41.13**	**870.1**	**166.1**
MOEDL_013	4.048	6	6	0	17.75	732.8	157.0
MOEDL_014	4.124	6	6	0	19.25	861.2	160.2
MOEDL_015	3.867	8	7	0	19.99	567.7	175.3
MOEDL_016	4.050	5	6	0	23.76	834.0	165.7
MOEDL_017	4.053	5	6	0	14.97	658.9	150.8
MOEDL_018	4.058	5	6	0	55.07	859.6	162.8
MOEDL_019	5.128	4	7	0	23.06	654.1	168.0
MOEDL_020	4.050	5	6	0	16.91	748.1	158.3

[a] SPECIFICITY is a logarithmic indicator of the expected discrimination for each query; N_HITS is the actual number of ligands hit by the model query; FEATS is the total number of features in the model query; PARETO indicates the Pareto rank of the each model; ENERGY is the total energy of the model; STERICS is the steric overlap for the model; HBOND is the pharmacophoric concordance; [b] The selected model (MODEL_012) is indicated in boldface.

The most significant pharmacophore hypothesis was characterized by the conflicting demands of maximizing pharmacophore consensus, maximizing steric consensus, and minimizing conformer potential energy [30]. We constructed a 3D plot to visualize the Pareto surface and select the best pharmacophore model (Figure 1). Considering only the ENERGY and STERICS criteria, the best model is shown in the upper left-hand corner of the graph in Figure 1b, where the ENERGY is low and the STERICS score is high. In terms of ENERGY and HBOND criteria, the best model is shown in the lower part of the graph in Figure 1c, where the ENERGY is low and the HBOND score is high. Finally, in terms of ENERGY and HBOND, the best model is shown in the upper part of the graph, where both scores are high (Figure 1d). Among the considered models, MODEL_012 (represented with a red cross in Figure 1) has the optimal position because it fulfills the three criteria and it has the highest Specificity value [31].

The best GALAHAD MODEL 012 is displayed in Figure 2. All of the aligned conformers represent low-energy conformations of the molecules, and the final alignment shows a satisfactory superimposition of the pharmacophoric points. Cyan, magenta, green and red spheres indicate hydrophobes, donor atoms, acceptor atoms and positive nitrogens, respectively. Model 012 includes 7 pharmacophore features: three hydrophobes (HY_1, HY_2 and HY_3), one donor atom (DA_4), one acceptor atom (AA_5) and two positive nitrogens (NP_6 and NP_7). The magenta sphere is covered by a green sphere because the donor atom and the acceptor atom are in the same position in this molecule.

Figure 1. Plot of the STERICS, ENERGY and HBOND values for the models with the top ten Specificity values. (**a**) 3D plot; (**b**) plot of STERICS *vs.* ENERGY; (**c**) plot of ENERGY *vs.* HBOND; (**d**) plot of STERICS *vs.* HBOND. The red cross represents MODEL_12.

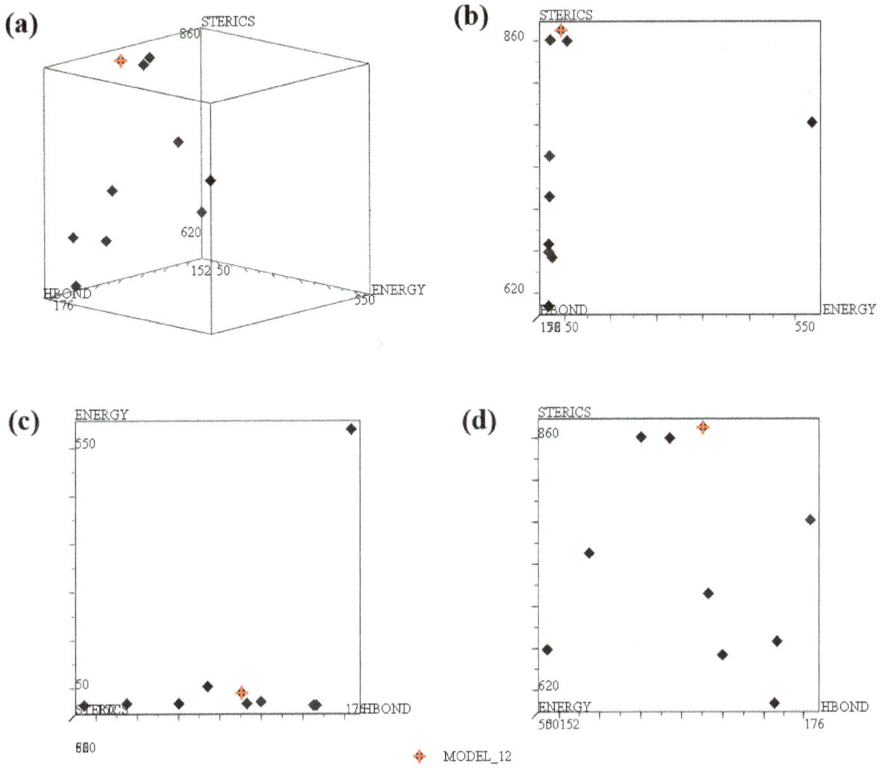

Figure 2. Selected pharmacophore MODEL_012 and the molecular alignment of the compounds used to elaborate the model.

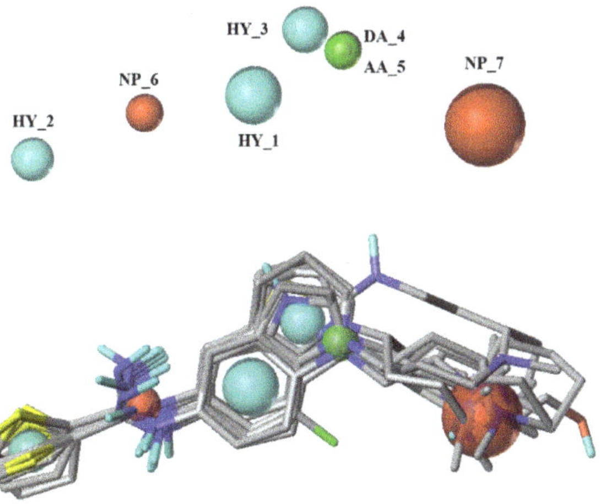

2.2. CoMFA (Comparative Molecular Field Analysis) Statistical Results

We used MODEL 012 as a template to align all molecules. The generated steric and electrostatic fields were scaled by the CoMFA-Standard scaling method in SYBYL with the default energy cutoff value. The CoMFA model yielded a good cross-validated correlation coefficient (q^2) of 0.513 with an optimized component value of 4, which suggests that the model should be a useful tool for predicting the IC_{50} values. A high non-cross-validated correlation coefficient (r^2_{ncv}) of 0.933 with a low standard error estimate (SEE) of 0.134 and an *f* value of 149.950 were obtained. The steric and electrostatic contributions were 45.1% and 54.9%, respectively. The predicted activities for the inhibitors are listed in Table 2 and the correlation between the predicted activities and the experimental activities is depicted in Figure 3. The predictive correlation coefficient (r^2_{pred}) was 0.742 for the test set. The statistical results indicate that the CoMFA model is a reliable predictor.

Table 2. Structure and biological values (pIC_{50}) of nNOS inhibitors.

No.		Structure	pIC_{50}	
			Observed	Predicted
		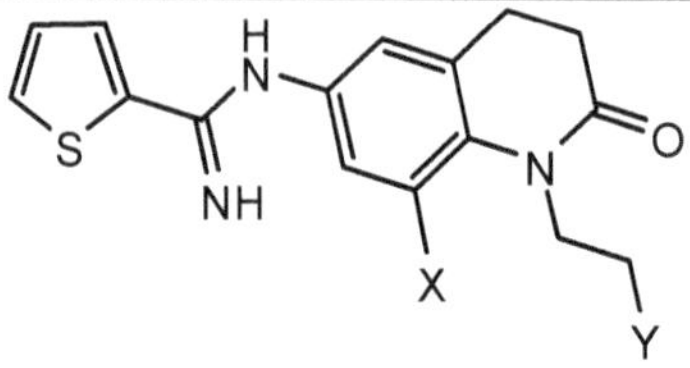 *series 1* [22]		
-	X	Y	-	-
1	H	$N(CH_3)_2$	6.237	6.089
2 *	H	$N(Et)_2$	5.656	5.750
3	H	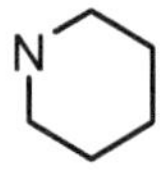	6.108	5.922
4	H	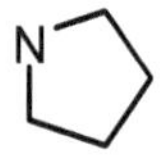	6.796	6.650
5	H	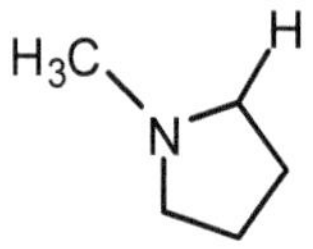	5.979	6.148
6	F	$N(CH_3)_2$	5.474	5.770
7	H	$CH_2N(CH_3)_2$	5.943	5.971
8	H	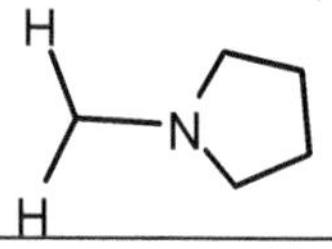	5.914	6.021
		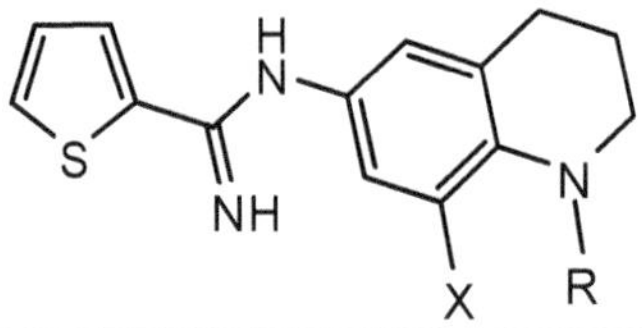 *series 2* [15,22]		
-	X	R	-	-
9 *	H	$-CH_2CH_2CH_2N(CH_3)_2$	6.569	6.588
10	H	$-CH_2CH_2NCH_3$	6.754	6.741
11 *	H	$-CH_2CH_2N\ CH_2CH_3$	6.857	6.694
12	H	$-CH_2CH_2NCH(CH_3)_2$	6.573	6.585
13	H	$-CH_2CH_2N(CH_3)\ (C_2H_5)$	7.013	6.987
14 *	H	$-CH_2CH_2N(CH_3)_2$	6.367	6.510
15	H	$-CH_2CH_2N(C_2H_5)_2$	6.585	6.642
16	F	$-CH_2CH_2N(C_2H_5)_2$	7.032	6.757
17	H	$-(CH_2)_3NCH_3$	6.629	6.736
18	H	$-CH_2CH_2N(CH_3)\ (CH_2)_2OH$	6.876	6.960
19	H	$-(CH_2)_2NH(CH_2)_2OH$	6.939	6.964

Table 2. *Cont.*

No.		Structure	pIC50 Observed	pIC50 Predicted
20	H	-$(CH_2)_3NH(CH_2)_2OH$	6.772	6.667
21	H	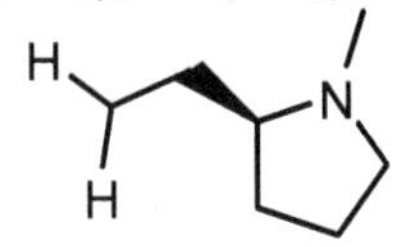	7.009	6.925
22	H	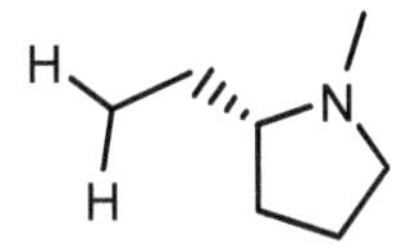	6.886	6.896
23 *	H	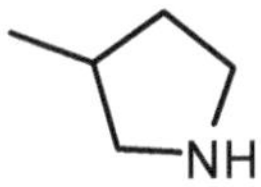	6.606	6.385
24	H	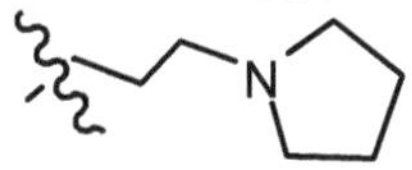	7.066	7.118
25	H	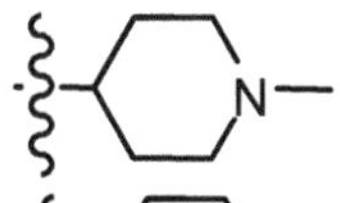	6.086	6.233
26	H	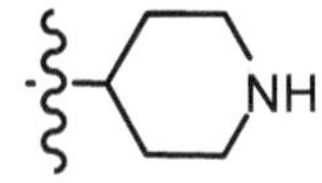	6.268	6.430
27 *	H	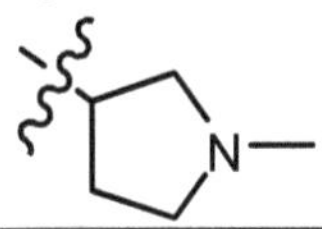	6.444	6.550
		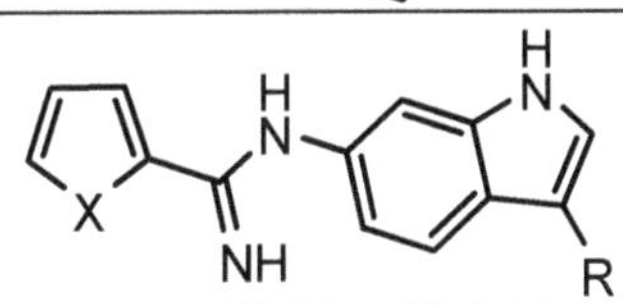 R *series 3* [21]		
-	X	R	-	-
28	S	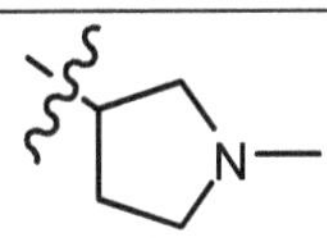	6.699	6.694
29	S	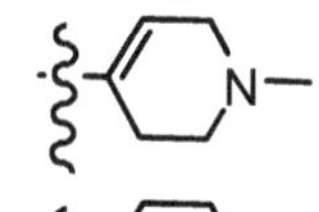	6.097	6.225
30	S	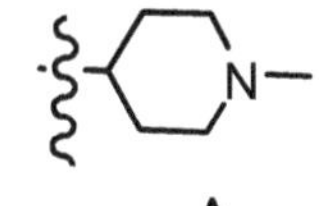	6.921	6.701
31	S	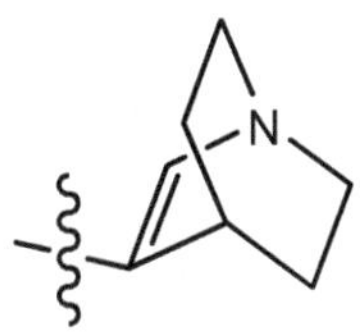	5.824	5.830
32	S	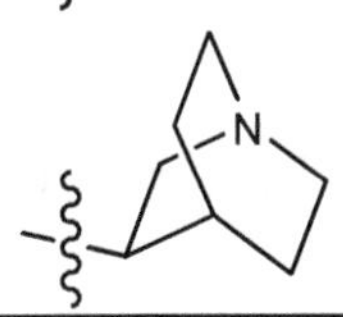	6.347	6.304

Table 2. *Cont.*

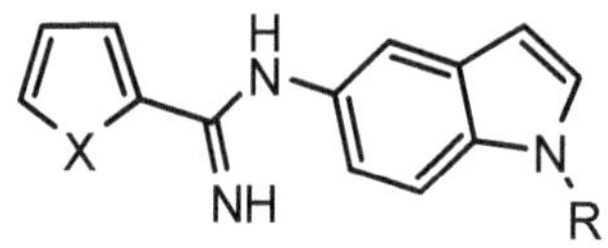

series 4 [17]

No.	X	R	pIC50 Observed	pIC50 Predicted
33	S	*N*-(1-(3-(dimethylamino)propyl)-	6.328	6.419
34 *	S	*N*-(1-(3-(cyclopropylamino)propyl)-	6.585	6.366
35	S	*N*-(1-(3-morpholinopropyl)-	6.181	6.120
36	S	*N*-(1-(3-((1-ethylpyrrolidin-2-yl)methylamino)propyl)-	6.886	6.700
37	S	*N*-(1-(3-adamantanaminopropyl)-	6.444	6.388
38	S	*N*-(1-(2-(dimethylamino)ethyl)-	6.770	6.736
39	S	*N*-(1-(2-(piperidin-1-yl)ethyl)-	6.770	6.930
40	S	*N*-(1-(2-(1-methylpiperidin-2-yl)ethyl)-	7.046	7.131
41	S	(*S*) *N*-(1-(2-(1-methylpyrrolidin-2-yl)ethyl)-	7.700	7.564
42	O	*N*-(1-(2-(1-methylpyrrolidin-2-yl)ethyl)-	6.602	6.824
43	S	*N*-(1-(1-methylazepan-4-yl)-	6.921	6.893
44	O	*N*-(1-(1-methylazepan-4-yl)-	6.367	6.443
45 *	S	*N*-(1-(8-methyl-8-azabicyclo[3.2.1]octan-3-yl)-	6.120	6.168
46	S	*N*-(1-(quinuclidin-3-yl)-	6.444	6.417
47	S	*N*-(1-(1-methylpiperidin-4-yl)-	6.387	6.286

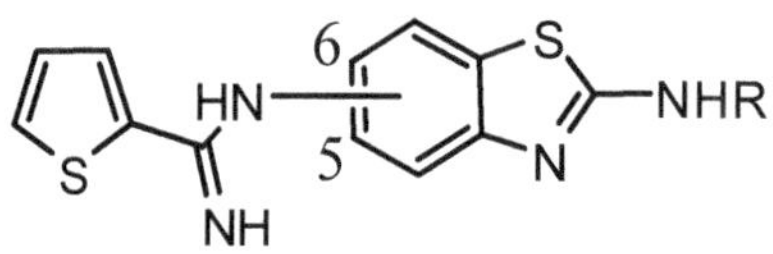

series 5 [16]

No.	Substituted	R	pIC50 Observed	pIC50 Predicted
48	5	2-(Pyridin-2-yl)ethyl	5.959	6.025
49	5	2-Morpholinoethyl	5.886	5.976
50 *	5	1-Benzylpiperidin-4-yl	6.398	6.281
51	5	1-(4-Fluorobenzyl)piperidin-4-yl	6.097	5.986
52	5	(±)-2-(1-Methylpyrrolidin-2-yl)ethyl	7.523	7.582
53	6	2-(Pyridin-2-yl)ethyl	5.886	5.83
54	6	2-Morpholinoethyl	5.699	5.676
55	6	1-Benzylpiperidin-4-yl	6.301	6.216
56	6	1-(4-Fluorobenzyl)piperidin-4-yl	6.699	5.779
57 *	6	2-(1H-Imidazol-5-yl)ethyl	6.523	6.789
58	6	4-Bromophenethyl	5.357	5.188
59	6	Tetrahydro-2H-pyran-4-yl	5.699	5.736

* Compounds taken for the test set.

Figure 3. Correlation between the experimental and CoMFA (Comparative Molecular Field Analysis) predicted activities of compounds.

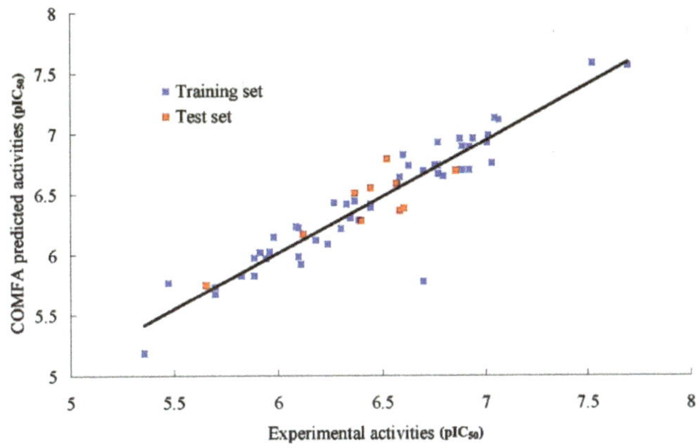

The CoMFA steric and electrostatic contour maps are shown in Figure 4 using compound 41 as a reference structure. In Figure 4a, the blue contour indicates regions in which an increase of positive charge enhances the activity, and the red contour indicates regions in which more negative charges are favorable for activity. The two large blue contours around the red sphere indicate that the substituent in this region should be electron deficient for increased binding affinity with a protein. Another small blue contour is found around the guanidine isosteric group indicating that a negatively charged substituent in this area is unfavorable. The CoMFA model showed the same result as the pharmacophore hypothesis. In Figure 4b, the steric field is represented by green and yellow contours, in which the green contours indicate regions where a bulky group is favorable and the yellow regions represent regions where a bulky group will decrease activity. In this case, the green contours around the substituent R demonstrated that bulky groups enhance the binding affinity of the nNOS. Most compounds with high activities in this dataset have the same such properties. The CoMFA contour maps and the predicted result further indicated that MODEL 012 can be used as a theoretical screening tool that is able to discriminate between active and inactive molecules [31].

Figure 4. (**a**) CoMFA steric contour maps and (**b**) CoMFA electrostatic contour maps.

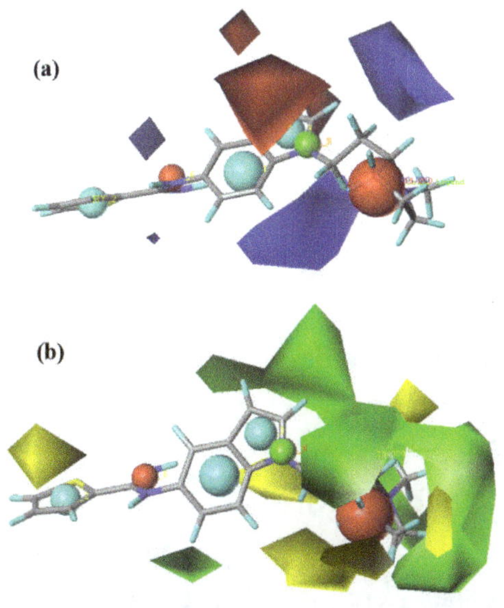

2.3. Virtual Screening

The pharmacophore based virtual screening was conducted to find potential nNOS inhibitors. A stepwise virtual screening procedure was applied, wherein the pharmacophore based virtual screening was followed by drug-likeness evaluation, screening of the pharmacophore query, QFIT (The QFIT score is a value between 0 and 100, where 100 is best and represents how close the ligand atoms match the query target coordinates within the range of a spatial constraint tolerance) scoring filtration, and a molecular docking study. The sequential virtual screening flowchart we employed is depicted in Figure 5, in which the reduction in the number of hits for each screening step is shown.

Figure 5. Virtual screening flowchart.

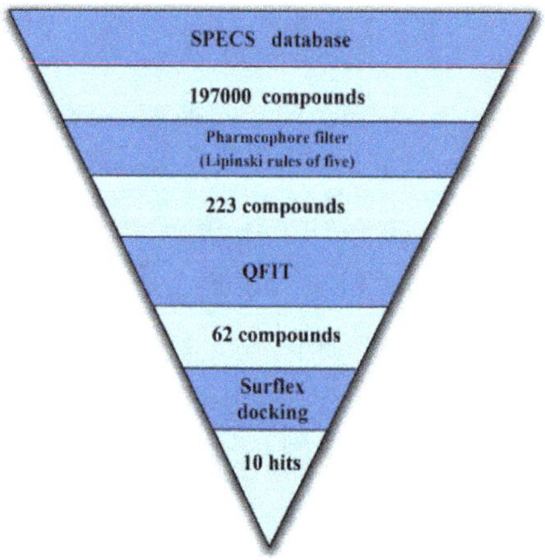

2.3.1. Database Searching

Flexible 3D screening was performed using the UNITY tool to screen the SPECS database [32], which contains approximately 197,000 compounds. The database query was generated based on the pharmacophore MODEL 012. The database was restricted with Lipinski's rule. In general, this rule describes molecules that have drug-like properties. Drug-likeness is a property that is most often used to characterize compound libraries such as combinatorial or screening libraries that are screened to find novel lead chemical compounds [33]. According to this rule, we used simple molecular descriptors, such as molecular weight ($\leq$500), hydrophobicity (MLogP $\leq$ 4.15) and the number of H-bond donor ($\leq$5) and acceptor atoms ($\leq$10), as the first filter to select the molecules with good absorption or permeation [34]. The remaining 223 compounds were further screened on the basis of QFIT to reduce the dataset, where QFIT is the pharmacophore match between the query and hit [35].

2.3.2. Molecular Docking

To predict the appropriate binding conformation for nNOS inhibitors and the reported hit compounds from virtual screening, Surflex Docking (Tripos Associates Inc., St. Louis, MO, USA) was used to generate an ensemble of docking conformations. The top 62 hit compounds with the highest QFIT score from screening after UNITY filtering were further screened using molecular docking into the binding site of nNOS to select the compounds with the ability to form favorable interactions with the active site. The docked compounds were filtered based on scoring function and interaction with the crucial residues [24] in the binding site. Finally, ten compounds were selected on the basis of the dock score and favorable interactions with the key residues. The results of the hit compounds with their dock score and QFIT values are shown in Table 3. Among the active compounds reported [24], AG_205/36953325 has a similar linker length and two aromatic ring centers on both ends. There is also a hydrogen bond donor in the aromatic ring center and at least one hydrogen bond donor on the linker. The phenolic hydroxyl makes a hydrogen bond with the NOS active site GLU592, which is conserved in all mammalian NOS isoforms [24], and the hydrophobic phenyl ring π-stacks with the heme (HEM801) next to the GLU. The long, flexible linker extending from the phenyl ring allows the 2-phenyl-2,3-dihydro-1H-pyrazole to reach and to π-stack with TYR706 (Figure 6). The binding mode of this hit compound is similar to that of the reported co-crystallized compound [24] and indicates that the identified hit compounds may have the same mechanism of action as known nNOS inhibitors.

Table 3. Chemical structures of the hit compounds and their dock scores and QFIT values.

SPECS ID	Structure	Dock Scores	QFIT
AG_205/36953325	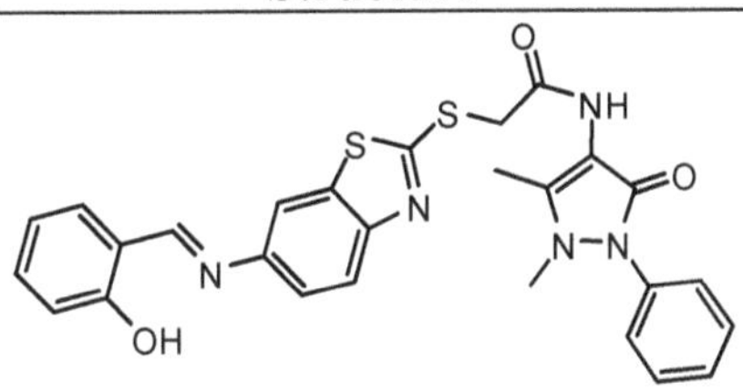	8.29	65.74
AG_205/11218159	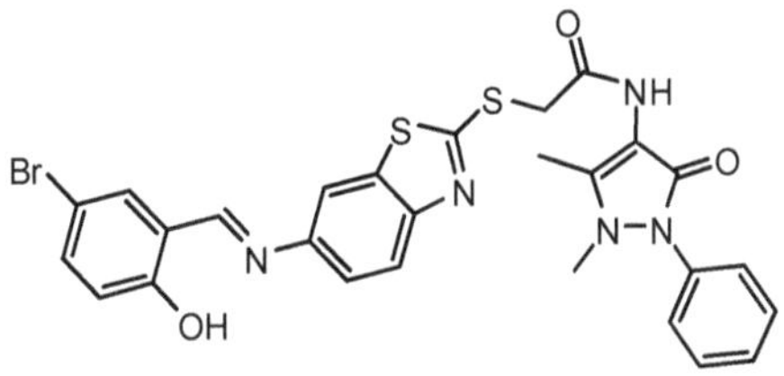	8.20	65.74
AG_205/11218337	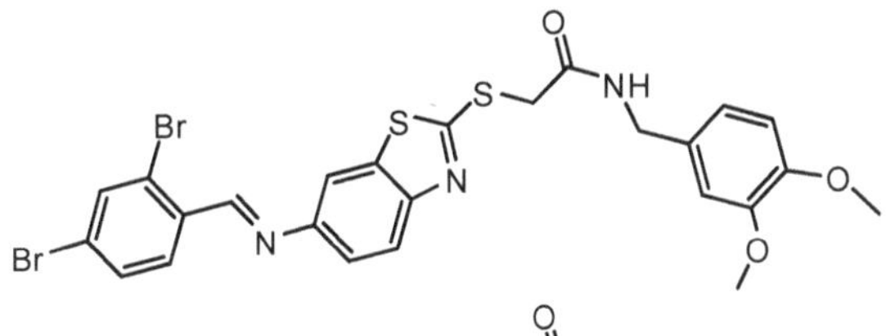	8.01	65.82
AG_205/11218321	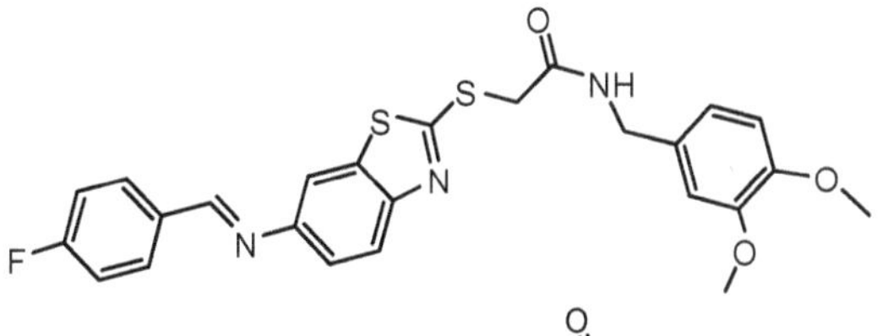	7.86	65.82
AG_205/36564022	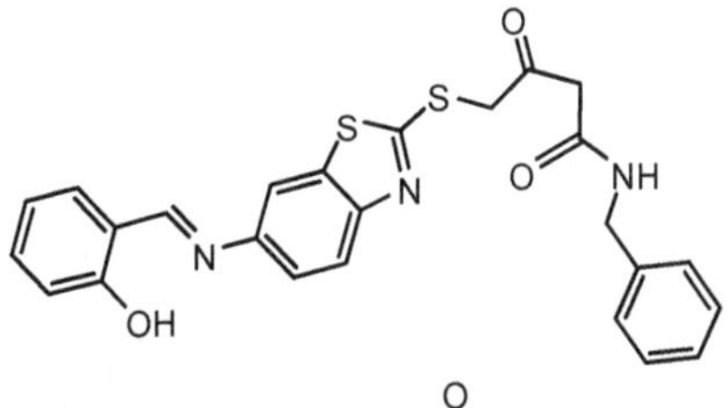	7.65	65.82
AG_205/36953138	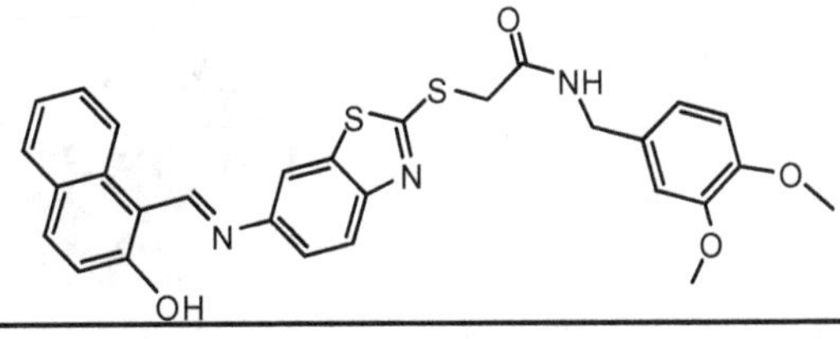	7.63	65.81

Table 3. *Cont.*

SPECS ID	Structure	Dock Scores	QFIT
AG_205/09949027	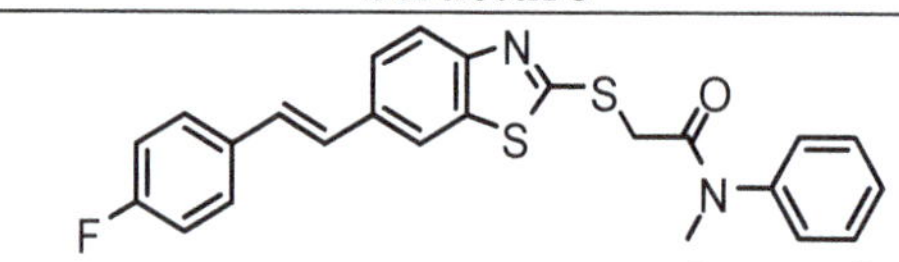	7.34	65.82
AG_205/36953406	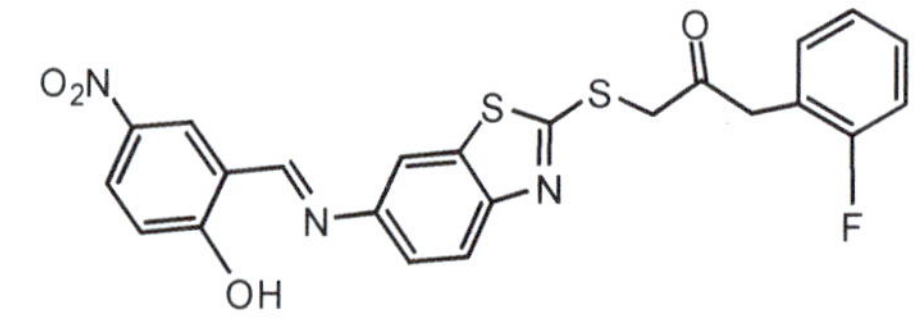	6.78	65.82
AG_205/36265063	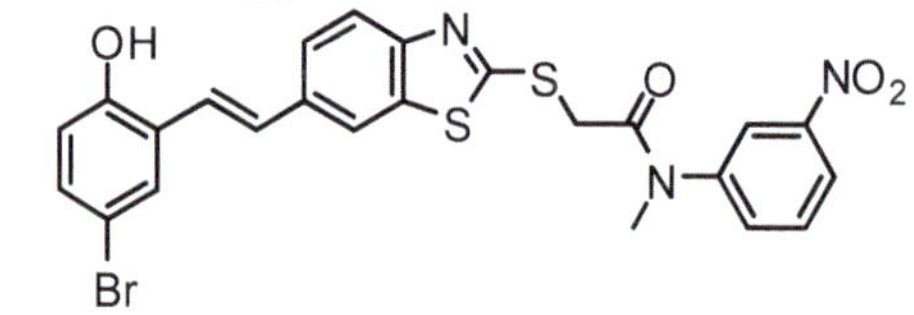	6.51	65.82
AG_205/36940042	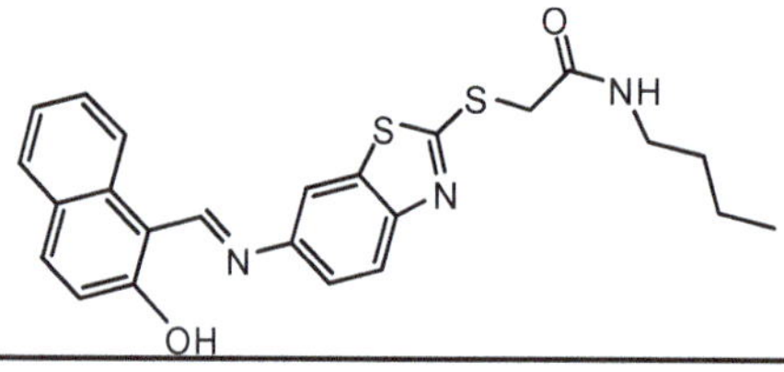	6.22	65.81

Figure 6. (**a**) Mapping of the hit molecule (AG_205/36953325) by MODEL 012 from SPECS databases; (**b**) The orientation of AG_205/36953325 in the active site of nNOS; (**c**) The secondary structure of the active site and AG_205/36953325; and (**d**) The MOLCAD (a software package of SYBYL) cavity depth potential surfaces structure of the binding site within AG_205/36953325. The cavity depth color ramp ranges from blue (outside of the pocket) to light red (cavities deep inside the pocket).

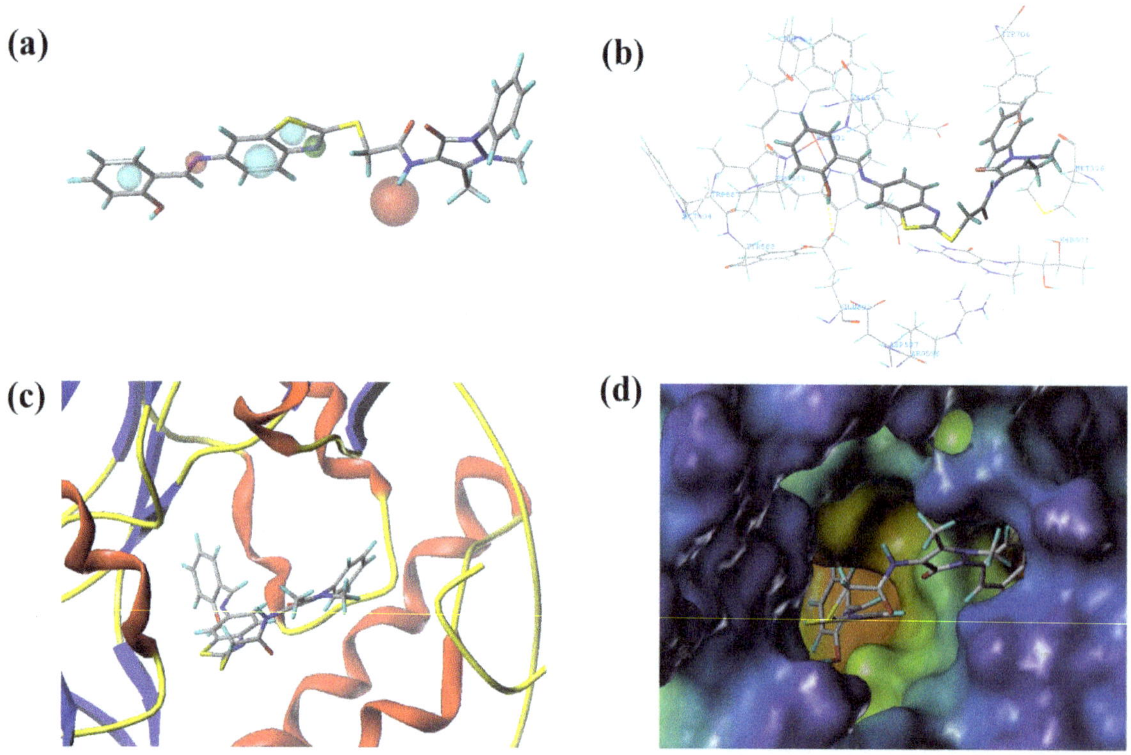

3. Experimental Section

3.1. Compounds and Biological Data

Fifty-nine novel nNOS inhibitors were taken from the literature [15–17,21,22] with their biological activities in terms of IC_{50} values; 49 compounds were used as a training set and the remaining 10 compounds were used as a test set, based on random selection. The compounds in the test set have a range of biological activity values similar to that of the training set. The IC_{50} values of the inhibitors were converted into pIC_{50} (log ($1/IC_{50}$)) and used as dependent variables in the Pharmacophore generation and CoMFA calculations. The structures of the compounds and their pIC_{50} values are given in Table 2. All molecular modeling calculations were conducted using SYBYL X 1.3 (Tripos Associates Inc.). Molecular building was performed with a molecule sketch program in the same software. The molecular geometry of each compound was first minimized using the standard Tripos molecular mechanics force field with 0.01 kcal/(mol A) energy gradient convergence criterion. Partial atomic charges were calculated by the Gasteiger-Hückel method and energy minimizations were performed using the Conjugate Gradient method with 1000 iterations [36,37].

3.2. Pharmacophore Generation

Pharmacophore models were generated and analyzed using the GALAHAD module. In this study, ten compounds (13, 16, 19, 21, 24, 30, 40, 41, 43, and 52) were selected to carry out the pharmacophore hypothesis, and the genetic algorithm was used to create conformers for all molecules. The compounds that were selected to generate the pharmacophore hypothesis are highly active. All of the ligands were aligned with a population size value of 60, a maximum generation value of 60 and a value of molecular required hitting of 5. Twenty models were generated with default parameters.

3.3. CoMFA Field Calculation Partial Least Square Analysis

The standard CoMFA procedure as implemented by SYBYL X 1.3 (Tripos Associates Inc.) was performed. Each set of aligned molecules was positioned inside a 3D cubic lattice with a grid spacing of 2.0 A (default distance) in all Cartesian directions and was generated to enclose the molecule aggregate. The fields generated were automatically scaled by the CoMFA standard in SYBYL. The partial least squares (PLS) methodology was used to derive a linear relationship for the CoMFA, and cross-validation was performed using the leave-one-out (LOO) method to choose the optimum number of components (ONC) and assess the statistical significance of each model. In PLS, the independent variables were the CoMFA descriptors, and the pIC_{50} values were used as dependent variables. The ONC was the number of components that led to the highest cross-validated correlated correlation coefficient q^2 (or r^2_{cv}). Non-cross-validation was performed to calculate conventional r^2_{ncv} using the same number of components [38–40].

3.4. Virtual Screening

The selected pharmacophore model was validated and converted into a UNITY query for pharmacophore guided virtual screening studies. The query was screened against the SPECS database.

The flex search option was implemented to perform virtual screening. Primary filters such as Lipinski's rule of five were applied to reduce the dataset. Further screening of the hits was carried out using the Surflex Dock in SYBYL.

The docking study was performed to validate the hits obtained from the virtual screening. The crystal structure of nNOS was retrieved from the RCSB Protein Data Bank (PDB code: 4EUX) [24]. The nNOS structure was utilized in subsequent docking experiments without energy minimization. Protein structures were prepared using the biopolymer module of SYBYL. Hydrogen atoms were added to the structure, atom types and charges were assigned using AMBER7 FF99 force field, and side chain amides were modified. The ligand method was used as the mode of construction for the protomol, threshold and bloat using default values to determine the extent of the protomol.

4. Conclusions

nNOS is a therapeutic target for central nervous system diseases that has attracted interest from pharmaceutical companies and researchers. Selective inhibition of nNOS activity represents an exciting drug approach for the development of new therapeutic agents to treat neurodegenerative diseases. In this study, we described a rational strategy for identifying novel nNOS inhibitors using a pharmacophore-based virtual screening protocol. The best pharmacophore model (MODEL 012) was established and showed good statistical parameters in the validation process. MODEL 012 was further employed as a 3D search query to screen the SPECS compound database. Molecular docking studies were also performed to improve the reliability and accuracy of the virtual screening. Ten hit compounds were identified as potential selective nNOS inhibitors and exhibited good search scoring, high docking scores, similar binding mode to experimentally proven compounds and favorable drug-like properties. The pharmacophore models developed in this work, and the information gained about the interactions between nNOS and the potential selective inhibitors, indicated that the combination of pharmacophore, molecular docking, and virtual screening efforts is a successful approach for identifying effective inhibitory compounds that may have an impact on future experimental studies in selective nNOS inhibition. The identified hit compounds were structurally different from available inhibitors and may serve as potential leads or starting points for structural optimization to identify novel nNOS inhibitors.

Acknowledgments

The authors gratefully acknowledge the support of this work by the Natural Science Foundation of China (No. 21172108), Natural Science Foundation of Jiangsu Education Committee (No. 12KJB350003) and Science and Technology Development Foundation of Nanjing Medical University (No. 2013NJMU023 and 2013NJMU098).

Author Contributions

G.X. performed all experiments and data treatments. Writing was done by G.X., Y.C., K.S., X.W. and F.L., and management and submission tasks were done by F.L., Y.H. and G.X.

References

1. Alderton, W.K.; Cooper, C.E.; Knowles, R.G. Nitric oxide synthases: Structure, function and inhibition. *Biochem. J.* **2001**, *357*, 593–615.
2. Stuehr, D.J. Structure-function aspects in the nitric oxide synthases. *Annu. Rev. Pharmacol. Toxicol.* **1997**, *37*, 339–359.
3. Gabriela, M.; Subhash, C.A.; Jailall, R.; Shawn, P.M.; Suman, R.; John, S.A.; Dongqin, Z.; Frank, P. First-in-class, dual-action, 3,5-disubstituted indole derivatives having human nitric oxide synthase (nNOS) and norepinephrine reuptake inhibitory (NERI) activity for the treatment of neuropathic pain. *J. Med. Chem.* **2012**, *55*, 3488–3501.
4. Mustafa, A.K.; Gadalla, M.M.; Snyder, S.H. Signaling by gasotransmitters. *Sci. Signal* **2009**, *2*, doi:10.1126/scisignal.268re2.
5. Hao, J.X.; Xu, X.J. Treatment of a chronic allodynia-like response in spinally injured rats: Effects of systemically administered nitric oxide synthase inhibitors. *Pain* **1996**, *66*, 313–319.
6. Moncada, S.; Palmer, R.M.; Higgs, E.A. Nitric oxide: Physiology, pathophysiology, and pharmacology. *Pharmacol. Rev.* **1991**, *43*, 109–142.
7. Vallance, P.; Leiper, J. Blocking NO synthesis: How, where and why? *Nat. Rev. Drug Discov.* **2002**, *1*, 939–950.
8. Calabrese, V.; Mancuso, C.; Calvani, M.; Rizzarelli, E.; Butterfield, D.A.; Stella, A.M. Nitric oxide in the central nervous system: Neuroprotection versus neurotoxicity. *Nat. Rev. Neurosci.* **2007**, *8*, 766–775.
9. Tanabe, M.; Nagatani, Y.; Saitoh, K.; Takasu, K.; Ono, H. Pharmacological assessments of nitric oxide synthase isoforms and downstream diversity of NO signaling in the maintenance of thermal and mechanical hypersensitivity after peripheral nerve injury in mice. *Neuropharmacology* **2009**, *56*, 702–708.
10. Miclescu, A.; Gordh, T. Nitric oxide and pain: "Something old, something new". *Acta Anaesthesiol. Scand.* **2009**, *53*, 1107–1120.
11. Gruber, H.J.; Bernecker, C.; Lechner, A.; Weiss, S.; Wallner-Blazek, M.; Meinitzer, A.; Höbarth, G.; Renner, W.; Fauler, G.; Horejsi, R.; *et al.* Increased nitric oxide stress is associated with migraine. *Cephalalgia* **2010**, *30*, 486–492.
12. Payne, J.E.; Bonnefous, C.; Symons, K.T.; Nguyen, P.M.; Sablad, M.; Rozenkrants, N.; Zhang, Y.; Wang, L.; Yazdani, N.; Shiau, A.K.; *et al.* Discovery of dual inducible/neuronal nitric oxide synthase (iNOS/nNOS) inhibitor development candidate 4-((2-cyclobutyl-1H-imidazo [4,5-b]pyrazin-1-yl)methyl)-7,8-difluoroquinolin-2(1H)-one (KD7332) part 2: Identification of a novel, potent, and selective series of benzimidazole-quinolinone iNOS/nNOS dimerization inhibitors that are orally active in pain models. *J. Med. Chem.* **2010**, *53*, 7739–7755.
13. Erdal, E.P.; Litzinger, E.A.; Seo, J.; Zhu, Y.; Ji, H.; Silverman, R.B. Selective neuronal nitric oxide synthase inhibitors. *Curr. Top. Med. Chem.* **2005**, *5*, 603–624.
14. Silverman, R.B. Design of selective neuronal nitric oxide synthase inhibitors for the prevention and treatment of neurodegenerative diseases. *Acc. Chem. Res.* **2009**, *42*, 439–451.
15. Ramnauth, J.; Renton, P.; Dove, P.; Annedi, S.C.; Speed, J.; Silverman, S.; Mladenova, G.; Maddaford, S.P.; Zinghini, S.; Rakhit, S.; *et al.* 1,2,3,4-Tetrahydroquinoline-based selective human

neuronal nitric oxide synthase (nNOS) inhibitors: Lead optimization studies resulting in the identification of *N*-(1-(2-(methylamino)ethyl)-1,2,3,4-tetrahydroquinolin-6-yl)thiophene-2-carboximidamide as a preclinical development candidate. *J. Med. Chem.* **2012**, *55*, 2882–2893.

16. Patman, J.; Bhardwaj, N.; Ramnauth, J.; Annedi, S.C.; Renton, P.; Maddaford, S.P.; Rakhit, S.; Andrews, J.S. Novel 2-aminobenzothiazoles as selective neuronal nitric oxide synthase inhibitors. *Bioorg. Med. Chem. Lett.* **2007**, *17*, 2540–2544.
17. Renton, P.; Speed, J.; Maddaford, S.; Annedi, S.C.; Ramnauth, J.; Rakhit, S.; Andrews, J. 1,5-Disubstituted indole derivatives as selective human neuronal nitric oxide synthase inhibitors. *Bioorg. Med. Chem. Lett.* **2011**, *21*, 5301–5304.
18. Maddaford, S.; Renton, P.; Speed, J.; Annedi, S.C.; Ramnauth, J.; Rakhit, S.; Andrews, J.; Mladenova, G.; Majuta, L.; Porreca, F. 1,6-Disubstituted indole derivatives as selective human neuronal nitric oxide synthase inhibitors. *Bioorg. Med. Chem. Lett.* **2011**, *21*, 5234–5238.
19. Annedi, S.C.; Maddaford, S.P.; Ramnauth, J.; Renton, P.; Speed, J.; Rakhit, S.; Andrews, J.S.; Porreca, F. 3,5-Disubstituted indole derivatives as selective human neuronal nitric oxide synthase (nNOS) inhibitors. *Bioorg. Med. Chem. Lett.* **2012**, *22*, 1980–1984.
20. Annedi, S.C.; Ramnauth, J.; Maddaford, S.P.; Renton, P.; Rakhit, S.; Mladenova, G.; Dove, P.; Silverman, S.; Andrews, J.S.; Felice, M.D.; *et al.* Discovery of *cis*-*N*-(1-(4-(methylamino)cyclohexyl)indolin-6-yl)thiophene-2-carboximidamide: a 1,6-disubstituted indoline derivative as a highly selective inhibitor of human neuronal nitric oxide synthase (nNOS) without any cardiovascular liabilities. *J. Med. Chem.* **2012**, *55*, 943–955.
21. Annedi, S.C.; Maddaford, S.P.; Mladenova, G.; Ramnauth, J.; Rakhit, S.; Andrews, J.S.; Lee, D.K.; Zhang, D.; Porreca, F.; Bunton, D.; *et al.* Discovery of *N*-(3-(1-methyl-1,2,3,6-tetrahydropyridin-4-yl)-1H-indol-6-yl) thiophene-2-carboximidamide as a selective inhibitor of human neuronal nitric oxide synthase (nNOS) for the treatment of pain. *J. Med. Chem.* **2011**, *54*, 7408–7416.
22. Ramnauth, J.; Speed, J.; Maddaford, S.P.; Dove, P.; Annedi, S.C.; Renton, P.; Rakhit, S.; Andrews, J.; Silverman, S.; Mladenova, G.; *et al.* Design, synthesis, and biological evaluation of 3,4-dihydroquinolin-2(1H)-one and 1,2,3,4-tetrahydroquinoline-based selective human neuronal nitric oxide synthase (nNOS) inhibitors. *J. Med. Chem.* **2011**, *54*, 5562–5575.
23. Xue, F.; Li, H.; Delker, S.L.; Fang J.; Martásek, P.; Roman, L.J.; Poulos, T.L.; Silverman, R.B. Potent, highly selective, and orally bioavailable gem-difluorinated monocationic inhibitors of neuronal nitric oxide synthase. *J. Am. Chem. Soc.* **2010**, *132*, 14229–14238.
24. Huang, H.; Ji, H.; Li, H.; Jing, Q.; Labby, K.J.; Martásek, P.; Roman, L.J.; Poulos, T.L.; Silverman, R.B. Selective monocationic inhibitors of neuronal nitric oxide synthase. Binding mode insights from molecular dynamics simulations. *J. Am. Chem. Soc.* **2012**, *134*, 11559–11572.
25. Delker, S.L.; Ji, H.; Li, H.; Jamal, J.; Fang, J.; Xue, F.; Silverman, R.B.; Poulos, T.L. Unexpected binding modes of nitric oxide synthase inhibitors effective in the prevention of a cerebral palsy phenotype in an animal model. *J. Am. Chem. Soc.* **2010**, *132*, 5437–5442.
26. Klebe, G. Virtual ligand screening: Strategies, perspectives and limitations. *Drug Discov. Today* **2006**, *11*, 580–594.
27. Cramer, R.D.; Patterson, D.E.; Bunce, J.D. Comparative molecular field analysis (CoMFA). 1. Effect of shape on binding of steroids to carrier proteins. *J. Am. Chem. Soc.* **1988**, *110*, 5959–5967.

28. Xu, G.; Chu, Y.; Jiang, N.; Yang, J.; Li, F. The Three Dimensional Quantitative Structure Activity Relationships (3D-QSAR) and docking studies of curcumin derivatives as androgen receptor antagonists. *Int. J. Mol. Sci.* **2012**, *13*, 6138–6155.
29. SYBYL®-X Suite. Molecular Modeling from Sequence through Lead Optimization. Available online: http://www.certara.com/products/molmod/sybyl-x (accessed on 12 May 2014).
30. Zhao, X.; Yuan, M.; Huang, B.; Ji, H.; Zhu, L. Ligand-based pharmacophore model of *N*-Aryl and *N*-Heteroaryl piperazine alpha 1A-adrenoceptors antagonists using GALAHAD. *J. Mol. Graph. Model.* **2010**, *29*, 126–136.
31. Caballero, J. 3D-QSAR (CoMFA and CoMSIA) and pharmacophore (GALAHAD) studies on the differential inhibition of aldose reductase by flavonoid compounds. *J. Mol. Graph. Model.* **2010**, *29*, 363–371.
32. The Specs.net Chemistry. Available online: http://www.specs.net (accessed on 12 May 2014).
33. Shaikh, M.S.; Mittal, A.; Bharatam, P.V. Design of fructose-2,6-bisphosphatase inhibitors: A novel virtual screening approach. *J. Mol. Graph. Model.* **2008**, *26*, 900–906.
34. Lipinski C.A.; Lombardo, F.; Dominy, B.W.; Feeney, P.J. Experimental and computational approaches to estimate solubility and permeability in drug discovery and development settings. *Adv. Drug Deliv. Rev.* **1997**, *23*, 3–25.
35. Gugan, K.; Thirumurthy, M.; Changdev, G.G.; Seung, J.C. A combined 3D QSAR and pharmacophore-based virtual screening for the identification of potent p38 MAP kinase inhibitors: An *in silico* approach. *Med. Chem. Res.* **2013**, *22*, 1773–1787.
36. Lan, P.; Sun, J.R.; Chen, W.N.; Sun, P.H.; Chen, W.M. Molecular modelling studies on d-annulated benzazepinones as VEGF-R2 kinase inhibitors using docking and 3D-QSAR. *J. Enzym. Inhib. Med. Chem.* **2011**, *26*, 367–377.
37. Clark, M.; Cramer, R.D.; Opdenbosch, N.V. Validation of the general purpose tripos 5.2 force field. *J. Comput. Chem.* **1989**, *10*, 982–1012.
38. Lan, P.; Chen, W.N.; Xiao, G.K.; Sun, P.H.; Chen, W.M. 3D-QSAR and docking studies on pyrazolo[4,3-h]qinazoline-3-carboxamides as cyclin-dependent kinase 2 (CDK2) inhibitors. *Bioorg. Med. Chem. Lett.* **2010**, *20*, 6764–6772.
39. Pirhadi, S.; Ghasemi, J.B. 3D-QSAR analysis of human immunodeficiency virus entry-1 inhibitors by CoMFA and CoMSIA. *Eur. J. Med. Chem.* **2010**, *45*, 4897–4903.
40. Xu, G.; Zhou, Z.; Li, F. Combined 3D-QSAR modeling and molecular docking studies on naphthoquinone analogs as proteasome inhibitors. *Lett. Drug Des. Discov.* **2013**, *10*, 129–144.

9

Perineural Dexmedetomidine Attenuates Inflammation in Rat Sciatic Nerve via the NF-κB Pathway

Yan Huang [†], Yi Lu [†], Lei Zhang, Jia Yan, Jue Jiang and Hong Jiang *

Department of Anesthesiology, School of Medicine, Shanghai Ninth People's Hospital Affiliated to Shanghai Jiao Tong University, Shanghai 200011, China; E-Mails: huangyan606@126.com (Y.H.); luyi077@163.com (Y.L.); weiymzhl@126.com (L.Z.); mzkyanj@163.com (J.Y.); jiangjue1136@sina.com (J.J.)

† These authors contributed equally to this work.

* Author to whom correspondence should be addressed; E-Mail: dr_jianghong@163.com

---

Abstract: Recent studies have shown that dexmedetomidine exerts an anti-inflammatory effect by reducing serum levels of inflammatory factors, however, the up-stream mechanism is still unknown. The transcription factor NF-κB enters the nucleus and promotes the transcription of its target genes, including those encoding the pro-inflammatory cytokines IL-6 and TNF-α. In this study, we established a rat model that simulates a clinical surgical procedure to investigate the anti-inflammatory effect of perineural administration of dexmedetomidine and the underlying mechanism. Dexmedetomidine reduced the sciatic nerve levels of IL-6 and TNF-α at both the mRNA and protein level. Dexmedetomidine also inhibited the translocation of activated NF-κB to the nucleus and the binding activity of NF-κB. The anti-inflammatory effect is confirmed to be dose-dependent. Finally, pyrrolidine dithiocarbamate also reduced the levels of IL-6 and TNF-α and the activation of NF-κB. In conclusion, dexmedetomidine inhibited the nuclear translocation and binding activity of activated NF-κB, thus reducing inflammatory cytokines.

Keywords: dexmedetomidine; NF-κB; IL-6; TNF-α; nerve block

---

1. Introduction

Dexmedetomidine, a highly selective α2-adrenoceptor agonist, is widely used in clinical anesthesia, intensive care unit (ICU) management and pain treatment as a sedative agent [1–3]. Recent studies found that dexmedetomidine has an anti-inflammatory effect through reducing the serum levels of inflammatory factors, which may extend its application in the clinic [4–6]. However, the upstream mechanism by which dexmedetomidine reduces inflammatory factors levels remains largely unknown.

The NF-κB family contains five members, RelA (also known as p65), RelB, c-Rel, p105/p50, and p100/p52, which make homo- and heterodimers. NF-κB is a transcription factor that recognizes a common consensus DNA sequence and regulates a large number of target genes, especially genes involved in inflammation, injury and stress [7]. Interleukin (IL)-6 and tumor necrosis factor (TNF)-α are cytokines that play essential roles in inflammation. Studies have shown that NF-κB exists as a p65 and p50 heterodimer in the cytoplasm. Activated NF-κB enters the nucleus, where it can promote the transcription of its target genes, including the pro-inflammatory cytokines IL-6 and TNF-α. Pyrrolidine dithiocarbamate (PDTC), a selective NF-κB inhibitor and antioxidant, can inhibit the NF-κB pathway by blocking the entrance of activated NF-κB to the nucleus and the binding of NF-κB to the promoter regions of IL-6 and TNF-α [8–10].

Peripheral nerve block is a common regional anesthetic technique performed everyday throughout the world as an alternative to general anesthesia and is performed for postoperative analgesia [11–13]. Dexmedetomidine is usually injected in the peripheral nerve to prolong the duration of the peripheral nerve block as an adjuvant for local anesthetics [14–17]. In this study, perineural administration of dexmedetomidine not only blocked NF-κB translocation to the nucleus and NF-κB binding activity but also reduced IL-6 and TNF-α levels in rats. PDTC, an NF-κB inhibitor, can also reduce IL-6 and TNF-α levels by inhibiting NF-κB activity following perineural administration. In summary, dexmedetomidine can inhibit inflammation through the NF-κB pathway.

2. Results

2.1. Perineural High Doses of Dexmedetomidine Reduced the IL-6 and TNF-α Levels in the Sciatic Nerve

Rats were anesthetized and injected perineurally with either a high dose of dexmedetomidine (D_H, 20 μg/kg) or normal saline (C). Sciatic nerves were harvested 30, 60 and 90 min after injection. Real-time PCR revealed that dexmedetomidine reduced the mRNA levels of both IL-6 and TNF-α at all of the examined time points (Figure 1A,B). The protein levels of both IL-6 and TNF-α were significantly decreased after perineural injection of dexmedetomidine at all time points, as shown by both ELISA (Figure 1C,D) and Western blotting (Figure 1E–G). These results suggested that perineural injection of 20 μg/kg dexmedetomidine reduces the sciatic nerve levels of IL-6 and TNF-α at the level of both mRNA and protein.

Figure 1. Perineural high doses (20 μg/kg) of dexmedetomidine reduced IL-6 and TNF-α levels in the sciatic nerve. (**A**,**B**) RT-PCR showed that high doses of dexmedetomidine reduced the IL-6 and TNF-α mRNA levels in the sciatic nerve; (**C**,**D**) ELISA showed that high dose of dexmedetomidine reduced the IL-6 and TNF-α protein levels in the sciatic nerve; (**E**–**G**) Western blotting showed that high dose of dexmedetomidine reduced IL-6 and TNF-α protein levels in the sciatic nerve.

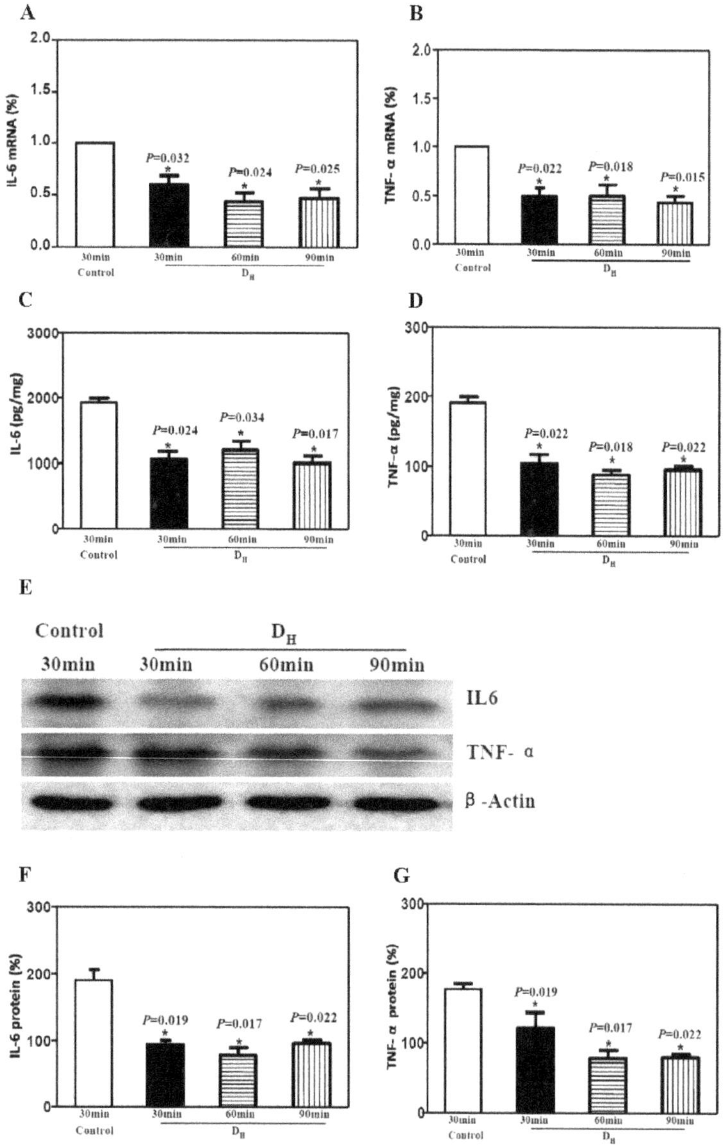

2.2. Perineural Dexmedetomidine Decreased NF-κB Translocation to the Nucleus and Transcriptional Binding Activity

As previous studies have shown [16–19], activated NF-κB should translocate to the nucleus and bind to the promoter region of multiple genes, including cytokine genes, inducing the expression of cytokine mRNA and protein. Thus, we assessed the effects of perineural administration of dexmedetomidine on the nuclear levels of NF-κB in sciatic nerve tissue. The sciatic nerve tissues were subjected to Western blot analysis for the total NF-κB protein level, and the nuclear extracts were assessed for the nuclear NF-κB protein level. The Western blot of NF-κB showed that perineural administration of dexmedetomidine decreased the nuclear level of NF-κB compared with the control group at 30, 60 and 90 min (Figure 2A,B), but no significant differences were detected in the total level of NF-κB (Figure 2A,C). These findings indicate that perineural administration of dexmedetomidine may prevent NF-κB translocation into the nucleus in the sciatic nerve and thus may decrease the subsequent expression of inflammatory factors.

Figure 2. Perineural administration of 20 μg/kg dexmedetomidine decreased the translocation to the nucleus and transcriptional binding activity of NF-κB. (**A**) Western blot showed that 20 μg/kg dexmedetomidine decreased NF-κB translocation into the nucleus; (**B**) Dexmedetomidine (20 μg/kg) decreased the nuclear NF-κB protein level; (**C**) Dexmedetomidine (20 μg/kg) did not alter the total NF-κB protein level; (**D**) EMSA showed that 20 μg/kg dexmedetomidine decreased the transcriptional binding activity of NF-κB (lane 3); PDTC also decreased NF-κB transcriptional binding activity (lane 5). NF-κB, nuclear factor-kappa B; PDTC, pyrrolidine dithiocarbamate.

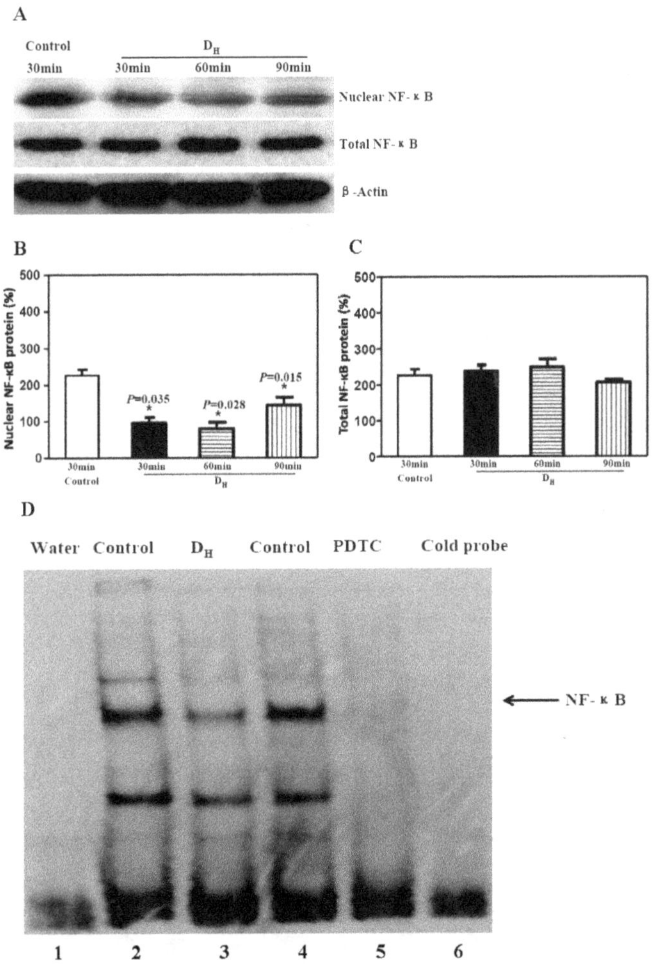

We then used EMSA to test the effect of dexmedetomidine on the transcriptional binding activity of NF-κB in nuclear extracts prepared from sciatic nerve tissues [20]. In Figure 2D, lane 1 is a negative control (double-distilled water), lane 2 represents the control group with perineural administration of normal saline, lane 3 represents the D_H group with perineural 20.0 μg/kg dexmedetomidine, and lane 6 shows the cold probe. We can clearly see that perineural administration of 20.0 μg/kg dexmedetomidine reduced the transcriptional binding activity of NF-κB compared with the control group.

2.3. Only High Dose Dexmedetomidine Attenuated the NF-κB Translocation to the Nucleus

Based on the above conclusions, we further tested whether different doses of dexmedetomidine have the same effect on attenuating the translocation of NF-κB. We further tested the D_M and D_L groups, which received a middle dose and a low dose of dexmedetomidine (10.0 and 5 μg/kg, respectively). Western blotting was used to analyze the total NF-κB protein level and the nuclear NF-κB protein level. The results showed that only the high dose of dexmedetomidine (D_H) attenuated NF-κB translocation to the nucleus, whereas the total and nuclear protein levels of NF-κB were unchanged in the D_M and D_L groups (Figure 3A–C). These results suggested that perineurally administered dexmedetomidine attenuates the inflammatory response above a certain threshold dose.

Figure 3. Only the high dose (20 μg/kg) of dexmedetomidine attenuated NF-κB translocation to the nucleus. (**A**) Western blotting showed that only the high dose of dexmedetomidine decreased NF-κB translocation to the nucleus; (**B**) The high dose of dexmedetomidine decreased the nuclear NF-κB protein level, but the middle doses (10 μg/kg) and low doses (5 μg/kg) did not have an effect; (**C**) Dexmedetomidine did not alter the total NF-κB protein level in any of the groups. NF-κB, nuclear factor-kappa B.

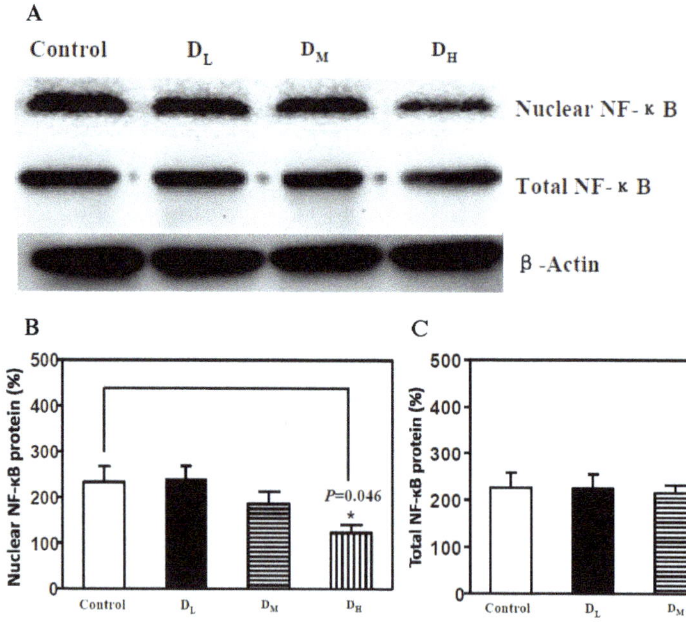

2.4. The Inflammation of the Sciatic Nerve Could Be Attenuated by PDTC via the NF-κB Pathway

PDTC, a selective NF-κB inhibitor and antioxidant, inhibits the NF-κB pathway by blocking the translocation of activated NF-κB to the nucleus [10]. Here, we assessed whether inflammation of the sciatic nerve could be attenuated by PDTC via the NF-κB pathway in a manner similar to that of dexmedetomidine. Western blot analysis confirmed that both the translocation of NF-κB to nucleus and the downstream expression of IL-6 and TNF-α protein were down-regulated by PDTC (Figure 4A–F).

RT-PCR (Figure 4G,H) and ELISA (Figure 4I,J) further confirmed the down-regulation of the inflammatory factors IL-6 and TNF-α. EMSA showed that the transcriptional binding activity of NF-κB was reduced by PDTC compared with the control group (Figure 2D, lane 5). These changes were in accordance with our results with dexmedetomidine and suggest that perineural administration of dexmedetomidine has a similar, or at least partly similar, anti-inflammatory effect as PDTC, via the NF-κB signalling pathway.

Figure 4. PDTC attenuated the inflammation of the sciatic nerve via the NF-κB pathway. (**A,C,D**) Western blotting showed that PDTC decreased NF-κB translocation into the nucleus; (**B,E,F**) Western blotting showed that PDTC reduced the IL-6 and TNF-α protein levels in the sciatic nerve; (**G,H**) RT-PCR showed that PDTC reduced the IL-6 and TNF-α mRNA levels in the sciatic nerve; (**I,J**) ELISA showed that PDTC reduced the IL-6 and TNF-α protein level in the sciatic nerve.

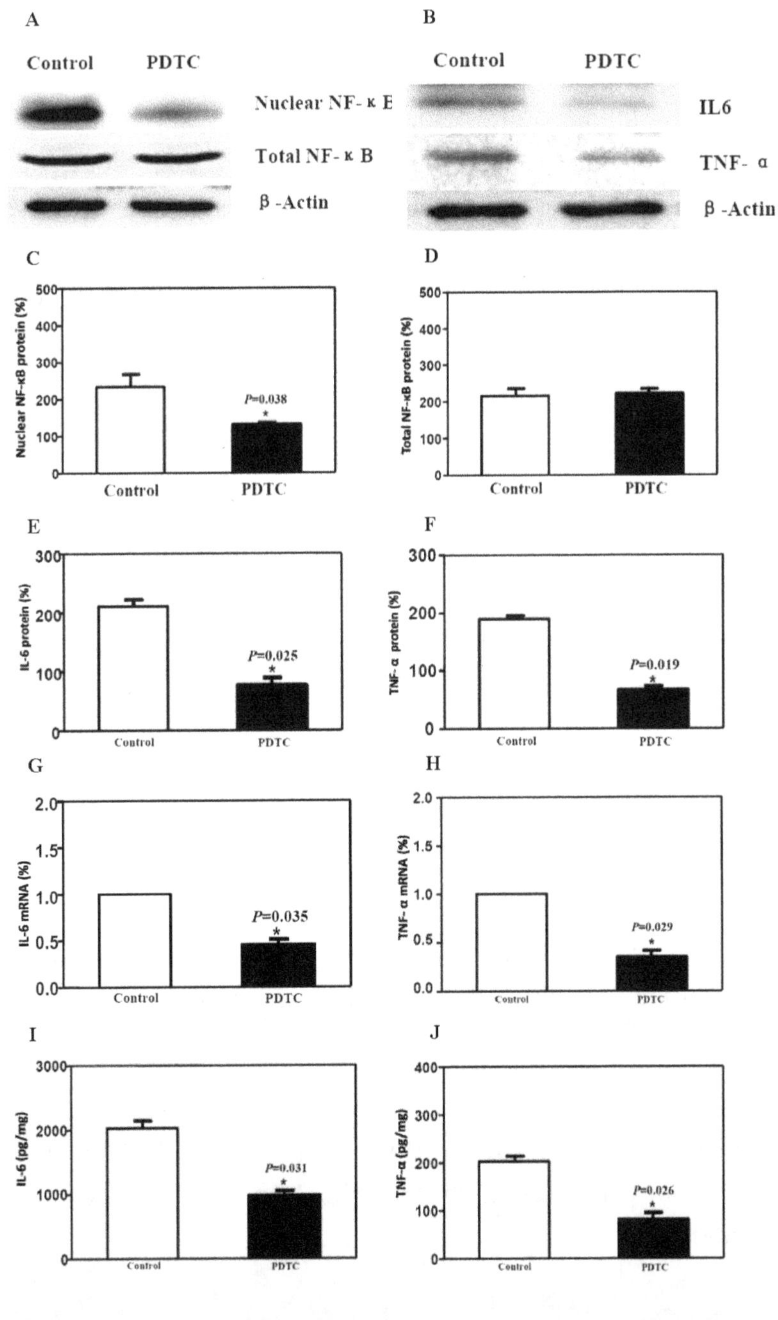

3. Discussion

Dexmedetomidine is widely used in clinical anesthesia as a most closely ideal sedative because of its analgesia and sedation effects without respiratory depression [18–21]. Recent studies found that dexmedetomidine has an anti-inflammatory effect by reducing the serum levels of inflammatory cytokines, however, the upstream mechanism is still unknown [4–6]. In the present study, we used a surgical procedure and perineural injection to induce a background inflammatory response (e.g., increasing IL-6 and TNF-α levels) in sciatic nerve tissue to investigate the anti-inflammatory effect of perineural administration of dexmedetomidine and the underlying mechanism. We found that, in the sciatic nerves of rats, perineural administration of 20 μg/kg dexmedetomidine reduced the level of IL-6 and TNF-α, prevented NF-κB translocation to the nucleus and decreased the transcriptional binding activity of NF-κB. These results, in accordance with perineural administration of the NF-κB pathway inhibitor PDTC, suggested that dexmedetomidine reduced inflammation by inhibiting the NF-κB signaling pathway.

Dexmedetomidine is usually intravenously administered during clinical anesthesia as a sedative agent. Currently, perineural administration of dexmedetomidine is widely used in peripheral nerve anesthesia as an adjuvant for local anesthetics to prolong the duration of a peripheral nerve block [3,17,22]. Here, we incised the skin and subcutaneous fat of rats to simulate the clinical surgical procedure. We then exposed the sciatic nerve and injected dexmedetomidine to investigate the inflammatory cytokine levels in the sciatic nerve tissue. As a result, we confirmed that perineural administration of dexmedetomidine inhibited the translocation of activated NF-κB to the nucleus and the binding activity of activated NF-κB, thus reducing the level of inflammatory cytokines. The anti-inflammatory effect of perineural administration of dexmedetomidine may extend its application in clinical anesthesia.

In a previous study [16], dexmedetomidine added to ropivacaine was shown to increase the duration of the sensory block in a dose-dependent fashion, varying from 0.5 to 20 μg/kg, in rats. Interestingly, in our study, NF-κB translocation to the nucleus was not inhibited in the D_M and D_L groups (which received dexmedetomidine doses of 10.0 and 5 μg/kg, respectively), but the D_H group (20 μg/kg) did show an effect. The results indicate that a dose threshold needs to be crossed before an anti-inflammatory effect occurs. Furthermore, Brummett's study confirmed that a high dose of dexmedetomidine, up to 40 μg/kg, was considered safe for rats because the histopathological evaluation showed that nerve axon and myelin were not altered by dexmedetomidine and there was no neurotoxicity or side-effects for the rats [15]. Similarly, there was no neurotoxicity or side-effect noted at 24 h or 14 days in our study. Based on these results, a high perineural dose of dexmedetomidine may be recommended for routine use as an adjuvant for local anesthetics owing to its anti-inflammatory and analgesia-prolonging effect.

4. Experimental Section

All of the investigators followed the Shanghai Ninth People's Hospital Animal Study Guidelines, and the study was approved by the Shanghai Ninth People's Hospital Committee for the Use and Care of Animals (Shanghai, China).

For blinding, all of the drug solutions were prepared in syringes without labels by an investigator other than the one performing the perineural sciatic injection. The investigators who harvested the tissue and performed the later Western blotting, real-time PCR, ELISA and EMSA were also blinded to the study groups.

4.1. Animals

Forty-eight Sprague-Dawley rats, weighing 180 to 220 g, were obtained from Shanghai Ninth People's Hospital SPF Animal Center (Shanghai, China). The rats were housed at 23 °C with a light-dark cycle and allowed free access to food and water.

4.2. Study Groups

The Sprague-Dawley rats were divided into four groups for further intervention. Control group rats received only normal saline. The D_H group received a high dose of dexmedetomidine (20.0 μg/kg), whereas the D_M and D_L groups received a middle dose and a low dose of dexmedetomidine (10.0 and 5 μg/kg, respectively).

4.3. Drug Preparation

An investigator who was not involved in either the perineural sciatic injection or the subsequent analysis prepared the drugs. Dexmedetomidine and normal saline were used to make final drug solutions. Each rat received a total volume of 0.2 mL for a perineural sciatic injection. The doses of dexmedetomidine were based on the individual rats' body weight for 20.0 μg/kg (D_H), 10.0 μg/kg (D_M), 5.0 μg/kg (D_L) respectively.

4.4. Animal Model and Perineural Injection

To investigate the anti-inflammatory effect of perineural administration of dexmedetomidine, we established a rat model of surgical-induced inflammation. Rats were anesthetized and maintained using 3.0% isoflurane. As previously described [15], an incision was made over the thigh, and the muscle and fascia were dissected to expose the sciatic nerve directly below the clear fascial covering. A total volume of 0.2 mL was injected into the perineural space below the clear fascia covering the nerve using a 30-gauge needle and tuberculin syringe. After injection, the muscle and skin of the thigh were sutured, and the isoflurane was discontinued. The animal model of surgical-induced inflammation was confirmed by increasing the inflammatory factor, such as IL-6 and TNF-α, after the surgical procedure.

4.5. Nuclear Extraction and Western Blotting

A nuclear extraction kit (Ab110168, Abcam, Cambridge, MA, USA) was used for the preparation of nuclear extracts from sciatic nerve tissues. For Western blotting, frozen rat sciatic nerve tissues were homogenized and the lysates were prepared in ice-cold lysis buffer. Nuclear extracts or total protein were collected and normalized for equal amounts of total protein measured by the bicinchoninic acid (BCA) method. Seventy micrograms of protein from each sample was separated on a sodium dodecyl sulfate polyacrylamide gel and transferred to PVDF membranes. The membranes were blocked with 5%

nonfat milk and incubated overnight with primary anti-NF-κB antibody (1:1000; sc-109, Santa Cruz, CA, USA), anti-IL-6 antibody (1:1000; ab6672, Abcam, Cambridge, MA, USA), anti-TNF-α antibody (1:1000; AB1837P; Millipore, Billerica, MA, USA), and anti-β-actin (1:5000, Sigma, St. Louis, MO, USA) at 4 °C, followed by incubation with the suitable HRP-conjugated secondary antibody for 4 h. β-actin protein was immunodetected as the internal standard.

4.6. Real-Time PCR and ELISA

The levels of IL-6 and TNF-α mRNA were detected by real-time polymerase chain reaction (RT-PCR) in the sciatic nerve tissues as described [11]. RNA was isolated following the protocol of the RNeasy Mini Kit (Qiagen, Inc., Valencia, CA, USA), while concentration determined using a NanoDrop ND-1000 Spectrophotometer (Thermo Scientific, Wilmington, DE, USA). Primers of Rat IL-6 is 5'-GACTGATGTTGTTGACAGCCACTGC-3'; 5'-TAGCCACTCCTTCTGTGACTCTAACT-3', TNF-α 5'-TTC TGT CTA CTG AAC TTC GGG GTG ATG GGT CC-3'; 5'-GTA TGA GAT AGC AAA TCG GCT GAC GGT GTG GG-3' and Rat GAPDH 5'-CCT TCA TTG ACC TCA ACT AC-3' ;5'-GGA AGG CCA TGC CAG TGA GC-3'. RT-PCR was carried out using the QuantiTect SYBR Green RT-PCR Kit (Qiagen). The quantity of the target mRNA was normalised against a house-keeping gene, GAPDH, which served as an internal control.

The levels of IL-6 and TNF-α proteins in the sciatic nerve were measured using ELISA kits according to the manufacturer's instructions. ELISA kits for TNF-α and IL-6 were obtained from R & D Systems (Minneapolis, MN, USA).

4.7. Electrophoretic-Mobility Shift Assay (EMSA)

An electrophoretic-mobility shift assay (EMSA) kit (GS-0030, Signosis, Santa Clara, CA, USA) was used to assess the transcriptional binding activity of NF-κB as a previous study described [11]. The nuclear extract (5 mg) was incubated with 1 μL poly d(I-C), 2.0 μL 5× Binding Buffer and 1.0 μL of transcription factor (TF) probe in a 0.5 mL microcentrifuge tube at 20–23 °C for 30 min in a PCR machine. We added 1.0 μL of cold TF probe into this reaction for the cold probe control. Samples were then loaded onto a 6.5% non-denaturing polyacrylamide gel and separated at 100 V, and the proteins were transferred to a membrane at 60 V for 1 h at 4 °C. The membrane was imaged using a chemiluminescence imaging system (Bio-Rad, Hercules, CA, USA).

4.8. Statistics

Data are shown as mean (SD). Student's *t*-test, one-way and two-way analysis of variance (ANOVA) were used to compare the differences among the experimental groups and the control group. $p < 0.05$ (*) was considered statistically significant. The significance testing was two-tailed. Normality tests showed that the data were normally distributed, and the GraphPad software Prism 5 (GraphPad Software Inc., San Diego, CA, USA) was used to analyze the data.

5. Conclusions

In conclusion, we have established a rat model that simulates a clinical surgical procedure to investigate the anti-inflammatory effect of perineural administration of dexmedetomidine and the underlying mechanism. Dexmedetomidine (20 μg/kg) inhibited the translocation of activated NF-κB to the nucleus and its binding activity, thus reducing inflammatory cytokine levels. These results suggest a potential application for dexmedetomidine as an adjuvant in peripheral nerve anesthesia. Future research should focus on finding clinical evidence to support the use of dexmedetomidine as an anti-inflammatory adjuvant for perineural administration in humans.

Acknowledgments

This work was supported by grants from National Natural Science Foundation of China (No. 81272083).

References

1. Niu, X.Y.; Ding, X.B.; Guo, T.; Chen, M.H.; Fu, S.K.; Li, Q. Effects of intravenous and intrathecal dexmedetomidine in spinal anesthesia: A meta-analysis. *CNS Neurosci. Ther.* **2013**, *19*, 897–904.
2. Friesen, R.H.; Nichols, C.S.; Twite, M.D.; Cardwell, K.A.; Pan, Z.; Pietra, B.; Miyamoto, S.D.; Auerbach, S.R.; Darst, J.R.; Ivy, D.D. The hemodynamic response to dexmedetomidine loading dose in children with and without pulmonary hypertension. *Anesth. Analg.* **2013**, *117*, 953–959.
3. Obayah, G.M.; Refaie, A.; Aboushanab, O.; Ibraheem, N.; Abdelazees, M. Addition of dexmedetomidine to bupivacaine for greater palatine nerve block prolongs postoperative analgesia after cleft palate repair. *Eur. J. Anaesthesiol.* **2010**, *27*, 280–284.
4. Tasdogan, M.; Memis, D.; Sut, N.; Yuksel, M. Results of a pilot study on the effects of propofol and dexmedetomidine on inflammatory responses and intraabdominal pressure in severe sepsis. *J. Clin. Anesth.* **2009**, *21*, 394–400.
5. Xianbao, L.; Hong, Z.; Xu, Z.; Chunfang, Z.; Dunjin, C. Dexmedetomidine reduced cytokine release during postpartum bleeding-induced multiple organ dysfunction syndrome in rats. *Mediat. Inflamm.* **2013**, *2013*, 627831.
6. Tüfek, A.; Kaya, S.; Tokgöz, O.; Firat, U.; Evliyaoğlu, O.; Çelik, F.; Karaman, H. The protective effect of dexmedetomidine on bupivacaine-induced sciatic nerve inflammation is mediated by mast cells. *Clin. Investig. Med.* **2013**, *36*, E95–E102.
7. Zhang, L.; Zhang, J.; Yang, L.; Dong, Y.; Zhang, Y.; Xie, Z. Isoflurane and sevoflurane increase interleukin-6 levels through the nuclear factor-kappa B pathway in neuroglioma cells. *Br. J. Anaesth.* **2013**, *110*, i82–i91.
8. Kim, K.S.; Oh da, H.; Choi, H.M.; Bang, J.S.; Ryu, C.J.; Kim, J.H.; Yoo, M.C.; Yang, H.I. Pyrrolidine dithiocarbamate, a NF-kappaB inhibitor, upregulates MMP-1 and MMP-13 in IL-1beta-stimulated rheumatoid arthritis fibroblast-like synoviocytes. *Eur. J. Pharmacol.* **2009**, *613*, 167–175.

9. Snyder, J.G.; Prewitt, R.; Campsen, J.; Britt, L.D. PDTC and Mg132, inhibitors of NF-kappaB, block endotoxin induced vasodilation of isolated rat skeletal muscle arterioles. *Shock* **2002**, *17*, 304–307.
10. He, H.J.; Zhu, T.N.; Xie, Y.; Fan, J.; Kole, S.; Saxena, S.; Bernier, M. Pyrrolidine dithiocarbamate inhibits interleukin-6 signaling through impaired STAT3 activation and association with transcriptional coactivators in hepatocytes. *J. Biol. Chem.* **2006**, *281*, 31369–31379.
11. McClure, J.H. Ropivacaine. *Br. J. Anaesth.* **1996**, *76*, 300–307.
12. Casati, A.; Fanelli, G.; Albertin, A.; Deni, F.; Anelati, D.; Antonino, F.A.; Beccaria, P. Interscalene brachial plexus anesthesia with either 0.5% ropivacaine or 0.5% bupivacaine. *Minerva Anestesiol.* **2000**, *66*, 39–44.
13. Casati, A.; Fanelli, G.; Aldegheri, G.; Berti, M.; Colnaghi, E.; Cedrati, V.; Torri, G. Interscalene brachial plexus anaesthesia with 0.5%, 0.75% or 1% ropivacaine: A double-blind comparison with 2% mepivacaine. *Br. J. Anaesth.* **1999**, *83*, 872–875.
14. Brummett, C.M.; Amodeo, F.S.; Janda, A.M.; Padda, A.K.; Lydic, R. Perineural dexmedetomidine provides an increased duration of analgesia to a thermal stimulus when compared with a systemic control in a rat sciatic nerve block. *Reg. Anesth. Pain Med.* **2010**, *35*, 427–431.
15. Brummett, C.M.; Norat, M.A.; Palmisano, J.M.; Lydic, R. Perineural administration of dexmedetomidine in combination with bupivacaine enhances sensory and motor blockade in sciatic nerve block without inducing neurotoxicity in rat. *Anesthesiology* **2008**, *109*, 502–511.
16. Brummett, C.M.; Padda, A.K.; Amodeo, F.S.; Welch, K.B.; Lydic, R. Perineural dexmedetomidine added to ropivacaine causes a dose-dependent increase in the duration of thermal antinociception in sciatic nerve block in rat. *Anesthesiology* **2009**, *111*, 1111–1119.
17. Esmaoglu, A.; Yegenoglu, F.; Akin, A.; Turk, C.Y. Dexmedetomidine added to levobupivacaine prolongs axillary brachial plexus block. *Anesth. Analg.* **2010**, *111*, 1548–1551.
18. Ramsay, M.A.; Luterman, D.L. Dexmedetomidine as a total intravenous anesthetic agent. *Anesthesiology* **2004**, *101*, 787–790.
19. Martin, E.; Ramsay, G.; Mantz, J.; Sum-Ping, S.T. The role of the alpha2- adrenoceptor agonist dexmedetomidine in postsurgical sedation in the intensive care unit. *J. Intensiv. Care Med.* **2003**, *18*, 29–41.
20. Ramsay, M.A.; Saha, D.; Hebeler, R.F. Tracheal resection in the morbidly obese patient: The role of dexmedetomidine. *J. Clin. Anesth.* **2006**, *18*, 452–454.
21. Venn, R.M.; Grounds, R.M. Comparison between dexmedetomidine and propofol for sedation in the intensive care unit: Patient and clinician perceptions. *Br. J. Anaesth.* **2001**, *87*, 684–690.
22. Marhofer, D.; Kettner, S.C.; Marhofer, P.; Pils, S.; Weber, M.; Zeitlinger, M. Dexmedetomidine as an adjuvant to ropivacaine prolongs peripheral nerve block: A volunteer study. *Br. J. Anaesth.* **2013**, *110*, 438–442.

10

DADS Suppresses Human Esophageal Xenograft Tumors through RAF/MEK/ERK and Mitochondria-Dependent Pathways

Xiaoran Yin [1,†], Jun Zhang [2,†], Xiaoning Li [1], Dong Liu [2], Cheng Feng [2], Rongrui Liang [3], Kun Zhuang [4], Chenlei Cai [2], Xinghuan Xue [1], Fuchun Jing [5], Xijing Wang [1], Jun Wang [6], Xinlian Liu [1] and Hongbing Ma [1,*]

[1] Department of Oncology, the Second Affiliated Hospital of Xi'an Jiaotong University, Xi'an 710004, China; E-Mails: yinxiaoran@163.com (X.Y.); qingcao0066@163.com (Xia.L.); xuexinghuan1962@163.com (X.X.); wangxijingxian@126.com (X.W.); liuxldoc@yeah.net (Xin.L.)

[2] Department of Digestion, the Second Affiliated Hospital of Xi'an Jiaotong University, Xi'an 710004, China; E-Mails: jun3z@163.com (J.Z.); liudong_doc@163.com (D.L.); fc_2004188@163.com (C.F.); cchenlei2007@163.com (C.C.)

[3] Department of Oncology, the First Affiliated Hospital of Soochow University, No. 188, Shizi Street, Suzhou 215006, China; E-Mail: lengbeng@hotmail.com

[4] Department of Digestion, Xi'an Central Hospital, Xi'an 710003, China; E-Mail: zhuanger6695@sohu.com

[5] Department of Digestive Diseases, Baoji People's Hospital, Baoji 721000, China; E-Mail: fleming7798@163.com

[6] Department of Gastroenterology, Xi'an Hospital of Traditional Chinese Medicine, Xi'an 710001, China; E-Mail: wangjuntaiji@126.com

[†] These authors contributed equally to this work.

[*] Author to whom correspondence should be addressed; E-Mail: mhbxian@126.com

---

Abstract: Diallyl disulfide (DADS) is a natural organosulfur compound isolated from garlic. DADS has various biological properties, including anticancer, antiangiogenic, and antioxidant effects. However, the anticancer mechanisms of DADS in human esophageal carcinoma have not been elucidated, especially *in vivo*. In this study, MTT assay showed that DADS significantly reduced cell viability in human esophageal carcinoma ECA109 cells, but was relatively less toxic in normal liver cells. The pro–apoptotic effect of DADS on ECA109 cells was detected by Annexin V-FITC/propidium iodide (PI) staining. Flow cytometry analysis showed that DADS promoted apoptosis in a dose-dependent manner and the apoptosis rate could be decreased by caspase-3 inhibitor Ac-DEVD-CHO. Xenograft study in nude mice showed that DADS treatment inhibited the growth of ECA109 tumor in both 20 and 40 mg/kg DADS groups without obvious side effects. DADS inhibited ECA109 tumor proliferation by down-regulating proliferation cell nuclear antigen (PCNA). DADS induced apoptosis by activating a mitochondria-dependent pathway with the executor of caspase-3, increasing p53 level and Bax/Bcl-2 ratio, and downregulating the RAF/MEK/ERK pathway in ECA109 xenograft tumosr. Based on studies in cell culture and animal models, the findings here indicate that DADS is an effective and safe anti-cancer agent for esophageal carcinoma.

Keywords: esophageal carcinoma; DADS; apoptosis; animal model

1. Introduction

Esophageal carcinoma is among the most common tumors in the world, ranking eighth in occurrence and sixth in mortality [1]. Approximately 70% of global esophageal carcinoma cases occur in China and the five–year survival rate is only 10% [2]. Generally, esophageal carcinoma patients in the primary stage can be cured by surgical resection. However, a majority of patients in the advanced stage eventually succumb to this disease [3]. Although surgery, radiotherapy and chemotherapy are regarded as important parts of the systemic therapy for metastatic esophageal carcinoma, the success of such treatments have been weakened by their severe systemic toxicities and local irritating effects. Therefore, in order to enhance efficacy and reduce toxicity, researchers have urgently tried to develop novel regimens with fewer side effects against esophageal carcinoma [4].

Plant-derived herbal medicines have been used in several Asian countries including China for a long time. Some plant compounds have anticancer activity with low toxicity and could be used as alternative chemotherapeutic agents for carcinomas [5]. Garlic, as an herbal medicine, has antimicrobial, antiplatelet, antithrombotic, antiarthritic and antitumorigenic properties [6]. Diallyl disulfide (DADS), $CH_2{=}CH{-}CH_2{-}S{-}S{-}CH_2CH{=}CH_2$, is a lipid–soluble organic compound isolated from garlic. Scientific investigations have shown that DADS reduces the risk of cardiovascular disease and diabetes [7], serves as anti-oxidant [8], fights against infections [9], and exhibits significant protection effects against malignancies [10–12]. Moreover, in human breast cancer MCF–7 cells, the apoptotic effect of DADS is even superior to chemotherapy agents such as 5F-dUMP (5-Fu) and cyclophosphamide (CTX) [13].

Considering limited data on DADS bioavailability, additional studies are warranted to check the effects of DADS in animal models of esophageal carcinoma [11,14]. Moreover, the molecular mechanisms of DADS on various carcinomas are still a matter of debate and the exact effects of DADS *in vivo* on esophageal carcinoma are still unclear. Therefore, in the present study, we used an

ECA109 xenograft model in nude mice to study the effect of DADS on tumor growth. Additionally, we investigated the potential biomarkers and associated molecular alterations in ECA109 xenograft tumor. This is the first study to evaluate the potential effects and mechanisms of DADS on human esophageal carcinoma *in vivo*.

2. Results and Discussion

2.1. Diallyl Disulfide (DADS) Inhibits Cell Viability

The MTT assay was used to detect the viability inhibitory effects of ECA109 cells and L02 cells incubated with various concentrations of DADS (10–60 μg/mL) for 24 h. DADS was dissolved in DMSO, and mixed with RPMI–1640 for experiments *in vitro*. The concentration of DMSO added to the medium of DADS was less than 0.01%. The medium with DMSO and in absence of DADS was used as the control group. In addition, we detected the difference of ECA109 cells incubated with DADS and *cis*-diammminedichloroplatinum (DDP) for 24 h. Our data showed that DADS obviously inhibited cell viability in a dose-dependent manner at concentrations of 10–60 μg/mL for 24 h ($p < 0.05$, Figure 1). Moreover, DADS had much lower cytotoxicity to L02 normal liver cells than ECA109 esophageal carcinoma cells ($p < 0.05$, Figure 1). Our data shows that DDP was more effective than DADS on ECA109 cells *in vitro* ($p < 0.05$, Figure 2); DDP was used as positive control for *in vivo* study.

Figure 1. Viability inhibitory effects of diallyl disulfide (DADS) on ECA109 cells and L02 cells. ECA109 and L02 cells were incubated with different doses of DADS (0, 10, 20, 30, 40, 50, 60 μg/mL) for 24 h respectively. Cell viability was detected by MTT assay and was represented as the percentage of relative absorbance. Data are expressed as the mean ± SD from five independent experiments (* $p < 0.05$, ** $p < 0.01$ compared with the control group, # $p < 0.05$, ## $p < 0.01$ ECA109 compared with L02).

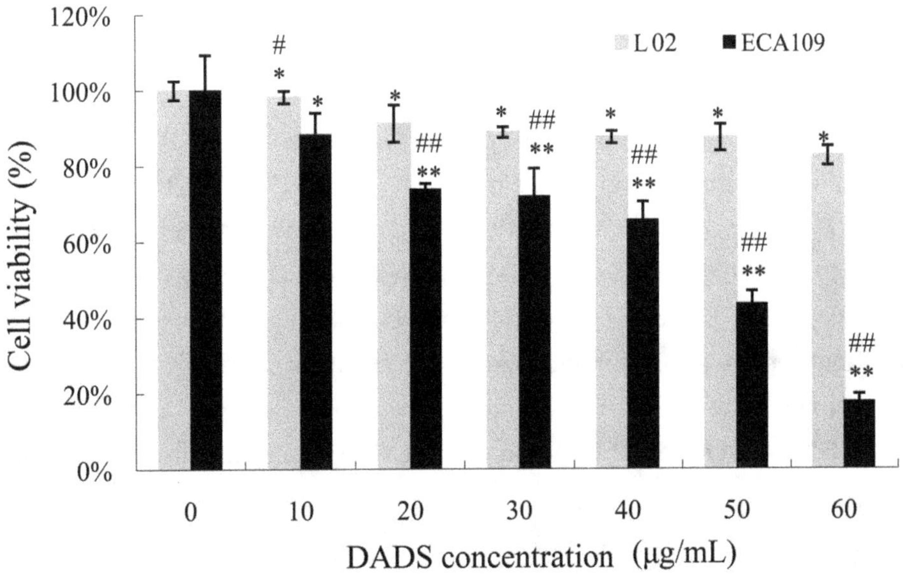

Figure 2. Viability inhibitory effects of DADS and *cis*-diammminedichloroplatinum (DDP) on ECA109 cells. ECA109 cells were incubated with different doses of DADS and DDP (0, 10, 20, 30, 40, 50, 60 μg/mL) for 24 h respectively. Cell viability was detected by MTT assay and was represented as the percentage of relative absorbance. Data are expressed as the mean ± SD from five independent experiments (* $p < 0.05$, ** $p < 0.01$ compared with the control group, ## $p < 0.01$ DDP compared with DADS).

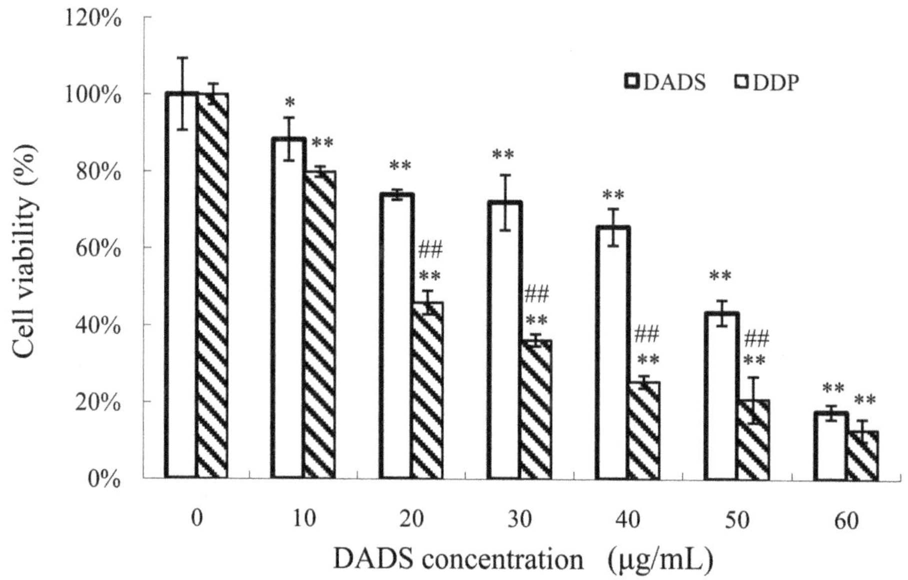

2.2. DADS-Induced Apoptosis

ECA109 cells were examined by phase contrast microscopy after being incubated with different concentrations of DADS (0, 20, 40, 80 μg/mL) for 24 h. The cells in the control group showed a typical intact appearance, whereas the DADS-treated cells displayed dose-dependent changes in cell shape. Membrane blebbing and formation of apoptotic bodies were found in 20 and 40 μg/mL DADS groups, while cellular shrinkage, poor adherence and floating shapes were found in the 80 μg/mL DADS group (Figure 3a).

As there were too many dead cells in the 80 μg/mL DADS group, we explored the apoptotic rate of ECA109 cells incubated with different concentrations of DADS (0, 20 and 40 μg/mL) for 24 h using Annexin V-FITC and propidium iodide (PI) staining and flow cytometry. Our data showed that the rate of apoptosis in the 0, 20 and 40 μg/mL DADS groups were (10.26 ± 1.45)%, (15.25 ± 2.99)% and (42.68 ± 4.08)% respectively. These results revealed that DADS induced the apoptosis of ECA109 cells in a dose-dependent manner ($p < 0.05$, Figure 3c). On the other hand, ECA109 cells were pretreated with caspase-3 inhibitor (Ac-DEVD-CHO) and then exposed to DADS for 24 h. Our results indicated that Ac-DEVD-CHO was able to protect ECA109 cells against DADS-induced apoptosis ($p < 0.05$, Figure 3d).

Figure 3. Apoptotic effects of DADS on ECA109 cells. (**a**) Morphology of ECA109 cells treated with different concentrations of DADS for 24 h and examined under phase contrast microscopy (×400); (**b**) DADS (0, 20 and 40 μg/mL) induced dose-dependent apoptosis in ECA109 cells. Ac-DEVD-CHO inhibited the apoptosis induced by DADS. Apoptosis was assessed using Annexin V-FITC/propidium iodide (PI) double staining; (**c**) Statistical analysis of the apoptosis rate of DADS; (**d**) Effects of Ac-DEVD-CHO against the apoptosis induced by DADS. Data are expressed as the mean ± SD from three independent experiments (* $p < 0.05$, ** $p < 0.01$ compared with the control group, # $p < 0.05$, ## $p < 0.01$ DADS + Ac-DEVD-CHO compared with DADS).

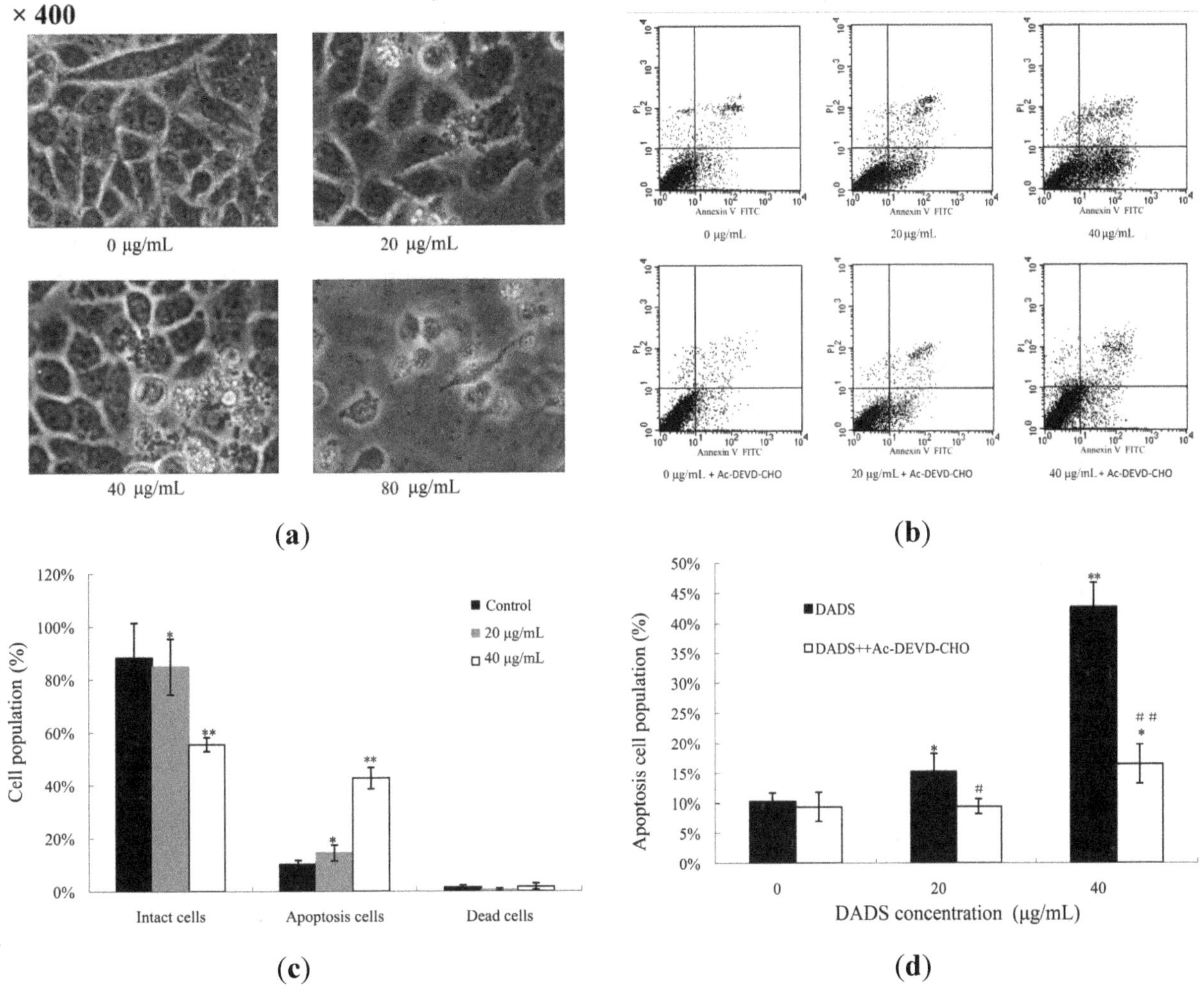

2.3. DADS Blocked the Growth of Xenograft Tumor

To evaluate the effect of DADS on the development of esophageal carcinoma *in vivo*, 5×10^6 ECA109 cells were injected into the flanks of nude mice. After three weeks, all the mice developed palpable tumors. The total of twenty-four mice were randomly divided into four groups ($n = 6$ per group). DADS was dissolved in DMSO, and mixed with phosphate buffered saline (PBS) for intraperitoneal injections in nude mice. The concentration of DMSO added to the medium was less than 0.01%. The PBS medium with DMSO in absence of DADS was utilized as the negative control group. Injections of DADS at 20 and 40 mg/kg body weight were done in therapy groups. Injections of

DDP at 2 mg/kg body wt were performed in the positive control group. These injections were made every three days, eight times. Compared with the negative control group, we observed significant difference of tumor weight in the 20 mg/kg DADS group ($p < 0.05$, Figure 4a), 40 mg/kg DADS group and DDP positive control group ($p < 0.01$, Figure 4a). At the end of the study, DADS decreased tumor volume from 292.02 ± 27.08 mm^3 per mouse in the negative control group to 211.95 ± 20.14, 179.08 ± 15.95 and 122.64 ± 12.62 mm^3 per mouse in 20 mg/kg DADS group ($p < 0.05$, Figure 4b), 40 mg/kg DADS group and DDP positive control group ($p < 0.01$, Figure 4b) respectively. In addition, there was no sign of possible changes of body weight in the DADS groups compared with the negative control group ($p > 0.05$, Figure 4c). However, the data showed that there was significant loss of body weight in DDP positive control group compared with the negative control group and DADS therapy groups ($p < 0.05$, Figure 4c).

Figure 4. Effects of DADS on ECA109 xenograft tumor. Nude mice were implanted with ECA109 cells. After the xenograft tumors became palpable, intraperitoneal injections were made eight times every three days, including the negative control group, 20 mg/kg DADS group, 40 mg/kg DADS group and 2 mg/kg DDP positive control group. Effects of DADS on (**a**) tumor volume; (**b**) tumor weight; and (**c**) body weight were recorded. Data shown in **a**–**c** are the average of six mice in each group, and are expressed as the mean ± SD (* $p < 0.05$, ** $p < 0.01$ compared with the control group).

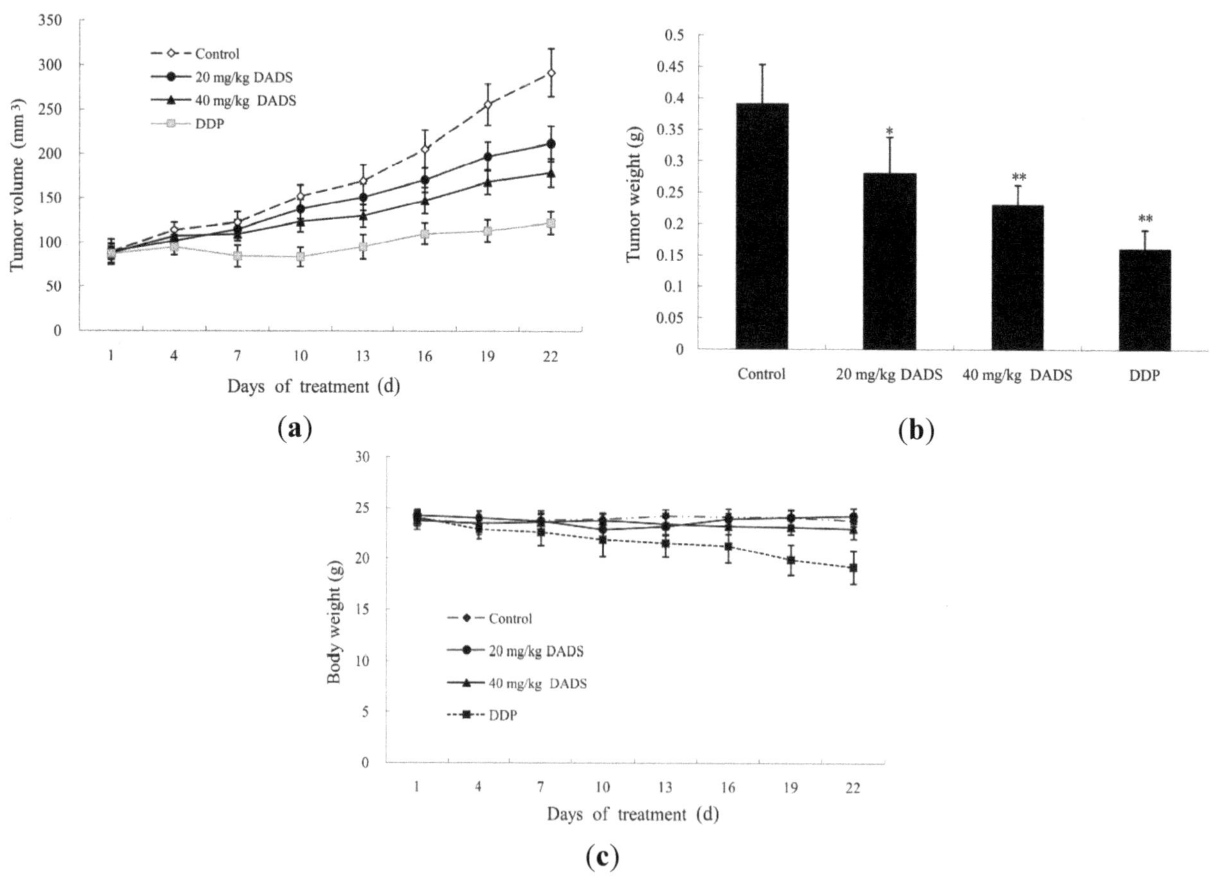

2.4. *DADS Inhibited Cell Proliferation and Induced Apoptosis in Xenograft Tumor*

We analyzed the effects of DADS on ECA109 tumor proliferation and apoptosis by immunohistochemical staining of proliferation cell nuclear antigen (PCNA) and caspase-3 respectively. By microscopic observation, a larger number of PCNA immunoreactive cells was observed in the negative control group (PBS medium with DMSO and in absence of DADS was utilized for intraperitoneal injections in nude mice) than in the 20 and 40 mg/kg DADS groups (Figure 5a), which accounted for 62.79% ± 9.58%, 32.31% ± 4.13% and 19.29% ± 6.49% respectively ($p < 0.01$, Figure 5b). However, more caspase-3 immunoreactive cells were observed in the DADS groups than the negative control group (Figure 5a). The quantification of caspase-3 immunoreactive cells was 11.84% ± 2.99% in the control group, and was significantly increased to 42.37% ± 7.39% and 54.28% ± 6.25% in the 20 mg/kg DADS group and 40 mg/kg DADS group, respectively ($p < 0.01$, Figure 5c).

Figure 5. Anti-proliferative and pro-apoptotic effects of DADS on ECA109 xenograft tumors. Tumors from the negative control group, 20 mg/kg DADS group and 40 mg/kg DADS group were processed for immunohistochemical staining of proliferation cell nuclear antigen (PCNA) (**a**,**b**) and caspase-3 (**a**,**c**). A representative picture had been shown for each case. Immunoreactive cells (yellow to brown) in xenograft tumors were enumerated and analyzed by Image-Pro Plus analysis system (Media Cybernetics, Bethesda, MD, USA) linked to an Olympus microscope (Olympus Corporation, Center Valley, PA, USA). The total number of cells was presented from all the samples in each group of five randomly selected microscopic fields. The data are expressed as the mean ± SD (×400) (** $p < 0.01$ compared with the control group).

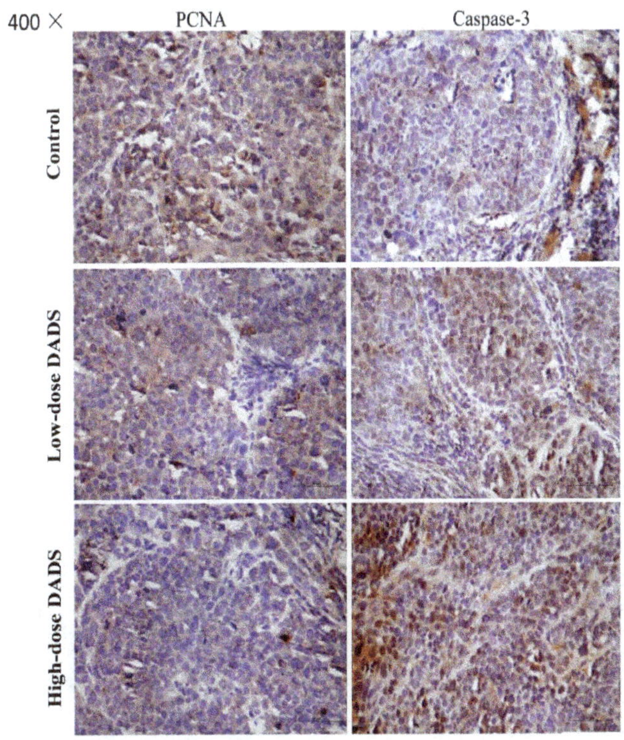

(**a**)

Figure 5. *Cont.*

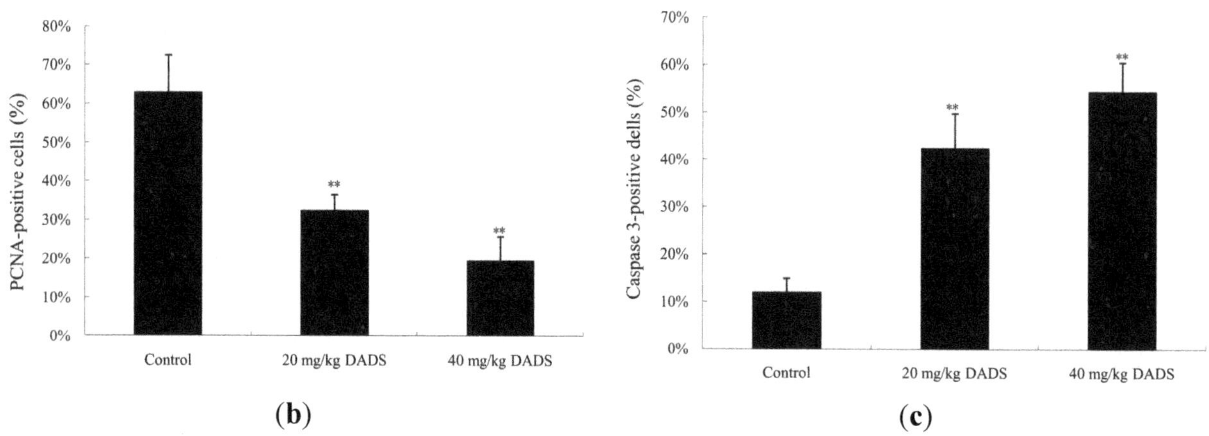

2.5. DADS Activated Mitochondria-Dependent Pathway and Up-Regulated Bax/Bcl-2 Ratio in Xenograft Tumors

It is well known that mitochondria–mediated apoptosis involves the release of cytochrome C, as well as the activation of caspase-9 and caspase-3. Our results from qPCR indicated that the levels of cytochrome C, caspase-9 and caspase-3 were stimulated in DADS groups ($p < 0.01$, Figure 6a). Moreover, DADS significantly increased the expression levels of active caspase-3 and active caspase-9 in total proteins, as well as the expression levels of cytochrome C in cytoplasm proteins in 20 and 40 mg/kg DADS groups by western blot analysis ($p < 0.01$, Figure 6c,e–g). However, DADS did not affect caspase-8 expression levels ($p > 0.05$, Figure 6a).

On the other hand, Bcl–2 and Bax are major proteins of the mitochondria apoptosis pathway. Our results of qPCR showed that the expression levels of Bcl-2 decreased in the DADS groups ($p < 0.05$, Figure 6a), whereas the expression level of Bax increased only in the 40 mg/kg DADS group ($p < 0.01$, Figure 6a). Therefore, there was a significant up-regulation of the Bax/Bcl-2 ratio in the 40 mg/kg DADS group ($p < 0.01$, Figure 6b). In addition, the results of qPCR and Western blot suggested that DADS enhanced the expression levels of p53 in the 40 mg/kg group ($p < 0.01$, Figure 6a,e).

2.6. DADS Alters the RAF/MEK/ERK Pathway in Xenograft Tumors

Western blot analysis was used to evaluate the effects of DADS on the protein levels of RAF1, MEK1, phosphor-MEK1 (p-MEK1), ERK1/2 and p-ERK1/2 in ECA109 xenograft tumors. Our results showed a significant down-regulation of RAF1, p-MEK1, ERK1/2 and p-ERK1/2 protein expressions in 20 and 40 mg/kg DADS groups ($p < 0.01$, Figure 7b,d–f). The expression level of MEK1 decreased in 40 mg/kg DADS group ($p < 0.01$, Figure 7c). These results suggested that DADS had a profound effect on the apoptosis in ECA109 xenograft tumor, which might be correlated with the RAF/MEK/ERK pathway.

Figure 6. DADS activated mitochondria-dependent pathway and shift in Bax/Bcl-2 ratio in ECA109 xenograft tumors. The mRNA and protein expression levels of caspase-3, caspase-8, caspase-9, cytochrome C, Bax, Bcl-2 and p53 from the negative control group, 20 mg/kg DADS group and 40 mg/kg DADS group were assessed by qPCR and western blot. (**a**) The mRNA expressions of caspase-3, caspase-8, caspase-9, cytochrome C, Bax, Bcl-2 and p53; (**b**) Bax/Bcl-2 ratio; (**c**) Representative blots; Densitometric analysis was made on the expressions of p53 (7F5) (**d**); active caspase-3 (**e**); active caspase-9 (**f**) and cytochrome C (**g**). β-Actin was used as the loading control. Data are expressed as the mean ± SD from three independent experiments (* $p < 0.05$, ** $p < 0.01$ compared with the control group).

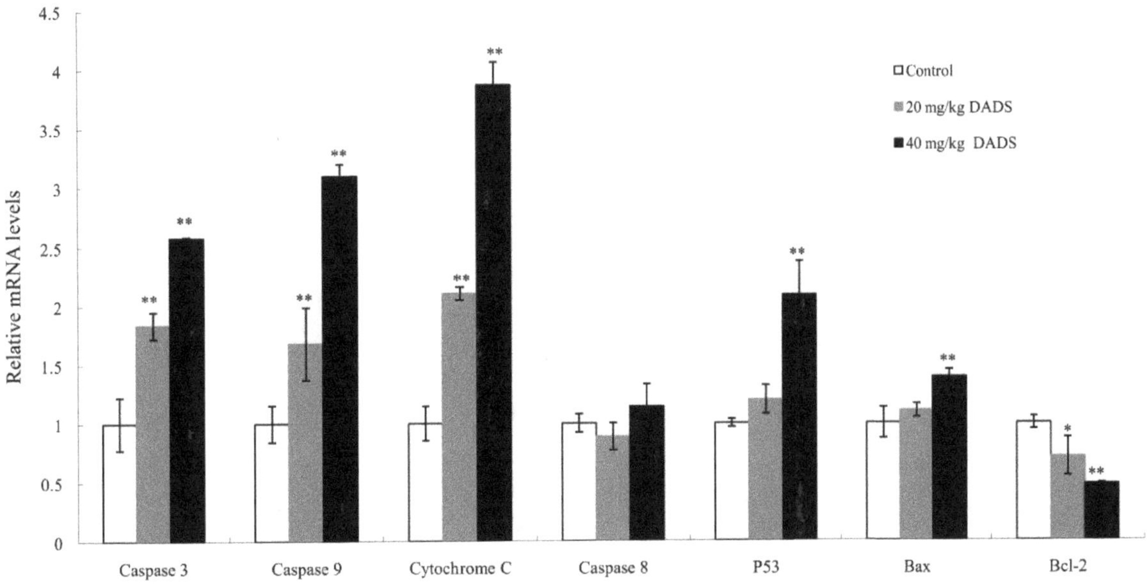

(**a**)

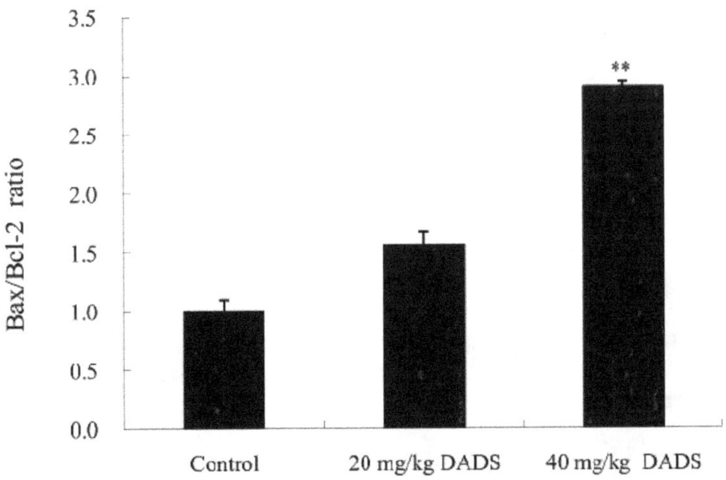

(**b**)

Figure 6. *Cont.*

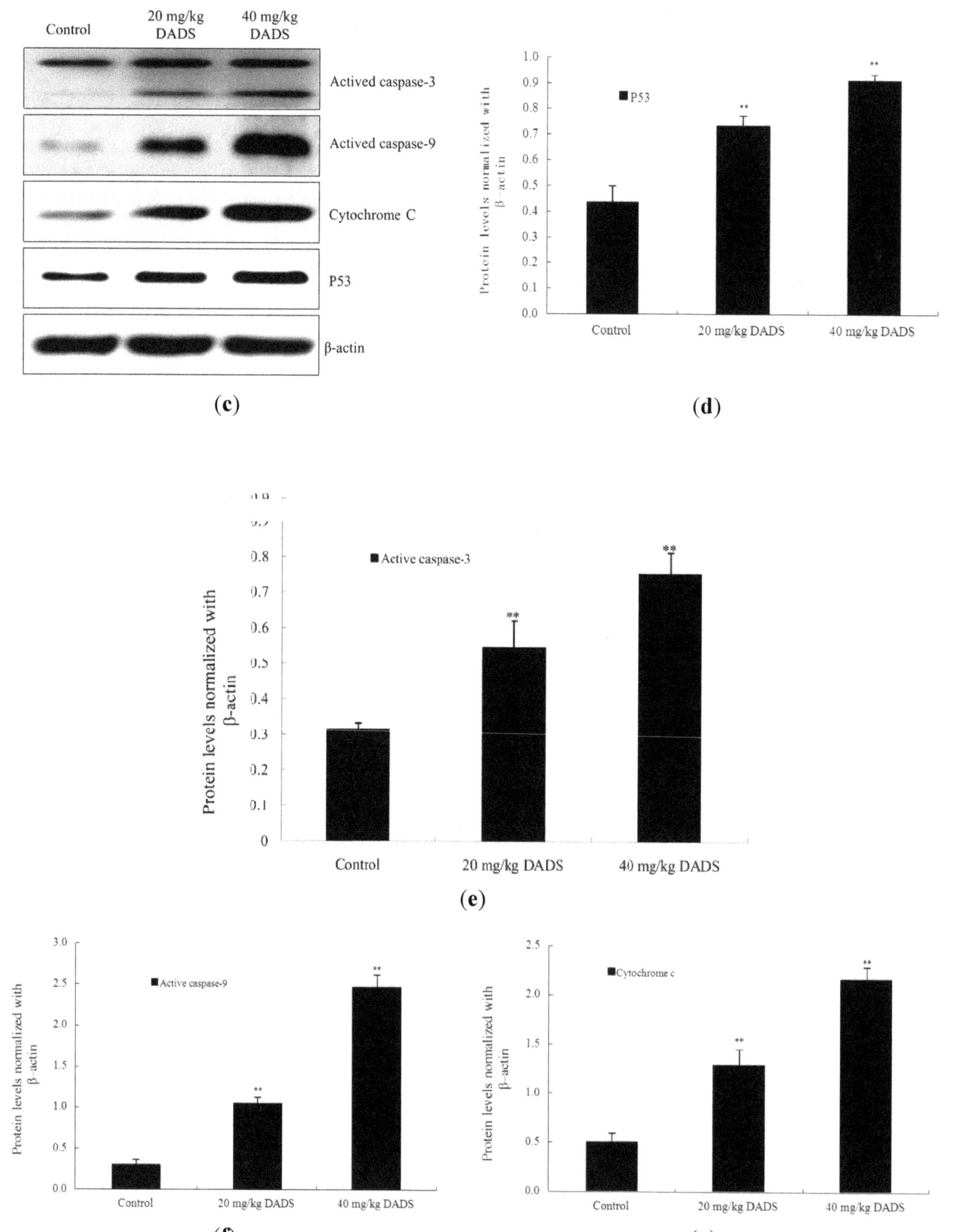

Figure 7. DADS down-regulated RAF/MEK/ERK pathway in ECA109 xenograft tumor. The protein expression levels of RAF1, MEK1, phosphor-MEK1 (p-MEK1), ERK1/2 and p-ERK1/2 from the negative control group, 20 mg/kg DADS group and 40 mg/kg DADS group were assessed by western blot analysis. (**a**) Representative blots. Densitometric analysis was made on the expressions of RAF1 (**b**); MEK1 (**c**); pMEK1 (**d**); ERK1/2 (**e**) and pERK1/2 (**f**). β-Actin was used as the loading control. Data are expressed as the mean ± SD from three independent experiments (** $p < 0.01$ compared with the control group).

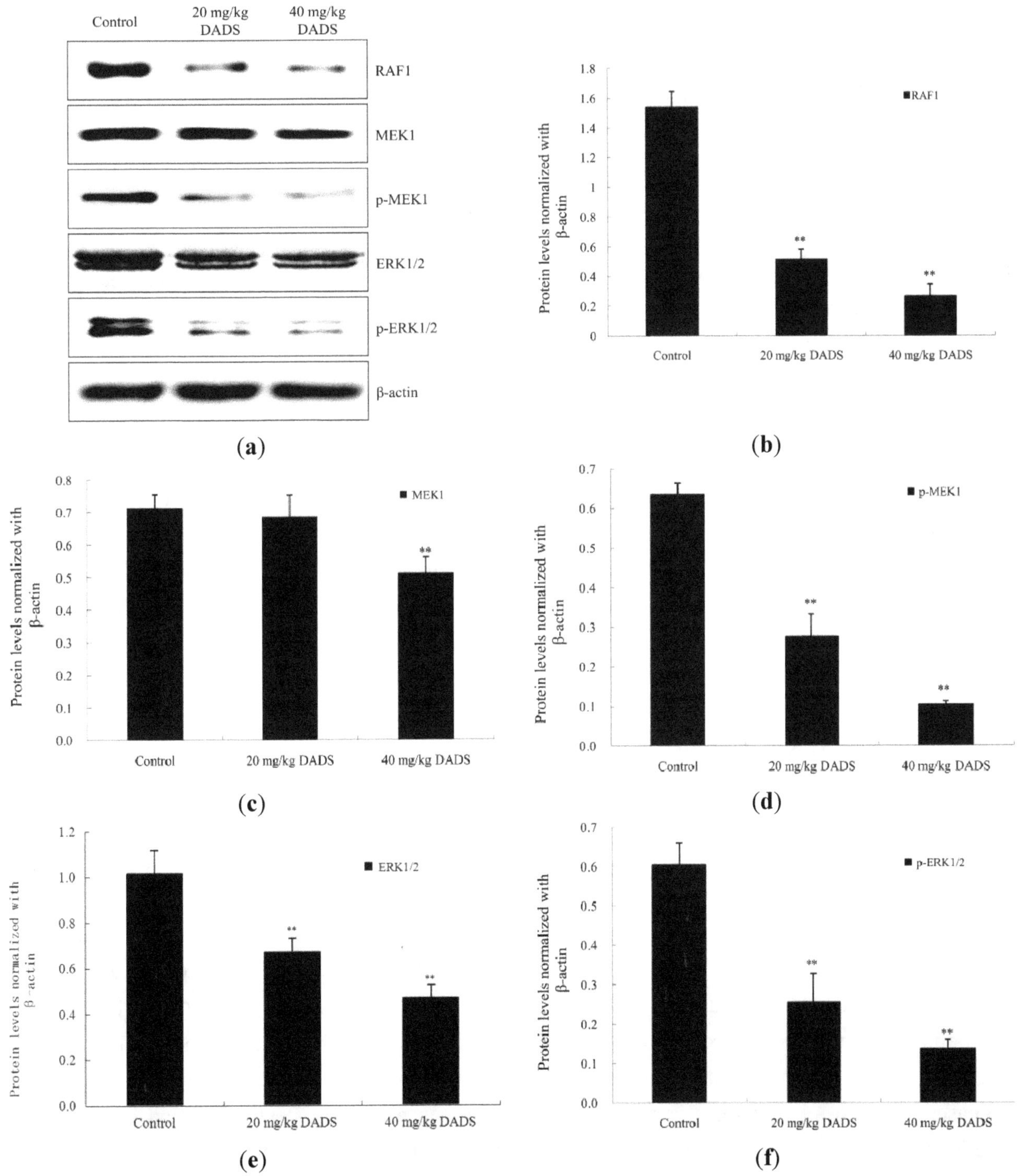

2.7. Discussion

DADS, a lipid-soluble organic compound isolated from garlic, is a potentially useful agent for cancer prevention and therapy, as it has the ability to reactivate the expression of genes in differentiation, cell cycle regulation, apoptosis and so on [10,12,15,16]. By using MTT assay, DADS showed a dose-dependent anti-viability effect on ECA109 cells *in vitro*. The viability inhibitory properties of DADS were attributed to its induction of apoptosis in human esophageal carcinoma ECA109 cells (Figures 1–3). Moreover, we demonstrated that DADS had much lower cytotoxicity to normal liver cells L02 in comparison with ECA109 carcinoma cells (Figure 1). In addition, as the data showed that DDP had greater effect on ECA109 cells than DADS *in vitro* (Figure 2), we used DDP as the positive control in an *in vivo* study.

Studies of xenograft tumors represent well-established preclinical animal models for evaluating anticancer effects of test agents *in vivo*. Therefore, additional studies are warranted to check the effects of DADS by using animal models [11,14,17–19]. Researchers have injected DADS in nude mice at 30–200 mg/kg body wt intraperitoneally [17–19]. Consistent with these data, we selected suitable doses of DADS at 20 and 40 mg/kg body weight. Our study showed that DADS treatment inhibited the growth of ECA109 tumors in volume and weight at the two dosages used (Figure 4a,b). Importantly, intraperitoneal injections of DADS for eight times showed no apparent signs of toxicity. However, the data indicated that there was a significant loss of body weight in the DDP positive control group compared with the negative control group and DADS therapy groups (Figure 4c). Although we did not find a stronger anti-cancer effect of DADS compared to the traditional chemotherapy agent DDP, our study indicated that DADS could suppress the growth of ECA109 xenograft tumor effectively and had fewer side effects than DDP. Moreover, our data showed that DADS decreased the expression of tumor proliferation biomarker PCNA in the 20 and 40 mg/kg DADS groups (Figure 5a,b). Therefore, we suggest that DADS might be a promising candidate drug for esophageal carcinoma patients.

Apoptosis is programmed cell death that plays a major role during cancer treatment [20]. DADS has the ability to induce apoptosis of some human tumor cells. However, the apoptosis induced by DADS involves different apoptotic genes and proteins depending on the cell types of different tumors [15,16]. The effects of DADS on esophageal carcinoma are still unclear, especially *in vivo*. Our study proved the apoptosis effect of DADS on ECA109 cells by using several methods. First, under light microscope, we observed morphology changes of apoptosis, such as membrane blebbing and formation of apoptotic bodies in the 20 and 40 μg/mL DADS groups, and cellular shrinkage, poor adherence and floating shapes in the 80 μg/mL DADS group (Figure 3a). Second, we detected the apoptosis rate by the double-staining of Annexin V-FITC and PI. Our results revealed that DADS induced the apoptosis of ECA109 cells in a dose-dependent manner (Figure 3b,c). In addition, the study indicated that DADS might inhibit the viability of ECA109 cells by promoting apoptosis.

Apoptosis signals are controlled by two distinct pathways, including the extrinsic pathway (death receptor pathway) and the intrinsic pathway (mitochondrial pathway) [21]. Caspases are cysteine proteases that play pivotal roles in apoptosis. Fourteen caspases have been identified based on their functions, which are divided into two groups (initiator caspases and effector caspases) [22]. Initiator caspases (caspase-2, -8, -9, and -10) are activated as a result of protein complex formation [23]. In the death receptor pathway, the activation of the death receptor leads to initiation of a caspase cascade by caspase-8. The mitochondrial pathway is characterized by the release of cytochrome C from mitochondria and the activation of a caspase cascade through caspase-9 [24]. Caspase-3, -6 and -7 function as executioners. Caspase-3 is a crucial executor that cleaves various substrates related to apoptosis [23,25]. Most of the apoptosis procedures induced by DADS are executed by caspase-3. However, some kinds of apoptosis are independent with caspase-3 [26–29]. In order to prove the apoptosis of DADS on ECA109 cells, we studied caspase-3 by qPCR and western blot *in vitro* and *in vivo*, as well as by immunohistochemical assay of xenograft tumor *in vivo*. Our results showed that the apoptosis of DADS was caspase-dependent, since caspase-3 was active during this procedure (Figures 5a,c and 6a,c,e) and that the pre–treatment with caspase-3 inhibitor (Ac-DEVD-CHO) could dramatically block the apoptosis induced by DADS (Figure 3b,d). Besides, many agents can activate cellular apoptotic programs through the mitochondria pathway, which triggers changes in regulatory factors [10]. Some soluble proteins including cytochrome C and Apaf-1, which can combine with caspase-9 to form the apoptosome, are released from the mitochondrial intermembrane space, and subsequently initiate an apoptosis cascade [30]. The mechanisms of apoptosis induced by DADS are different in various cells of different carcinomas. DADS induces apoptosis and promotes the activities of caspase-8 and caspase-9 in human colon cancer cell line (COLO 205) [26]. However, in the present study, our results of qPCR and western blot indicated that the activations of caspase-9 and caspase-3 as well as the release of cytochrome C from mitochondria to cytoplasm were stimulated in DADS groups (Figure 6a,c,f,g), which were involved in the typical mitochondrial apoptosis pathway [24]. Hence, these data suggested that the apoptosis effect induced by DADS on ECA109 cells was caspase-dependent *in vitro* as well as *in vivo*. In addition, our results indicated that one central mechanism of the apoptosis inducing by DADS in esophageal xenograft tumor was the activation of the mitochondrial pathway, but not the death receptor pathway.

The activation of caspases has a close relationship with the transduction of apoptosis signalling. P53 is known to inhibit cell proliferation and induce caspase-mediated apoptosis. Bax is a key target of p53 transcription factor in apoptosis [31]. Bcl-2, an antiapoptotic protein, is able to bind and inactivate Bax to modulate tumor cells responding apoptosis [32]. P53 and the Bax/Bcl-2 ratio play important roles in the apoptotic process. The molecular mechanisms of DADS on various carcinomas are still a matter of debate. DADS could up-regulate the p53 level to take part in the apoptotic processes of melanoma in the B16F-10 cell line and human cervical cancer Ca Ski cell line [33,34]. However, the effect of DADS is independent of p53 activity in the osteosarcoma Saos-2 cell line [35]. Moreover, p53 is increased in the colon cancer COLO 205 cell line, and is decreased in the colon cancer SW480 cell line by DADS treatment [26,36]. These experiments have indicated that DADS has various peculiarities in the treatment of different carcinomas. Moreover, even different cell lines of the same carcinoma are probably not alike under DADS treatment. P53 has been found to mutate in 83% esophageal squamous cell carcinomas [2], while p53 is highly expressed in the ECA109 cell line [37]. In the present study, our results of qPCR and Western blot suggested that DADS could enhance p53 expression levels in the two dosages of DADS groups, especially in the 40 mg/kg DADS group (Figure 6a,c,d). By qPCR assay, we found that mRNA expression levels of Bcl-2 were down-regulated in the two DADS groups, whereas the expression level of Bax was up-regulated in the 40 mg/kg DADS group (Figure 6a). Moreover, our data indicated the significant increase of the Bax/Bcl-2 ratio in the 40 mg/kg DADS group (Figure 6b), leading to the pro-apoptosis of ECA109 cells. Based on these observations, our study showed that the up-regulations of p53 expression levels and the Bax/Bcl-2 ratio were involved in DADS-induced cell death.

The RAF/mitogen-activated protein kinase/extracellular signal-regulated kinase (RAF/MEK/ERK) pathway plays a prominent role in the regulation of cell growth [38]. The RAF/MEK/ERK pathway can be affected by the activation of p53 [39]. ERK is a downstream component of conserved signaling module activated by the serine/threonine kinase, RAF. RAF can be recruited to the cellular membrane and activate MEK, which phosphorylates and activates ERK in turn [38]. ERK phosphorylation may control transcription by targeting several different regulators such as transcription factors and histone proteins, which result in proliferation, differentiation and protection against apoptosis [40]. DADS has been shown to be a histone deacetylase (HDAC) inhibitor, which has the ability to affect the growth and survival of tumor cells [12]. Although some studies have indicated that DADS inhibits the phosphorylation of ERK1/2 during the apoptotic processes of the human leukemia HL-60 cell line and human colon cancer COLO 205 cell line [16,41], other studies have shown that DADS activates ERK1/2 in human non-small cell lung cancer H1299 cell line and human nasopharyngeal carcinoma CNE2 cell line [15,42]. Moreover, DADS has no influence on ERK1/2 in apoptosis of the human prostate carcinoma DU145 cell line [10]. In the present study, our western blot results showed that the expression levels of RAF1, phosphor-MEK1 (p-MEK1), ERK1/2 and p-ERK1/2 were inhibited in both the 20 and 40 mg/kg DADS groups (Figure 7a,b,d–f), and that the expression level of MEK1 was down-regulated in the 40 mg/kg DADS group (Figure 7a,c). Based on these findings, it seemed that the down-regulation of the RAF/MEK/ERK signaling pathway contributed to the apoptosis induced by DADS in the ECA109 xenograft tumor. Moreover, the RAF/MEK/ERK pathway might be a valuable therapy target for esophageal carcinoma in the future.

3. Experimental Section

3.1. Reagents and Antibodies

ECA109 human esophageal carcinoma cell line and L02 human normal liver cell line were purchased from the Chinese Academy of Shanghai Institute of Cell Biology. DADS and DDP were purchased from Sigma–Aldrich Chemical Company, St. Louis, MO, USA. DMSO, MTT, propidium iodide (PI), phosphate buffered saline (PBS) were purchased from Sigma–Aldrich. Fetal bovine serums (FBS), RPMI-1640 medium and 0.25% trypsin were purchased from Hyclone Company, Logan, UT, USA. Trizol was purchased from Invitrogen, Grand Island, NY, USA. Annexin V-FITC apoptosis kit was purchased from Roche Technology Company, Branchburg, NJ, USA. PrimeScript™ RT Master Mix kit and SYBR® Premix Ex Taq II kit were purchased from Takara Technology Company, Sakado-shi, Saitama, JAPAN. Enhanced chemiluminescence (ECL) kit was purchased from Amersham Life Science, Arlington Heights, UK. Materials and chemicals used for electrophoresis were obtained from Bio-Rad Laboratories, Hercules, CA, USA. ProteoJET cytoplasmic Protein Extraction kit was purchased from Fermentas, Pittsburgh, PA, USA. Antibodies to RAF1, MEK1, phosphor-MEK1 (p-MEK1), ERK1/2, phosphor-ERK1/2 (p-ERK1/2), p53 (7F5), caspase-3, active caspase-3, caspase-9, active caspase-9, cytochrome C and proliferation cell nuclear antigen (PCNA) were purchased from Cell Signaling Technology Company, Danvers, MA, USA. The β-actin antibody was purchased from Santa Cruz Biotechnology, Dallas, TX, USA. Horseradish peroxidase- (HRP-) coupled goat anti-mouse IgG and anti-rabbit IgG (secondary antibody) were purchased from Santa Cruz Biotechnology.

3.2. Cell Culture

Human esophageal carcinoma cell line ECA109 and human normal liver cell line L02 were cultured in RPMI-1640 supplemented with 10% FBS under standard culture condition (37 °C, 95% humidified air and 5% CO_2). Exponentially growing ECA109 cells were used for all assays.

3.3. Cell Viability Assay

Cell viability was tested by MTT assay. ECA109 cells and L02 cells were seeded in 96-well plates at 1×10^4 cells/well and incubated with DADS or DDP (10–60 μg/mL) in five replicates for 24 h. Cells treated with PBS with DMSO and in absence of DADS were used as the negative control. After the incubation, 5 mg/mL MTT reagent (20 μL) was added into each well, followed by the addition of 150 μL DMSO. The plates were measured at 570 nm (A570) by spectrophotometer. The percentage of cell viability inhibition rate was calculated according to the following formula:

$$\text{Cell viability (\%)} = 1 - [(\text{A570 (control)} - \text{A570 (sample)}/\text{A570 (control)}] \times 100\% \tag{1}$$

3.4. Apoptosis Assay

The apoptosis rate was determined by using an Annexin V-FITC detection kit. ECA109 cells of 5×10^5 were incubated with different concentrations of DADS (0, 20, 40 μg/mL) and 10 μM caspase-3 inhibitor (Ac-DEVD-CHO) with DADS for 24 h. The cells were resuspended in 100 μL binding buffer at 1×10^6 cells/mL, and incubated with 5 μL Annexin V-FITC and 10 μL PI for 15 min in the dark. Then, these cells were added into 400 μL binding buffer and measured by flow cytometer. Apoptosis was analyzed by Cell Quest software (BD Biosciences, San Jose, CA, USA).

3.5. Xenograft Tumor Assay in Vivo

Female BALB/c nude mice (4–6 weeks old) were purchased from Beijing Experimental Animal Center. These mice were handled according to the Guidelines for the Care and Use of Laboratory Animals with the approval of the Medical Ethics Committee of the Second Affiliated Hospital of Xi'an Jiaotong University (ID: 2012120, 01 November 2012). Exponentially growing ECA109 cells of 5×10^6 were suspended in 200 μL RPMI–1640 and injected subcutaneously into the flank of each mouse. After growth for three weeks, all the mice developed palpable tumors. Twenty-four mice were randomly divided into four groups ($n = 6$ per group). The intraperitoneal injections of PBS with DMSO and in absence of DADS as the negative control group, DADS at 20 and 40 mg/kg body weight as therapy groups, DDP at 2 mg/kg body weight as the positive control group were made every three days for eight times. Tumors were monitored every three days by measuring length and width with a vernier caliper (tumor volume = $0.5 \times L \times W^2$). All the mice were sacrificed three days after the last injection and the xenograft tumors were observed and measured.

3.6. Immunohistochemical Staining

Tumor samples were formalin-fixed and paraffin-embedded. Paraffin blocks were cut serially at 5 μm thick. The sections were incubated with a specific primary antibody, such as PCNA (1:100) and caspase-3 (1:100), for 1 h at 37 °C followed by the overnight incubation at 4 °C in humidity chamber. Then, they were incubated with an appropriate biotinylated secondary antibody (1:200–1:400) followed by conjugated horseradish peroxidase–streptavidin and 3,3'-diaminobenzidine working solution, and then counterstained with hematoxylin. Immunoreactive cells (yellow to brown) were enumerated and analyzed by Media Cybernetics Image-Pro Plus analysis system linked to Olympus microscope. The total number of cells was presented from five randomly selected microscopic fields of every sample in each group (×400).

3.7. Quantitative Real-Time PCR

Total RNA was extracted from each tumor sample by Trizol method, and the quantity of RNA was assessed by spectrophotometry. The cDNA was obtained by reverse transcription with 1 μg total RNA by using PrimeScript™ RT Master Mix kit. qPCR was made with SYBR Premix Ex Taq™ II Perfect Real Time kit. All the reactions were performed on ABI qPCR System. The individual value was normalized by the loading control, β-actin. The mRNA expression was expressed as fold, and comparative cycle threshold (C_t) method was used to study the relative quantification of gene expression. Sequences of gene primers were listed in Table 1.

3.8. Western Blot Assay

ECA109 xenograft tumors of the negative control group and the two DADS groups were washed with cold PBS and homogenized in RIPA lysis buffer. The homogenates were centrifuged at 10,000× *g* for 10 min at 4 °C, and supernatants were collected as total proteins. Moreover, cytoplasmic proteins were prepared by using ProteoJET cytoplasmic Protein Extraction kit according to the manufacturer's instruction.

The proteins were separated by 8%–12% sodium dodecyl sulfate-polyacrylamide gel electrophoresis (SDS-PAGE), transferred to polyvinylidene difluoride (PVDF) membrane, and probed with a specific primary antibody, such as RAF1 (1:1000), MEK1 (1:1000), p-MEK1 (1:500), ERK1/2 (1:1000), p-ERK1/2 (1:300), caspase-3 (1:1000), active caspase-3 (1:500), caspase-9 (1:1000), active caspase-9 (1:500), cytochrome C, p53 (7F5) (1:1000) and β-actin (1:1000), followed by an appropriate peroxidase–conjugated secondary antibody (1:5000–1:10,000). The individual value was normalized by the loading control, β-actin. Antigen-antibody complex signals were visualized using BeyoECL Plus (Amersham Life Science). In addition, densitometric analysis was performed by Image J software (National Institutes of Health, Bethesda, MD, USA).

3.9. Quantification and Statistic Analysis

Quantitative data were expressed as the mean ± SD from at least three independent experiments. The two-tailed student's *t*-test was performed for paired samples, and one-way ANOVA or two-factor factorial ANOVA was used for multiple groups. The p value less than 0.05 was considered significant. Statistical analyses were performed by SPSS 17.0 statistics software (IBM, Armonk, NY, USA).

4. Conclusions

In summary, the present study demonstrated that DADS suppresses esophageal tumors without any apparent signs of toxicity, which is in agreement with a strong increase of apoptosis both *in vitro* and *in vivo*. DADS inhibits ECA109 tumor proliferation through the down-regulation of PCNA. Moreover, DADS induces apoptosis by activating the mitochondria-dependent pathway executed by caspase-3, increasing p53 expression level and the Bax/Bcl-2 ratio, and down-regulating the RAF/MEK/ERK pathway in ECA109 xenograft tumors. Overall, our studies of DADS in cell culture and animal models indicate that DADS is a potentially effective and safe anti-cancer agent for esophageal carcinoma treatment.

Acknowledgments

This study was supported by the Fund for Science and Technology Program of Shaanxi Province (No. 2010K01-141 and No. 2011K13-02-05) and the Important Clinic Project of the Chinese Ministry of Health (No. 2007353). This work was supported by the Research Center of the Second Affiliated Hospital of Xi'an Jiaotong University. The authors are grateful to Zongfang Li and Ke Li for their technical assistances.

Author Contributions

Xiaoran Yin, Cheng Feng and Dong Liu performed the majority of the experiments; Jun Zhang and Xiaoning Li provided vital reagents and analytical tools, as well as revised the manuscript; Xiaoran Yin and Hongbing Ma designed the study and wrote the manuscript.

References

1. Liu, R.; Peng, Y.; Li, X.; Wang, Y.; Pan, E.; Guo, W.; Pu, Y.; Yin, L. Identification of plasma metabolomic profiling for diagnosis of esophageal squamous-cell carcinoma using an UPLC/TOF/MS platform. *Int. J. Mol. Sci.* **2013**, *14*, 8899–8911.
2. Song, Y.; Li, L.; Ou, Y.; Gao, Z.; Li, E.; Li, X.; Zhang, W.; Wang, J.; Xu, L.; Zhou, Y.; *et al.* Identification of genomic alterations in oesophageal squamous cell cancer. *Nature* **2014**, *509*, 91–95.
3. Cui, X.; Zhao, Z.; Liu, D.; Guo, T.; Li, S.; Hu, J.; Liu, C.; Yang, L.; Cao, Y.; Jiang, J.; *et al.* Inactivation of miR-34a by aberrant CpG methylation in Kazakh patients with esophageal carcinoma. *J. Exp. Clin. Cancer Res.* **2014**, *33*, 20.
4. Shen, Z.T.; Wu, X.H.; Li, B.; Shen, J.S.; Wang, Z.; Li, J.; Zhu, X.X. Nedaplatin concurrent with three-dimensional conformal radiotherapy for treatment of locally advanced esophageal carcinoma. *World J. Gastroenterol.* **2013**, *19*, 9447–9452.

5. Yeruva, L.; Elegbede, J.A.; Carper, S.W. Methyl jasmonate decreases membrane fluidity and induces apoptosis through tumor necrosis factor receptor 1 in breast cancer cells. *Anti-Cancer Drugs* **2008**, *19*, 766–776.
6. Eswar, K.; Venkateshbabu, N.; Rajeswari, K.; Kandaswamy, D. Dentinal tubule disinfection with 2% chlorhexidine, garlic extract, and calcium hydroxide against *Enterococcus faecalis* by using real-time polymerase chain reaction: *In vitro* study. *J. Conserv. Dent.* **2013**, *16*, 194–198.
7. Truong, D.; Hindmarsh, W.; O'Brien, P.J. The molecular mechanisms of diallyl disulfide and diallyl sulfide induced hepatocyte cytotoxicity. *Chem. Biol. Interact.* **2009**, *180*, 79–88.
8. Lee, I.C.; Kim, S.H.; Baek, H.S.; Moon, C.; Kim, S.H.; Kim, Y.B.; Yun, W.K.; Kim, H.C.; Kim, J.C. Protective effects of diallyl disulfide on carbon tetrachloride-induced hepatotoxicity through activation of Nrf2. *Environ. Toxicol.* **2013**, doi:10.1002/tox.21930. Available online: http://onlinelibrary.wiley.com/doi/10.1002/tox.21930/abstract;jsessionid=1C5EEE912870EFFD9CEB32D9B9CFC1D2.f02t04?deniedAccessCustomisedMessage=&userIsAuthenticated=false (accessed on 1 December 2013).
9. Alam, M.; Zubair, S.; Farazuddin, M.; Ahmad, E.; Khan, A.; Zia, Q.; Malik, A.; Mohammad, O. Development, characterization and efficacy of niosomal diallyl disulfide in treatment of disseminated murine candidiasis. *Nanomed. Nanotechnol. Biol. Med.* **2013**, *9*, 247–256.
10. Shin, D.Y.; Kim, G.Y.; Lee, J.H.; Choi, B.T.; Yoo, Y.H.; Choi, Y.H. Apoptosis induction of human prostate carcinoma DU145 cells by diallyl disulfide via modulation of JNK and PI3K/AKT signaling pathways. *Int. J. Mol. Sci.* **2012**, *13*, 14158–14171.
11. Tang, H.; Kong, Y.; Guo, J.; Tang, Y.; Xie, X.; Yang, L.; Su, Q.; Xie, X. Diallyl disulfide suppresses proliferation and induces apoptosis in human gastric cancer through Wnt-1 signaling pathway by up-regulation of miR-200b and miR-22. *Cancer Lett.* **2013**, *340*, 72–81.
12. Myzak, M.C.; Dashwood, R.H. Histone deacetylases as targets for dietary cancer preventive agents: Lessons learned with butyrate, diallyl disulfide, and sulforaphane. *Curr. Drug Targets* **2006**, *7*, 443–452.
13. Jun, Z.; Suzuki, M.; Xiao, J.; Wen, J.; Talbot, S.G.; Li, G.C.; Xu, M. Comparative effects of natural and synthetic diallyl disulfide on apoptosis of human breast-cancer MCF-7 cells. *Biotechnol. Appl. Biochem.* **2009**, *52*, 113–119.
14. Lai, K.C.; Kuo, C.L.; Ho, H.C.; Yang, J.S.; Ma, C.Y.; Lu, H.F.; Huang, H.Y.; Chueh, F.S.; Yu, C.C.; Chung, J.G. Diallyl sulfide, diallyl disulfide and diallyl trisulfide affect drug resistant gene expression in colo 205 human colon cancer cells *in vitro* and *in vivo*. *Phytomed. Int. J. Phytother. Phytopharmacol.* **2012**, *19*, 625–630.
15. Hui, C.; Jun, W.; Ya, L.N.; Ming, X. Effect of Allium sativum (garlic) diallyl disulfide (DADS) on human non-small cell lung carcinoma H1299 cells. *Trop. Biomed.* **2008**, *25*, 37–45.
16. Tan, H.; Ling, H.; He, J.; Yi, L.; Zhou, J.; Lin, M.; Su, Q. Inhibition of ERK and activation of p38 are involved in diallyl disulfide induced apoptosis of leukemia HL-60 cells. *Arch. Pharm. Res.* **2008**, *31*, 786–793.
17. Liao, Q.J.; Su, J.; Zhou, X.T.; Tang, H.L.; Song, Y.; Su, Q. Inhibitory effect of diallyl disulfide on proliferation of human colon cancer cell line SW480 in nude mice. *Chin. J. Cancer* **2007**, *26*, 828–832. (In Chinese)
18. Xiang, S.L.; Xiao, X.L.; Ling, H.; Liao, Q.J.; Zhou, X.T.; Dong, L.; Su, Q. Antitumor effect of

diallyl disulfide on human gastric cancer MGC803 cells xenograft in nude mice. *Chin. J. Cancer* **2005**, *24*, 940–944. (In Chinese)

19. Zhao, J.; Huang, W.G.; He, J.; Tan, H.; Liao, Q.J.; Su, Q. Diallyl disulfide suppresses growth of HL-60 cell through increasing histone acetylation and p21WAF1 expression *in vivo* and *in vitro*. *Acta Pharmacol. Sin.* **2006**, *27*, 1459–1466.
20. Haneji, T.; Hirashima, K.; Teramachi, J.; Morimoto, H. Okadaic acid activates the PKR pathway and induces apoptosis through PKR stimulation in MG63 osteoblast-like cells. *Int. J. Oncol.* **2013**, *42*, 1904–1910.
21. Ozoren, N.; El-Deiry, W.S. Cell surface death receptor signaling in normal and cancer cells. *Semin. Cancer Biol.* **2003**, *13*, 135–147.
22. Jin, Z.; El-Deiry, W.S. Overview of cell death signaling pathways. *Cancer Biol. Ther.* **2005**, *4*, 139–163.
23. Olsson, M.; Zhivotovsky, B. Caspases and cancer. *Cell Death Differ.* **2011**, *18*, 1441–1449.
24. Thomas, S.A.; Vasudevan, S.; Thamkachy, R.; Lekshmi, S.U.; Santhoshkumar, T.R.; Rajasekharan, K.N.; Sengupta, S. Upregulation of DR5 receptor by the diaminothiazole DAT1 [4-amino-5-benzoyl-2-(4-methoxy phenyl amino) thiazole] triggers an independent extrinsic pathway of apoptosis in colon cancer cells with compromised pro and antiapoptotic proteins. *Apoptosis Int. J. Program. Cell Death* **2013**, *18*, 713–726.
25. Zheng, T.S.; Hunot, S.; Kuida, K.; Momoi, T.; Srinivasan, A.; Nicholson, D.W.; Lazebnik, Y.; Flavell, R.A. Deficiency in caspase-9 or caspase-3 induces compensatory caspase activation. *Nat. Med.* **2000**, *6*, 1241–1247.
26. Yang, J.S.; Chen, G.W.; Hsia, T.C.; Ho, H.C.; Ho, C.C.; Lin, M.W.; Lin, S.S.; Yeh, R.D.; Ip, S.W.; Lu, H.F.; *et al.* Diallyl disulfide induces apoptosis in human colon cancer cell line (COLO 205) through the induction of reactive oxygen species, endoplasmic reticulum stress, caspases casade and mitochondrial-dependent pathways. *Food Chem. Toxicol.* **2009**, *47*, 171–179.
27. Nagaraj, N.S.; Anilakumar, K.R.; Singh, O.V. Diallyl disulfide causes caspase-dependent apoptosis in human cancer cells through a Bax-triggered mitochondrial pathway. *J. Nutr. Biochem.* **2010**, *21*, 405–412.
28. Altonsy, M.O.; Habib, T.N.; Andrews, S.C. Diallyl disulfide-induced apoptosis in a breast-cancer cell line (MCF-7) may be caused by inhibition of histone deacetylation. *Nutr. Cancer* **2012**, *64*, 1251–1260.
29. Gayathri, R.; Gunadharini, D.N.; Arunkumar, A.; Senthilkumar, K.; Krishnamoorthy, G.; Banudevi, S.; Vignesh, R.C.; Arunakaran, J. Effects of diallyl disulfide (DADS) on expression of apoptosis associated proteins in androgen independent human prostate cancer cells (PC-3). *Mol. Cell. Biochem.* **2009**, *320*, 197–203.
30. Sun, K.W.; Ma, Y.Y.; Guan, T.P.; Xia, Y.J.; Shao, C.M.; Chen, L.G.; Ren, Y.J.; Yao, H.B.; Yang, Q.; He, X.J. Oridonin induces apoptosis in gastric cancer through Apaf-1, cytochrome c and caspase-3 signaling pathway. *World J. Gastroenterol.* **2012**, *18*, 7166–7174.
31. Liu, J.; Qin, C.K.; Lv, W.; Zhao, Q.; Qin, C.Y. OSU-03012, a non-Cox inhibiting celecoxib derivative, induces apoptosis of human esophageal carcinoma cells through a p53/Bax/cytochrome c/caspase-9-dependent pathway. *Anti-Cancer Drugs* **2013**, *24*, 690–698.
32. Produit-Zengaffinen, N.; Pournaras, C.J.; Schorderet, D.F. Retinal ischemia-induced apoptosis is

associated with alteration in Bax and Bcl-x(L) expression rather than modifications in Bak and Bcl-2. *Mol. Vis.* **2009**, *15*, 2101–2110.

33. Pratheeshkumar, P.; Thejass, P.; Kutan, G. Diallyl disulfide induces caspase-dependent apoptosis via mitochondria-mediated intrinsic pathway in B16F-10 melanoma cells by up-regulating p53, caspase-3 and down-regulating pro-inflammatory cytokines and nuclear factor-kappabeta-mediated Bcl-2 activation. *J. Environ. Pathol. Toxicol. Oncol.* **2010**, *29*, 113–125.
34. Lin, Y.T.; Yang, J.S.; Lin, S.Y.; Tan, T.W.; Ho, C.C.; Hsia, T.C.; Chiu, T.H.; Yu, C.S.; Lu, H.F.; Weng, Y.S.; *et al.* Diallyl disulfide (DADS) induces apoptosis in human cervical cancer Ca Ski cells via reactive oxygen species and Ca^{2+}-dependent mitochondria-dependent pathway. *Anticancer Res.* **2008**, *28*, 2791–2799.
35. Masuelli, L.; Marzocchella, L.; Focaccetti, C.; Tresoldi, I.; Palumbo, C.; Izzi, V.; Benvenuto, M.; Fantini, M.; Lista, F.; Tarantino, U.; *et al.* Resveratrol and diallyl disulfide enhance curcumin-induced sarcoma cell apoptosis. *Front. Biosci.* **2012**, *17*, 498–508.
36. Liao, Q.J.; Su, J.; He, J.; Song, Y.; Tang, H.L.; Su, Q. Effect of diallyl disulfide on cell cycle arrest of human colon cancer SW480 cells. *Chin. J. Cancer* **2009**, *28*, 138–141. (In Chinese)
37. Wang, T.T.; Wang, S.K.; Huang, G.L.; Sun, G.J. Luteolin induced-growth inhibition and apoptosis of human esophageal squamous carcinoma cell line Eca109 cells *in vitro*. *Asian Pac. J. Cancer Prev.* **2012**, *13*, 5455–5461.
38. Ciccarelli, A.; Giustetto, M. Role of ERK signaling in activity-dependent modifications of histone proteins. *Neuropharmacology* **2014**, *80C*, 34–44.
39. Bhalla, S.; Evens, A.M.; Dai, B.; Prachand, S.; Gordon, L.I.; Gartenhaus, R.B. The novel anti-MEK small molecule AZD6244 induces BIM-dependent and AKT-independent apoptosis in diffuse large B-cell lymphoma. *Blood* **2011**, *118*, 1052–1061.
40. Lv, C.; Sun, W.; Sun, H.; Wei, S.; Chen, R.; Wang, B.; Huang, C. Asperolide A, a marine-derived tetranorditerpenoid, induces G2/M arrest in human NCI-H460 lung carcinoma cells, is mediated by p53–p21 stabilization and modulated by Ras/Raf/MEK/ERK signaling pathway. *Mar. Drugs* **2013**, *11*, 316–331.
41. Lai, K.C.; Hsu, S.C.; Kuo, C.L.; Yang, J.S.; Ma, C.Y.; Lu, H.F.; Tang, N.Y.; Hsia, T.C.; Ho, H.C.; Chung, J.G. Diallyl sulfide, diallyl disulfide, and diallyl trisulfide inhibit migration and invasion in human colon cancer colo 205 cells through the inhibition of matrix metalloproteinase-2, -7, and -9 expressions. *Environ. Toxicol.* **2013**, *28*, 479–488.
42. Zhang, Y.W.; Wen, J.; Xiao, J.B.; Talbot, S.G.; Li, G.C.; Xu, M. Induction of apoptosis and transient increase of phosphorylated MAPKs by diallyl disulfide treatment in human nasopharyngeal carcinoma CNE2 cells. *Arch. Pharm. Res.* **2006**, *29*, 1125–1131.

11

Effects of the Novel Compound DK223 ([1*E*,2*E*-1,2-Bis(6-methoxy-2*H*-chromen-3-yl)methylene]hydrazine) on Migration and Proliferation of Human Keratinocytes and Primary Dermal Fibroblasts

Manh Tin Ho [1], Hyun Sik Kang [2], Jung Sik Huh [3], Young Mee Kim [1], Yoongho Lim [4] and Moonjae Cho [1,5,*]

[1] Department of Biochemistry, School of Medicine, Jeju National University, Jeju 690-756, Korea; E-Mails: homanhtin@gmail.com (M.T.H.); biochem310@jejunu.ac.kr (Y.M.K.)

[2] Department of Pediatrics, School of Medicine, Jeju National University, Jeju 690-756, Korea; E-Mail: medyapsb@naver.com

[3] Department of Urology, School of Medicine, Jeju National University, Jeju 690-756, Korea; E-Mail: urohjs@jejunu.ac.kr

[4] Division of Bioscience and Biotechnology, Konkuk University, Seoul 143-701, Korea; E-Mail: yoongho@konkuk.ac.kr

[5] Institute of Medical Science, Jeju National University, Jeju 690-756, Korea

* Author to whom correspondence should be addressed; E-Mail: moonjcho@jejunu.ac.kr

---

Abstract: Wound healing plays an important role in protecting the human body from external infection. Cell migration and proliferation of keratinocytes and dermal fibroblasts are essential for proper wound healing. Recently, several studies have demonstrated that secondary compounds produced in plants could affect skin cells migration and proliferation. In this study, we identified a novel compound DK223 ([1*E*,2*E*-1,2-bis(6-methoxy-2*H*-chromen-3-yl)methylene]hydrazine) that concomitantly induced human keratinocyte migration and dermal fibroblast proliferation. We evaluated the regulation of epithelial and mesenchymal protein markers, such as E-cadherin and Vimentin, in human keratinocytes, as well as extracellular matrix (ECM) secretion and metalloproteinase families in dermal fibroblasts. DK223 upregulated keratinocyte migration and significantly increased the epithelial marker E-cadherin in a time-dependent manner. We also found that reactive oxygen species (ROS) increased significantly in keratinocytes after 2 h of DK223 exposure, returning to normal levels after 24 h, which indicated that DK223 had an early shock effect on ROS production. DK223 also stimulated fibroblast proliferation, and induced significant secretion of ECM proteins, such as collagen I, III, and fibronectin. In dermal fibroblasts, DK223 treatment induced TGF-β1, which is involved in a signaling pathway that mediates proliferation. In conclusion, DK223 simultaneously induced both keratinocyte migration via ROS production and fibroblast proliferation via TGF-β1 induction.

Keywords: wound healing; keratinocyte migration; fibroblast proliferation; scar formation; skin regeneration

---

1. Introduction

As the outer sheath of the human body, the skin absorbs initial damage from injuries or wounds. Disruption of the normal anatomic structure and loss of organ function lead to the repair process known as wound healing. Wound healing integrates different types of dermal cells and immune cells, such as keratinocytes and dermal fibroblasts, to mediate hemostasis, coagulation, and inflammation [1,2]. Wound healing begins with inflammation and immune cell recruitment to protect tissue from foreign invaders, such as bacteria and viruses. The next phase resurfaces the skin by stimulating regeneration and repair through proliferation of fibroblasts, re-epithelialization of keratinocytes, and other mechanisms. The final phase involves scar formation, which can cause concern for some patients when the scar is not aesthetically pleasing. Therefore, several studies have investigated methods to enhance the regeneration process, which is a specific substitution of the damaged tissue, and to reduce skin repair, which causes fibrosis and scar formation [1].

Herbal plants, such as garlic and curcuma, have been used traditionally for wound healing, and it is known that their effects are due to secondary compounds, such as flavonoids, saponins and alkaloids [3]. For example, Lopez-Jornet *et al.* showed that potassium apigenin and other flavonoids present in verbena extract possess powerful anti-inflammatory properties [4]. In addition, Duarte *et al.* demonstrated the use of chamomile extract ointment for stimulating oral mucosa re-epithelialization and formation of collagen fibers after 10 days of treatment [5]. Moreover, these compounds were demonstrated to influence expression of extracellular matrix (ECM) proteins in skin, including collagen and elastin, which are markers of skin wrinkle [6]. Galicka *et al.* reported increased collagen synthesis upon exposure to apigenin glycoside 7-*O*-glucuronide, a flavonoid glycoside, which also promoted procollagen transformation into collagen [7].

Furthermore, wound healing was controlled by matrix metalloproteinases (MMPs), enzymes that degrade the epidermal layer of the ECM, and are related to the cellular migration, invasion and metastasis processes [8]. MMPs, such as MMP1, MMP8, MMP13, play a specific role in mediating collagen degradation to reduce scar formation in wound healing. For example, Dang *et al.* reported upregulation of MMP1 expression to double normal levels, resulting in scarless wounds in fetal rat skin [9]. The role of MMPs in skin remodeling is well known, they are secreted extra-cellularly and regulated ECM protein accumulation in the wound healing process [10]. Notably, it has been reported that bioactive compounds regulate the expression and activity of MMPs. Catanzaro *et al.* demonstrated the effects of a sturgeon-based bioactive compound on the expression of the tumor necrosis factor-alpha, MMPs, and type-10 collagen genes in human chondrocytes [11]. Application of bioactive compounds may offer a potential therapy for controlling the wound healing or skin aging process.

Natural secondary metabolites have been demonstrated to have several potential capabilities in gene expression regulation for skin repair. Based on the knowledge of the original structures, drug development science can be used to synthesize compounds that are conformationally modified to improve their activities [12]. In that way, novel compounds have been synthesized using innovative chemical techniques that expand on the original conformation. In this study, we examined the hypothesis that the novel compound DK223 ([1*E*,2*E*-1,2-bis(6-methoxy-2*H*-chromen-3-yl)methylene]hydrazine) could induce keratinocyte migration, fibroblast proliferation, anti-wrinkle gene expression, and enhance the regeneration of skin, rather than mediate scar formation.

2. Results

2.1. DK223 Promoted the Migration but not the Proliferation of HaCaT Cells

To investigate the ability of DK223 to induce migration of human keratinocytes, we treated HaCaT cells with different concentrations of DK223 in a 48 h scratch wound-healing assay. The results showed that DK223 at 2 μM significantly enhanced migration of HaCaT (167%), whereas other concentrations did not produce marked effects (Figure 1A). In order to confirm these results, we performed the migration assay with the ECIS system using other concentrations of DK223. In this assay, during cell growth, the current is impeded based on the number of cells covering the electrode, which indicates the velocity of cell movement. The results were collected as impedance *versus* time. As expected, 2 μM DK223 significantly enhanced the migration velocity of keratinocytes after 24 h compared with the control (Figure 1B).

We used the MTT assay to assess proliferation of HaCaT cells in response to DK223, and the results demonstrated that there was a significant increase in keratinocyte growth with 2 μM DK223 after 48 h (Figure 1C). Whereas the mRNA and protein expression of p53, p21, p27, cyclin D, and cyclin E did not significantly change in 24 h compared with the untreated cells (Figure 1D,E). These observations indicate that DK223 could induce cell migration, as well as proliferation of human keratinocytes.

2.2. DK223 Did not Induced Epithelial–Mesenchymal Transition (EMT) in HaCaT Cells

EMT is critical for wound healing, and tissue regeneration has been shown to induce keratinocyte migration [13]. Thus, we examined the mRNA and protein expression of EMT markers, such as vimentin, E-cadherin, and Slug after DK223 treatment to investigate whether DK223-induced migration affected the EMT process. As shown by Western blot in Figure 2A, two mesenchymal markers, vimentin and Slug, were down-regulated in a time-dependent manner, whereas the adherents junction protein E-cadherin was increased significantly, peaking 24 h after treatment. These results correlated with the changes in mRNA expression measured by RT-PCR (Figure 2B). This suggested that DK223 did not induced EMT, processes in HaCaT cells.

Figure 1. Effect of DK223 on the migration and proliferation of HaCaT cells. (**A**) Cells were seeded at a density of 3 × 10^4/mL 24 h before the scratch test. Scratch widths were measured 48 h after DK223 treatment. Data represent the mean width percentage ± SD for at least three replicates, * $p < 0.05$; (**B**) Cells were seeded at a density of 3 × 10^4/mL 24 h before treatment. The impedances were measured and analyzed at 24 h after treatment using the ECIS system software. The line data indicate the migration velocity of cells treated with different concentrations of DK223; (**C**) Cells were seeded overnight before treatment with varying concentrations of DK223 for 48 h. Cells were then incubated with MTT for 4 h at 37 °C, and the absorbance was measured at 570 nm; (**D**,**E**) The expression of cell cycle-related proteins in HaCaT cells induced by 2 μM DK223 for 24 h. Protein expression was examined by Western blot analysis with the specific antibodies indicated, and mRNA expression was assessed by RT-PCR with the gene-specific primers indicated. A histogram depicting the ImageJ data analysis results is shown. Values represent means ± SD of three independent experiments, * $p < 0.05$ compared with the control in all under experiments.

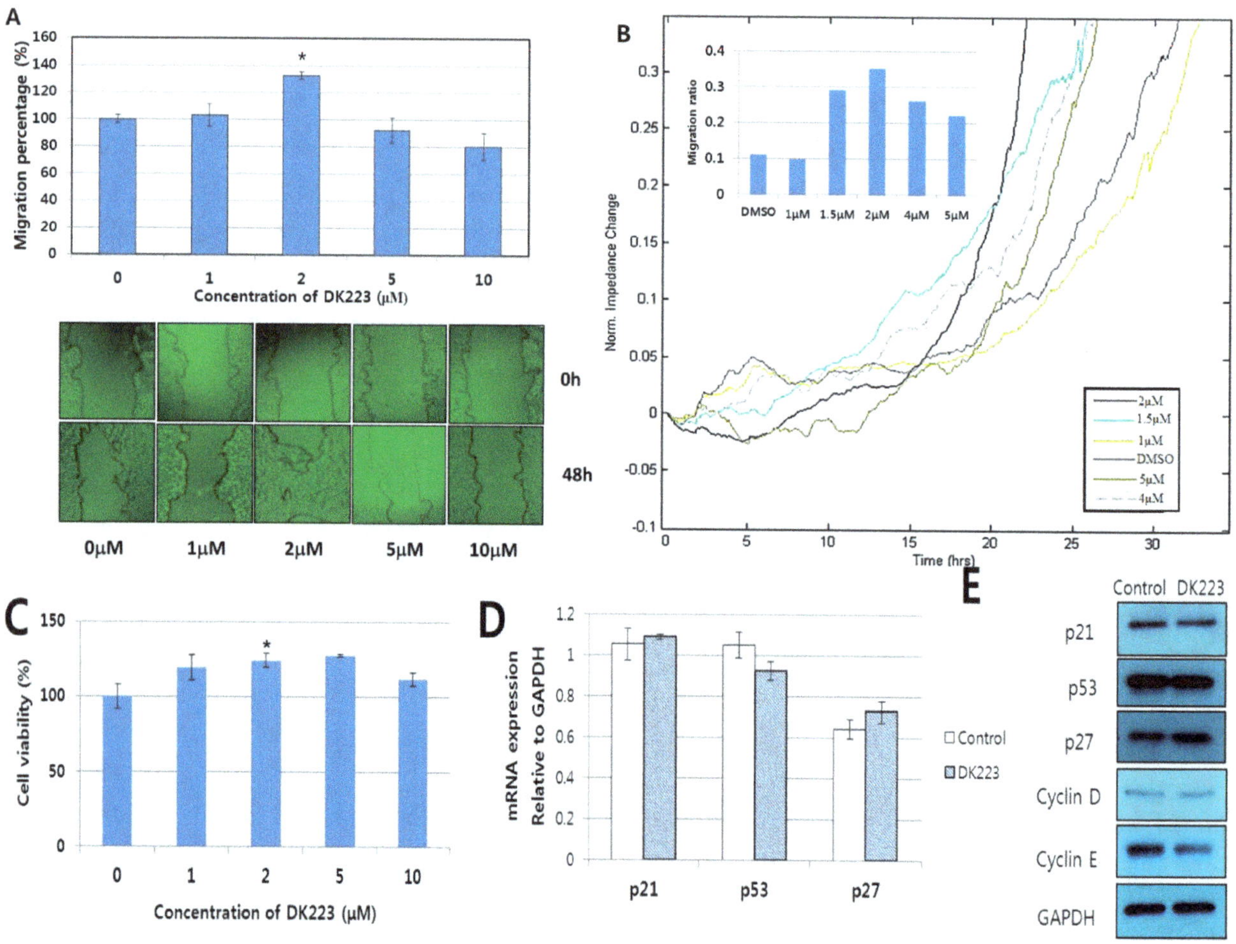

Figure 2. Time-dependent expression of EMT-related genes in HaCaT cells after treatment with DK223. (**A**) Protein expression was examined in HaCaT cells treated with 2 μM DK223 for different time periods using Western blot analysis with the specific antibodies indicated (**B**) mRNA expression was investigated by RT-PCR with the specific primers indicated.

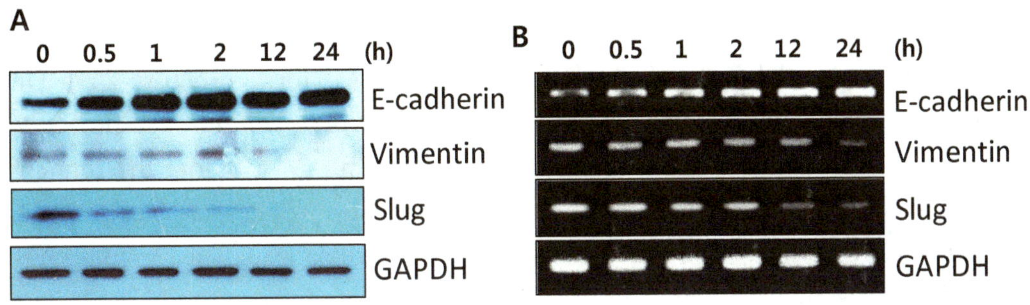

2.3. DK223 Induced NADPH Oxidase Expression and ROS Accumulation

To gain insight into the mechanism of keratinocyte migration induced by DK223, we assessed NADPH oxidase expression and ROS accumulation, as well as the signaling pathways related to cell migration. As demonstrated in Figure 3B,C, NADPH oxidase 4 mRNA and protein expression increased in a time-dependent manner, peaking 2 h after treatment. This correlated with an up-regulation in ROS accumulation, which also peaked at 2 h (Figure 3A), as well as with the effects on cellular signaling pathways. Phosphorylation of AKT was down-regulated at an early time point, while phosphorylation of ERK and JNK increased after 30 min of treatment (Figure 3D–F). These findings suggest a relationship between the early increase in ROS accumulation at 2 h and concomitant changes in intracellular signaling pathways.

2.4. DK223 Affected Signaling Pathways and Cell Migration via ROS Accumulation

To explore the mechanism mediating the effects of DK223 on signaling pathways and ROS accumulation, we pretreated cells with the NADPH inhibitor diphenylene iodonium (DPI) or the ROS scavenger *N*-acetylcysteine (NAC) prior to treatment with DK223 for 2 h. As expected, NADPH oxidase 4 was inhibited by DPI and NAC pretreatment. NAC also reduced DK223-induced phosphorylation of JNK and ERK. Interestingly, the activation of AKT, which was down-regulated by DK223 at 2 h, was also attenuated significantly in the presence of NAC and DPI (Figure 3G). These results indicated that DK223 induced the phosphorylation of JNK and ERK at 2 h via ROS accumulation. Interestingly, DK223-induced migration was inhibited significantly by NAC and DPI (Figure 3H), which indicated that the migration induced by DK223 might be regulate by ROS accumulation.

Figure 3. Time-dependent expression of NAPDH oxidase, ROS accumulation and signaling pathways in HaCaT cells after treatment with DK223. (**A**) Time- dependent ROS generation was detected in treated HaCaT cells using the DCF-DA assay. Cells were treated with 2 μM DK223 at different times and then stained with DCF-DA to detect ROS generation, as described previously. H_2O_2 was used as a positive control; (**B**,**C**) The expression of NAPDH oxidase 4 was examined by Western blot and RT-PCR, as described previously; (**D**–**F**) Signaling pathways were examined by Western blot with the specific antibodies indicated; (**G**) Cells were pretreated with 10 μM DPI or 20 μM NAC for 2 h before 24 h DK223 incubation. Signaling pathways were examined by Western blot with the specific antibodies indicated; (**H**) Cells were seeded at a density of 3 × 10^4/mL 24 h before the scratch test. Scratch widths were measured 48 h after DK223 treatment only or co-treatment with 10 μM DPI or 20 μM NAC. A histogram shows the results of ImageJ data analysis. Values represent means ± SD of three independent experiments, * $p < 0.05$ in all under experiments.

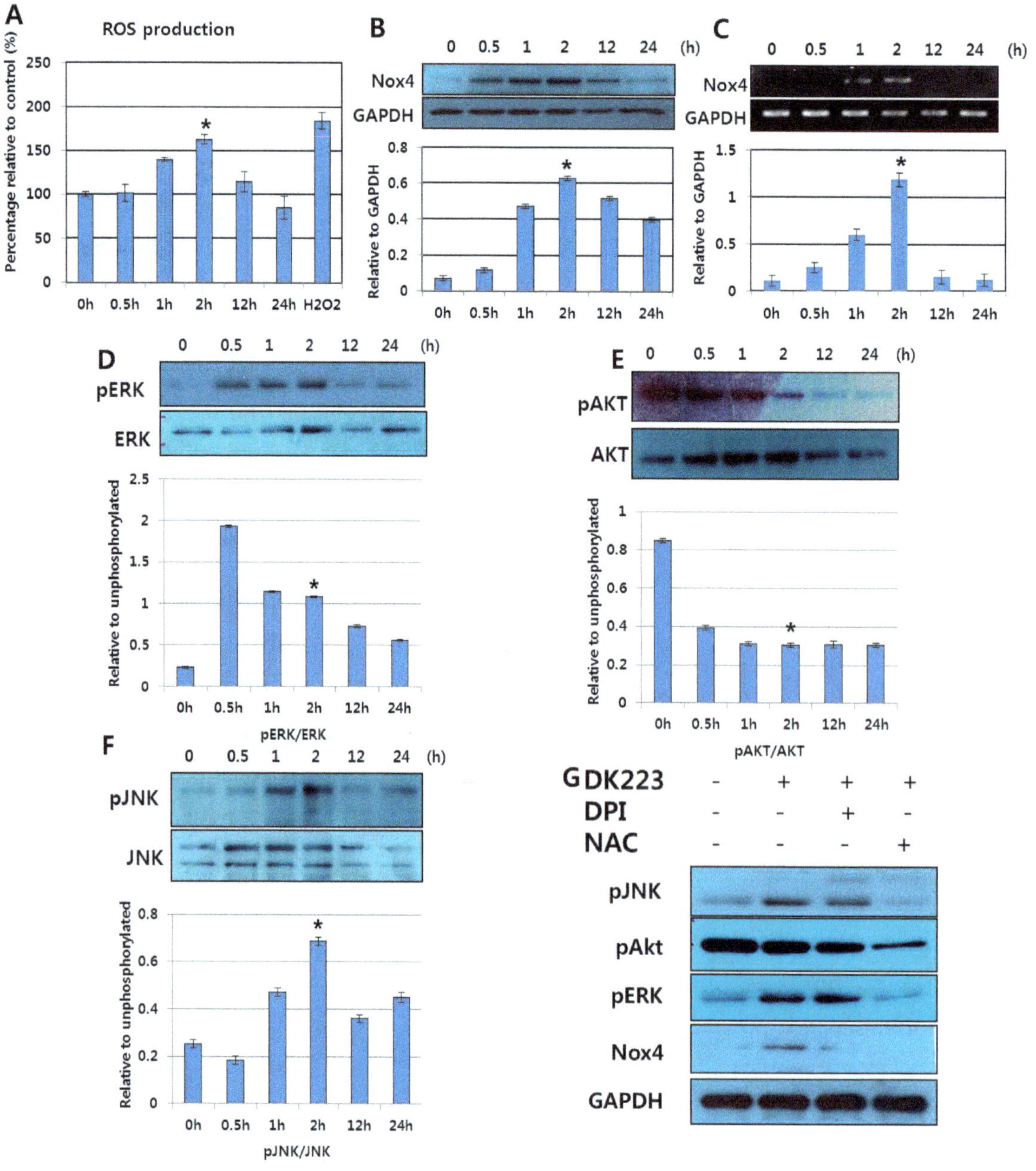

Figure 3. *Cont.*

H

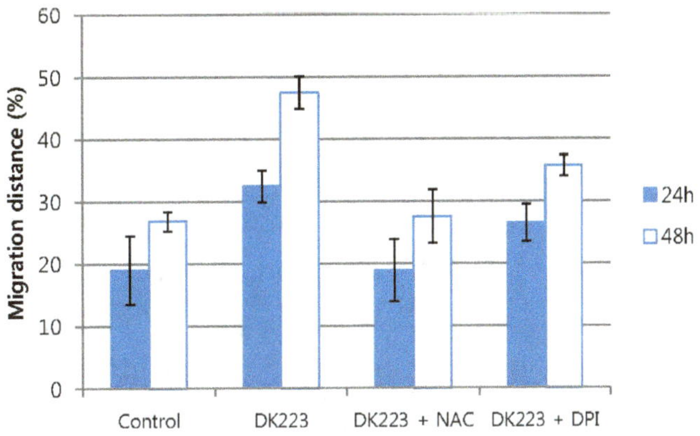

2.5. Migration-Related Proteins Are Down-Regulated by DK223 Treatment in HaCaT Cells

Because the EMT process did not appear to involve DK223-induced migration, we investigated other migration-related proteins, including the MMPs and collagen I and III in serum-free media which was concentrated by protein filter centrifugation (serum could block the filter). It has been demonstrated recently that these proteins could regulate the migration and proliferation of keratinocytes [14,15]. We observed a significant down-regulation in the mRNA and protein expression of collagen I and III after 24 h of DK223 treatment (Figure 4A–C), while the levels of MMP-1 were increased (Figure 4C) [14]. Thus, high levels of this proteinase might degrade collagen I and III upon DK223 treatment. Moreover, another ECM protein, fibronectin, was highly expressed (Figure 4A–C) with DK223 treatment, which might be associated with the down-regulation of MMP7 (Figure 4D). MMP7 is also known as a matrilysin, since it can use fibronectin as a cleavage substrate [15].

Alternatively, the mRNA expression of two other metalloproteinases, MMP2 and MMP9, also increased slightly compared with the control (Figure 4D), which correlated with results from the zymography assay for gelatinase activity of MMP2 and MMP9 (Figure 4E,F). These results indicate that the effects of DK223 on keratinocyte migration could be mediated by the degradation of collagen via a highly expressed collagenase.

2.6. DK223 Ameliorates Proliferation of Human Dermal Fibroblasts

Tissue formation, which is the second phase of wound healing, is characterized by migration and proliferation of different cell types. After the initiation of keratinocyte migration, fibroblasts tend to proliferate [2]. Therefore, we investigated the effects of DK223 on human dermal fibroblasts. We initially examined the proliferation of dermal fibroblasts in response to DK223 for 24 and 48 h using the MTT assay. These results demonstrated that DK223 induced dermal fibroblast proliferation in a dose-dependent manner in both 24 and 48 h (Figure 5A). There was no significant difference between 2 and 5 μM concentrations of DK223; thus, we used 2 μM in subsequent experiments.

To confirm the enhanced proliferation of fibroblasts treated with DK223, we evaluated the mRNA and protein expression of cell cycle-related genes. As shown by Western blot in Figure 5B, the protein levels of p21, p27 and p53 were down-regulated significantly after a 24 h exposure to 2 μM DK223, while cyclin D and cyclin E were increased. These results correlated with changes in mRNA expression measured by RT-PCR (Figure 5C) except for p27 expression, which was increased after DK223 treatment. These data further indicate that the proliferation of fibroblasts increased with 2 μM DK223 after 24 h.

In addition, the migration results showed that DK223 at 2 and 5 μM significantly enhanced migration of fibroblast in both 24 and 48 h, whereas other concentrations did not give high effects (Figure 5D).

Figure 4. Expression of extracellular matrix proteins and migration-related genes in HaCaT cells treated with DK223. (**A**) mRNA expression was examined in HaCaT cells treated with 2 μM DK223 for 24 h using RT-PCR with the specific primers indicated; (**B**) Cells were treated with 2 μM DK223 in serum-free media. Conditioned media were removed and concentrated using Amicon centrifugation. Proteins in the media were analyzed by Western blot for collagen I, III, and fibronectin using the specific antibodies indicated; (**C**) Proteins in the media was analyzed by Western blot for MMP1 using the specific antibodies indicated; (**D**) mRNA expression was examined in HaCaT cells treated with 2 μM DK223 for 24 h using RT-PCR with the specific primers indicated; (**E**,**F**) Zymograph assay of the conditioned media from HaCaT cells treated with 2 μM DK223 for 24 h. Conditioned media were removed and concentrated using Amicon centrifugation. Proteins in the media were analyzed by a gelatin zymograph, as described previously. A histogram shows the results of ImageJ data analysis. Data are represented as the mean percentage of distance ± SD from at least three replicates, * $p < 0.05$ in all under experiments.

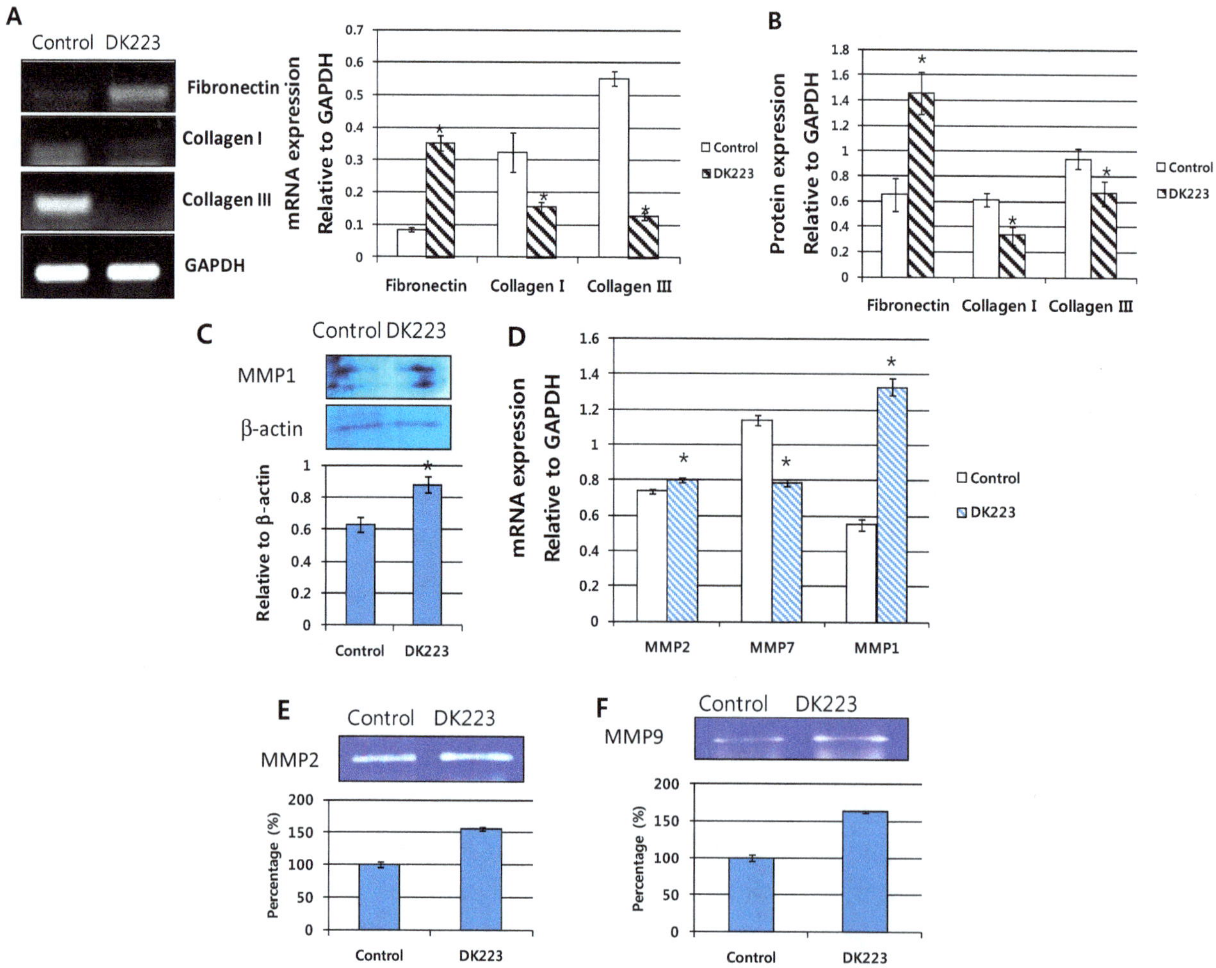

Figure 5. Proliferation and migration of dermal fibroblasts treated with DK223 and expression of cell- cycle-related genes in dermal fibroblasts after incubation with DK223. (**A**) Human dermal fibroblasts were seeded at a density of 3×10^4/mL for 24 and 48 h before treatment. MTT assay was performed as described previously; (**B,C**) The expressions of cell cycle-related genes, such as p21, p53, p27, cyclin E, cyclin D, were examined by Western blot and RT-PCR in 24 h as described previously; (**D**) Cells were seeded at a density of 3×10^4/mL 24 h before the scratch test. Scratch widths were measured 48 h after DK223 treatment. A histogram shows the results of ImageJ data analysis. Data are represented as the mean distance percentages ± SD from at least three replicates, * $p < 0.05$ in all under experiments.

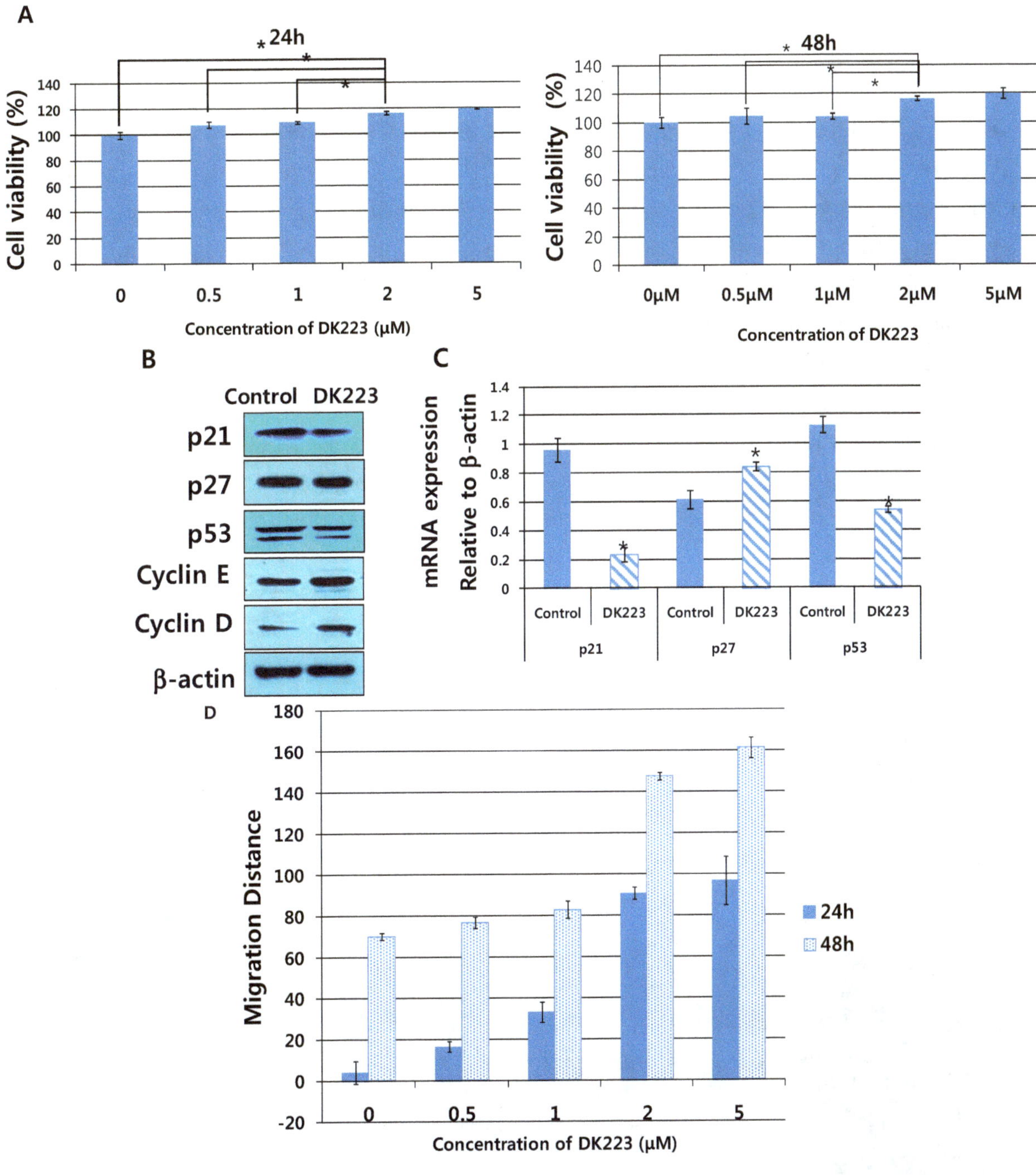

2.7. Dermal Fibroblasts Promote DK223-Induced ECM Deposition

The ECM contains components essential to wound healing, including collagen I, III, and fibronectin [16]. Therefore, we examined ECM protein secretion from fibroblasts induced by DK223 for 24 h. Western blot analysis revealed high levels of collagen I, III and fibronectin with DK223 treatment (Figure 6A), which correlated with mRNA expression (Figure 6B). Another mesenchymal marker, vimentin, was augmented significantly compared with the control, indicating myofibroblast differentiation and possible migration (Figure 6B). Notably, MMP1, a collagenase protein, was inhibited markedly when treated with DK223 (Figure 6B), which could explain the high levels of collagen I and III in DK223-treated fibroblasts. However, differential effects were seen between MMP2 and MMP9, also known as gelatinase A and gelatinase B. MMP2 was up-regulated in DK223 treatment, while MMP9 was down-regulated (Figure 6C,D). Thus, correlating the expression of these MMPs with our results requires further investigation.

Figure 6. Expression of extracellular matrix proteins and metalloproteinase genes. (**A**) Dermal fibroblasts were treated with 2 μM DK223 in serum-free media. Conditioned media were removed and concentrated using Amicon centrifugation. Proteins in the media were analyzed by Western blot for collagen I, III, fibronectin, MMP1, and vimentin with the specific antibodies indicated; (**B**) mRNA expression was examined in human dermal fibroblast cells treated with 2 μM DK223 for 24 h using RT-PCR and the specific primers indicated; (**C**,**D**) Zymograph assay of conditioned media from dermal fibroblasts treated with 2 μM DK223 for 24 h. Conditioned media were removed and concentrated using Amicon centrifugation. Proteins in the media were analyzed by a gelatin zymograph as described previously. A histogram shows the results of ImageJ data analysis. Data are represented as the mean distance percentages ± SD from at least three replicates, * $p < 0.05$.

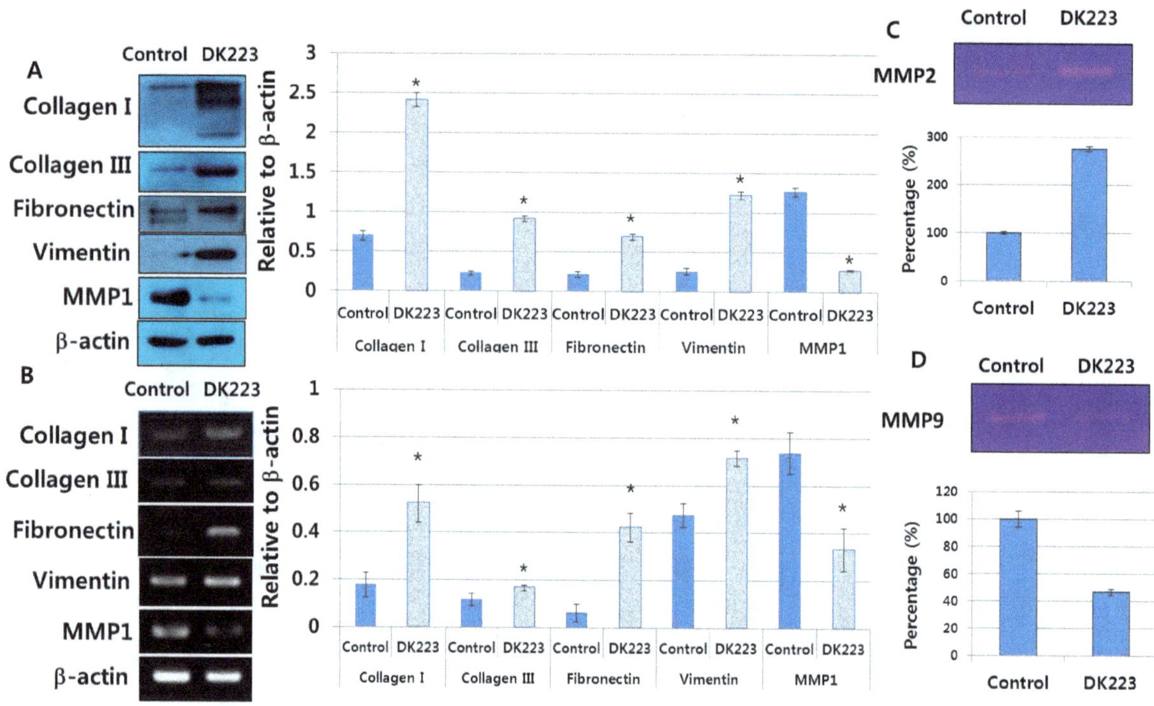

2.8. DK223 Induces TGF-β11 Secretion in Fibroblasts

Fibroblasts have a key role in wound healing because they secrete growth factors and cytokines, such as TGF-β1, connective transforming growth factor (CTGF), IL-6 and IL-8 [17]. We investigated the production of TGF-β1 in DK223-treated fibroblasts to determine whether proliferation could be correlated with collagen deposition in fibroblasts. We found that DK223 significantly increased TGF-β1 mRNA expression (Figure 7A).

Figure 7. The effect of DK223 on TGF-β1 expression and on dermal fibroblast signaling pathways in response to a TGF-β1 receptor inhibitor. (**A**) Dermal fibroblasts were treated with 2 μM DK223 in serum-free media. TGF-β1 mRNA expression was examined in fibroblast cells treated with 2 μM DK223 for 48 h using RT-PCR with specific primers; (**B**,**D**) Dermal fibroblasts were treated with 2 μM DK223 in serum-free medium for different time periods; (**C**,**E**) Dermal fibroblasts were pretreated with 10 μM TGF-β1 receptor inhibitor (TGFRI)—LY2157299 before incubating with DK223 for 6 h. Signaling pathways were examined by Western blot with the specific antibodies indicated. A histogram shows the results of ImageJ data analysis. Values represent the means ± SD of three independent experiments, * $p < 0.05$ compared with the control in all under experiments.

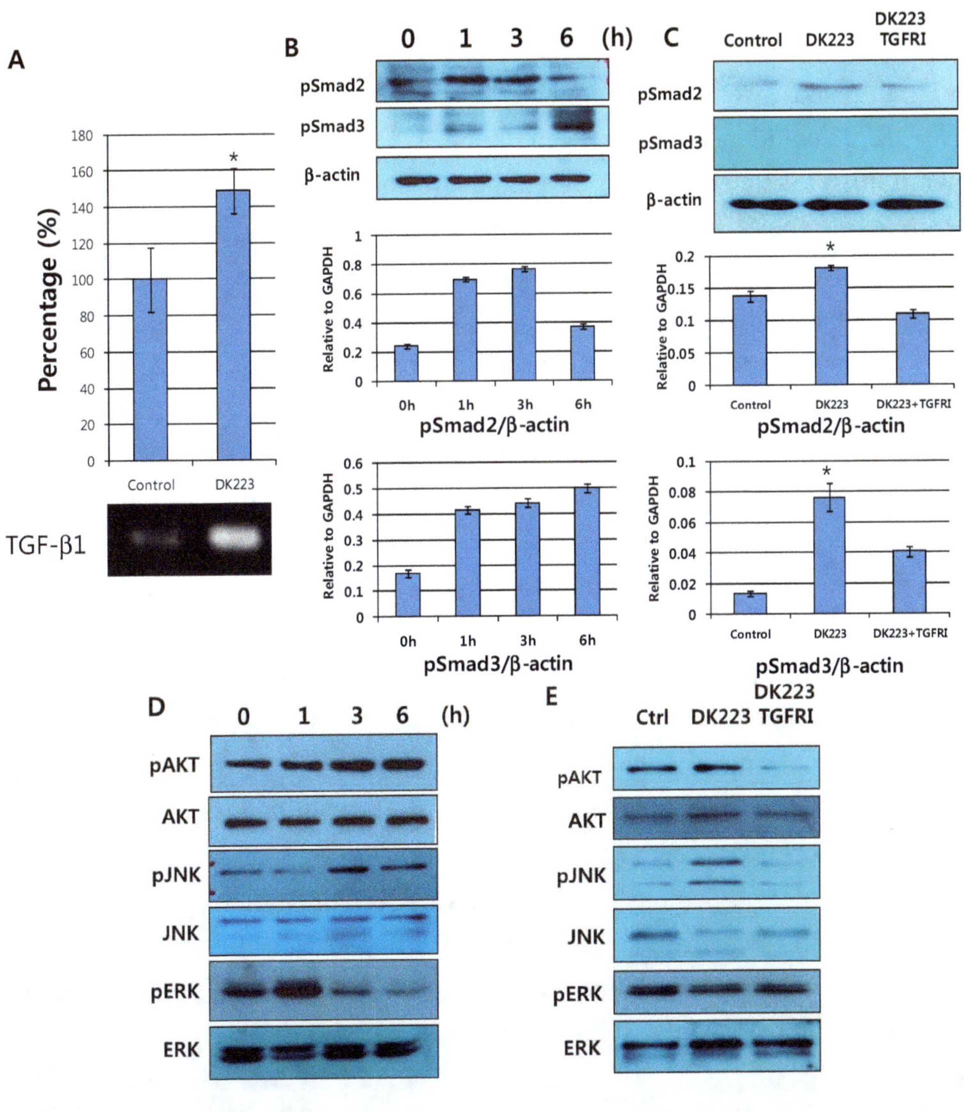

It has been suggested that TGF-β1 might promote fibroblast proliferation [18]. Thus, we investigated the correlations between DK223-induced TGF-β1 cellular changes in fibroblasts by examining the activation of various signaling pathways. The results demonstrated that the phosphorylation of AKT, a potential oncogene, was elevated in a time-dependent manner (Figure 7D). In addition, we observed early activation of pSmad2 at 1 h and increased phosphorylation of pSmad3 (Figure 7B) accompanied by the significant activation of JNK at 6 h (Figure 7D). These events indicate that DK223 activates the JNK/pSmad3L/c-Myc oncogenic pathway that mediates increased proliferation of fibroblasts. Interestingly, ERK phosphorylation was down-regulated below basal levels after an initial early increase at 1 h (Figure 7D). This could be the mechanism underlying the anti-proliferative response of the Ras/Raf/MEK/ERK signaling pathway that was previously reported in primary human fibroblasts [19,20]. Taken together, these results suggest that TGF-β1 signaling pathways mediate fibroblast proliferation in response to DK223.

To confirm the involvement of TGF-β1, we treated cells with a TGF-β1 receptor inhibitor (TGFRI), which significantly inhibited pSmad2, pSmad3, JNK, and Akt phosphorylation (Figure 7C,E). Furthermore, TGFRI pretreatment restored ERK phosphorylation to normal levels (Figure 7E). In summary, our results indicate that DK223 modified cellular signaling pathways by elevating TGF-β1 secretion.

3. Discussion

The wound repair process protects the human body from infections and fluid loss; yet, it results in scar formation. In this study, we investigated the effects of DK223 on wound healing processes with the expectation that DK223 could induce skin regeneration.

Skin regeneration is characterized by a re-epithelialization process that covers the wound surface and stimulates re-angiogenesis [21]. After the wound has been blocked by a blood clot, fibroblasts begin secreting ECM proteins, such as collagen III and fibronectin. These proteins reorganize the base structure under the blood clot to aid in keratinocyte migration [1]. We have studied this phenomenon by treating human keratinocytes with different concentrations of DK223 *in vitro*. While DK223 did not promote keratinocyte cell growth, migration was enhanced significantly. Mesenchymal markers, such as Vimentin and Slug, were down-regulated in a time-dependent manner, whereas the epithelial marker E-cadherin was increased markedly. This indicates that keratinocytes did not induce the EMT process and that the cells were bound together more tightly as migration increased. This phenomenon was compatible with our previous report of increased keratinocyte migration and higher levels of junction and adherent proteins, such as E-cadherin [22]. This was also reported by Li *et al.*, who showed that a whole sheet of epithelial cells could migrate while maintaining tight cell-cell adhesion, a phenomenon they called "collective migration" [23]. As shown in Figure 3, DK223 significantly up-regulated E-cadherin, which plays an important role in re-epithelialization since adherent junctions prevent the epithelial barrier from further damage after wounding [23]. This indicates that DK223 was able to induce collective migration to protect the epithelial barrier from wounds.

In a recent study, Kim *et al.* demonstrated that HaCaT keratinocyte migration was induced by the EGF-like ligand neuregulin, which was activated via Rac1 and Nox-driven ROS accumulation [24]. In our study, DK223 also significantly increased HaCaT cell migration via intracellular signaling pathways. Our results demonstrated that ROS accumulation peaked at 2 h, along with signaling proteins, such as AKT and ERK. In recent studies, AKT2 was shown to induce cell migration [25] and ERK/MAPK phosphorylation might be activated by ROS [26,27]. In addition, ERK/MAPK phosphorylation ameliorated keratinocyte migration [28]. In light of these results, we propose that DK223 induces keratinocyte migration by modulating intracellular signaling pathways via ROS accumulation.

Dermal fibroblasts are the primary ECM-producing cell type in the skin [29]. Once the wound has formed a blood clot via fibrin, dermal fibroblasts proliferate and infiltrate under the wound [16]. These cells secrete collagen and fibronectin, which replace the clot fibrin to accelerate wound closure [16]. Nevertheless, ECM accumulation in instances of excessive healing may cause unaesthetic scars [2]. In this study, DK223 induced keratinocyte migration and promoted the fibroblast-to-myofibroblast transition to help the wound heal more rapidly [30], with the evidence that vimentin was upregulated in fibroblasts, whereas it modulated ECM production in keratinocytes and fibroblasts. Furthermore, DK223 treatment increased fibronectin expression in both fibroblasts and keratinocytes. It is well known that fibronectin, which is normally produced in the first stage of wound healing, acts as the scaffold for collagen deposition and assists in cell migration to promote the wound healing process [31,32]. Collagens I and III are the main products of the wound healing process. Production of these collagens is necessary for wound healing; however, collagen deposition can promote scar formation. Thus, collagen production must be controlled for ideal wound healing. The DK223 effect resulted in increased collagen in fibroblasts, whereas a reduction in keratinocytes was seen. Correspondingly, levels of the collagenase MMP1 were also increased in keratinocytes and reduced in fibroblasts. These observations suggest a regulatory role for DK223 in maintaining the balance of ECM production in skin repair. Similarly, Xie *et al.* reported that basic fibroblast growth factor (bFGF) improved wound healing by regulating the balance of ECM synthesis and degradation [33]. These simultaneous effects balance ECM production in the wound healing process and might prevent keloid scar formation. Thus, DK223 differentially modulates MMPs and ECM production in keratinocytes and fibroblasts to regulate individual cell functions during wound healing.

According to our data, DK223 affects both keratinocyte migration and fibroblast proliferation to accelerate the wound healing process. It has been previously demonstrated that other novel compounds also exhibit similar effects. Lee *et al.* reported that heat-processed ginseng (sun ginseng) protected against UVB-induced damage in keratinocytes and fibroblasts by restoring Bcl-2 and Bcl-xL mRNA levels in keratinocytes to reduce UVB-induced apoptosis, and promote procollagen production in dermal fibroblasts by inhibiting MMP-1 gene expression [34]. Werner *et al.* also reported that the keratinocyte-fibroblast interaction is also important for wound healing as keratinocytes modulate fibroblast to myofibroblast differentiation by secreting the growth factor-like TGF-β1, which increases production of myofibroblasts in ECM [35]. Moreover, Singh *et al.* suggested an alternative approach for wound healing by focusing on the effects of traditional medicines on keratinocytes and fibroblasts. Their bioactive compound increased both types of skin cells and reduced free-radical production to support the wound closure process [36].

TGF-β1 can participate in the wound healing process by inducing fibroblast migration and proliferation [37], activating the MMP family [38] and stimulating re-epithelialization [37]. It has been demonstrated that TGF-β1 expression was elevated significantly by excessive wound healing, leading to keloid scarring [39,40]. In our study, DK223 slightly increased TGF-β1 expression in fibroblasts, indicating that it did not promote scarring.

4. Materials and Methods

4.1. Reagent

The DK223 (Figure 1A) compound was synthesized and kindly provided by Youngho Lim in the Division of Bioscience and Biotechnology, Konkuk University, Seoul, Korea. K_2CO_3 (5 mmol, 692 mg) was dissolved in a solution of 2-hydroxy-5-methoxybenzaldehyde (**I**, 5 mmol, 760 mg) and acrolein (**II**, 7 mmol, 0.5 mL) in 1,4-dioxane (50 mL) and the reaction mixture was refluxed for 6 h. The solvent was evaporated and residue was extracted with diethyl ether (100 mL) and water (50 mL). Combined organic layers were dried over $MgSO_4$. Filtration and evaporation produced aldehyde (**III**, 86%, m.p. 48–50 °C), which was used for next step without further purification. *p*-Nitroacylhydrazine (**IV**, 2 mmol, 334 mg) and 6-methoxy-2*H*-chromene-3-carbaldehyde (**III**, 3 mmol, 570 mg) were dissolved in ethanol (30 mL) and a catalytic volume of conc. HCl was added. The resulting mixture was refluxed for 2 h. The reaction formed intermediates **V** and **VI**, which eventually produced DK233. A similar reaction has been reported previously [41]. After cooling to room temperature, the resulting precipitate was filtered and washed with ethanol. Recrystallization of crude solid resulted in pure DK223 (355 mg, 50%, m.p. 246–250 °C; (Figure 8B)).

Figure 8. (**A**) Chemical structure of DK223; (**B**) Method of DK223 synthesis, as described in the Materials and Methods section.

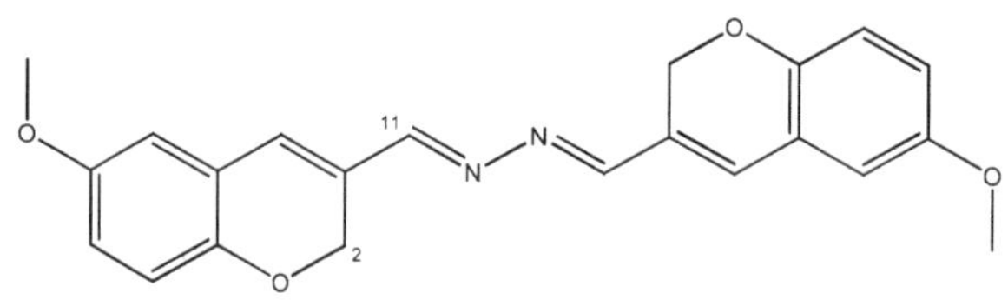

(1*E*,2*E*)-1,2-bis((6-methoxy-2*H*-chromen-3-yl)methylene)hydrazine

(A)

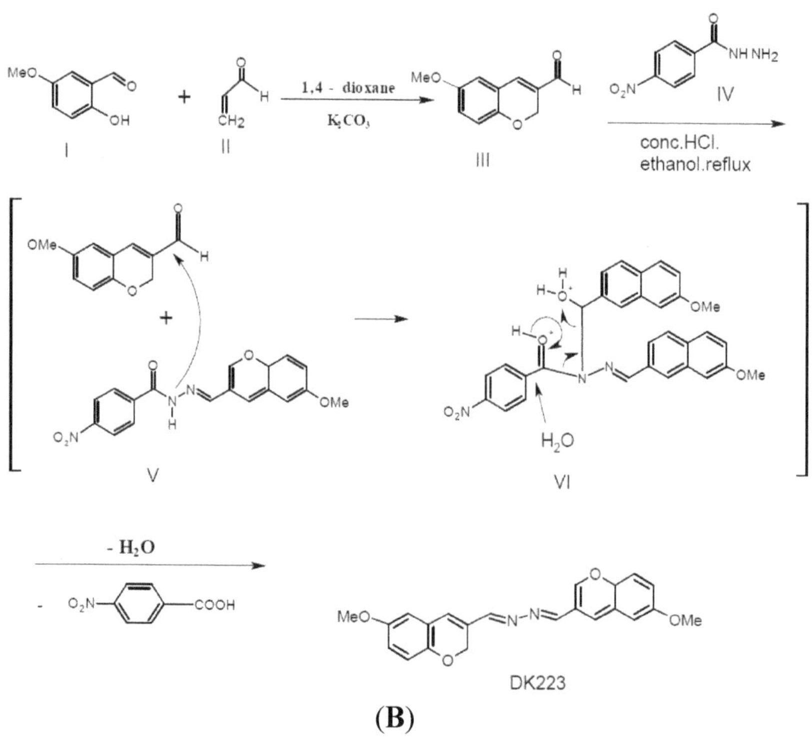

(B)

4.2. Cell Culture

In this study, we used the spontaneously immortalized keratinocyte cell line (HaCaT) and human dermal fibroblasts. HaCaT cells were cultured in RPMI medium (GIBCO, Grand Island, NY, USA) supplemented with 10% fetal bovine serum (FBS; GIBCO) and 1% penicillin/streptomycin (PAA Laboratories GmBH, Strasse, Austria). Human dermal fibroblast cells were cultured in DMEM media supplemented with 10% FBS (GIBCO) and 1% penicillin/streptomycin (PAA). Cells were incubated in a humidified atmosphere at 37 °C with 5% CO_2.

4.3. Scratch Wound Healing Assay

HaCaT cells were seeded in a 48-well plate before a 24 h wound healing scratch assay [42]. The scratch wound was made using a sterile 200 µL pipette tip to scratch a line across the bottom of the culture dish. Culture media was then removed and replaced with fresh media supplemented with DK223 or dimethyl sulfoxide (DMSO) (Amresco, Solon, OH, USA) as a control. Photographs were taken at 4× magnification using an OLYMPUS IX70 microscope equipped with a digital camera before treatment and 48 h after treatment. The width of the scratch was measured by the distance from the both edge of scratch by ImageJ software (National Institutes of Health, Bethesda, MD, USA). Each scratch was measured 60 times across the span of wound scratch and calculated the average to compare the migration after 24 or 48 h. The experiments were repeated 3 dependent times.

4.4. Migration Assay with the Electric Cell-Substrate Impedance Sensing (ECIS) System

ECIS® (Electric Cell-substrate Impedance Sensing) is a real-time, label-free, impedance-based method of assessing the activities of cells grown in tissue culture. When cells are added to the ECIS Arrays and attached to the electrodes, they act as insulators and increase the impedance. As cells grow and cover the electrodes, the current is impeded in a manner related to the number of cells covering the electrode, the morphology of the cells, and the nature of the cell attachment. When cells are stimulated to change their function, the accompanying changes in cell morphology alter the impedance. Data are generated as impedance *versus* time.

Electrode plates (eight wells, Applied Biophysics, Troy, NY, USA) were induced with an electrode-stabilizing solution provided by the manufacturer 10 min prior to seeding with HaCaT cells overnight. Cells were then treated with different concentrations of DK223. After 24 h, the electrode plates were placed in the ECIS apparatus in the incubator for migration analysis using the ECIS system software, according to the manufacturer's instructions (Applied Biophysics, Troy, NY, USA).

4.5. MTT Assay

Cells were seeded in a 96-well plate at a density of 3×10^4/mL. HaCaT cells were treated with DK223 or DMSO for 24 h, while dermal fibroblasts were treated for 48 h. MTT solution 5 mg/mL (Amresco, OH, USA) was added to each well and incubated at 37 °C for 4 h. The medium was then gently removed and replaced with 150 µL DMSO, followed by shaking for 30 min to dissolve the precipitate, and the absorbance was measured at 570 nm.

4.6. Western Blot

Cells were treated with DK223 or DMSO in a time- and dose-dependent manner. Cells lysate proteins were then harvested using a cell scraper and lysed in RIPA buffer. The protein concentration was determined using the bicinchoninic (BCA) assay (Thermo Scientific, Rockford, IL, USA). The protein in conditioned media (serum free media after treated cell with DK223) was concentrated by Amicon (Milipore, Darmstadt, Germany) centrifuge following manufacture instruction. The protein in media after centrifugation was determined the concentration using the Bardford assay (Bio-Rad, Hercules, CA USA). The proteins were separated by SDS-PAGE, followed by Western blot using the appropriate antibodies.

All antibodies for Western blot were purchased commercially and prepared according to the manufacturer's protocol. p21 (2947), AKT (9272), phosphorylated AKT (9271S), ERK (4695), Slug (9585S), and GAPDH (2118) were obtained from Cell Signaling (Danvers, MA, USA). E-cadherin (610181) was purchased from BD Science Transduction (San Jose, CA, USA). Cyclin E (sc-247), cyclin D1 (sc-246), p53 (sc-126), phosphorylated ERK (sc-7383), collagen I (sc-25974), collagen III (sc-28888), and fibronectin (sc-9068) were purchased from Santa Cruz Biotechnologies (Santa Cruz, Dallas, TX, USA). MMP1 (444209) was purchased from Calbiochem (Hessen, Darmstadt, Germany). We used anti-mouse (PI-2000, Vector Labs Inc., Burlingame, CA, USA), anti-rabbit (PI-1000, Vector Labs), and anti-goat (AP-107P, Millipore, Billerica, MA, USA) secondary antibodies. Differences were confirmed using ImageJ software to determine the relative ratio of changes in the target protein levels to those of the DMSO control.

4.7. RT-PCR

Total RNA from treated cells was extracted using TRIzol reagent (Invitrogen, Grand Island, NY, USA). Equal amounts of total RNA in each treatment group were used to synthesize cDNA using a reverse transcriptase kit (Promega, Seoul, Korea). The resulting cDNA was used for RT-PCR using the G-Taq kit (Cosmo Genetech, Seoul, Korea) based on the manufacturer's protocols.

RT-PCR was performed using the following gene-specific primers designed using the Blast Primer website: GAPDH, forward primer 5'-GAAGGTGAAGGTCGGAGTC-3', reverse primer 5'-GAAGATGGTGATGGATTTC-3'; p53, forward primer 5'-ACACGCTTCCCTGGATTGG-3', reverse primer 5'-CTGGCATTCTGGGAGCTTCA-3'; p21, forward primer 5'-GTCAGTTCCTTG AGCCG-3', reverse primer 5'-GAAGGTAGAGCTTGGGCAGG-3'; and MMP1, forward primer 5'-AGGGGAGATCATCGGGAC-3', reverse primer 5'-GGCTGGACAGGATTTTGG-3'; MMP2, forward primer 5'-AACACCTTCTATGGCTGCCC-3', reverse primer 5'-ACGAGCAAAGGCATC ACCA-3'; MMP7, forward primer 5'-TACAGTGGGAACAGGCTAGG-3', reverse primer 5'-GGCACTCCACATCTGGGC-3'. ImageJ software was used to analyze the results and the relative ratio of changes in the target gene to those of the DMSO control.

4.8. MMP Zymograph Assay

An MMP zymograph assay was performed according to the method described by Gogly *et al.* and modified with use of 8% sodium dodecyl sulfate (SDS) gels mixed with gelatin (0.01 mg/mL). The SDS in the gels was removed by two 30 min incubations in 200 mL 2.5% Triton X-100 at 4 °C, and the gel slabs were incubated at 37 °C overnight in incubation buffer. The gels were subsequently fixed and stained for 1 h in 0.05% Coomassie Blue R-250. The molecular weight protein marker was clearly visible as light blue bands against the blue background. Gelatinase activity was detected as clear zones of negative staining against the blue background. The gels were scanned as permanent records of the results [43].

4.9. ROS Generation Analysis

Accumulation of ROS was measured based on ROS-dependent oxidation of the oxidation-sensitive fluorescent probe 2'7'-dichlorofluorescin diacetate (DCFH-DA) to DCF [44]. Cells were seeded in a 96-well plate (3×10^4 cells/mL) for 24 h before flavonoid treatment and then treated with 2 μM DK223 for 0, 0.5, 1, 2, 12, and 24 h. H_2O_2 was used as a positive control. The cells were washed with PBS before removing medium, 200 μL of DCFH-DA (100 μM in PBS containing 1% FBS) were added, and the cells were incubated for 30 min at 37 °C in the dark. Intracellular ROS accumulation was measured using DCFH-DA with a DCF-DA microplate assay. A spectrofluorometer (SPECTRAFLUOR, Tecan, Männedorf, Switzerland) was used to assess ROS generation by measuring the fluorescence intensities from 10,000 cells/well at an excitation wavelength of 485 nm and an emission wavelength of 530 nm.

4.10. Statistics

The results were expressed as means ± standard deviation (S.D.). Group comparisons were performed using the SPSS v.16.0 software (SPSS Inc., Chicago, IL, USA) with one-way analysis (ANOVA) and Student's *t*-test. $p < 0.05$ was considered to indicate statistical significance. All experiments were repeated at least in triplicate.

5. Conclusions

In conclusion, the novel compound DK223 has potent capabilities in wound healing and skin regeneration. It induced keratinocyte migration and fibroblast proliferation, while maintaining balance among ECM proteins, such as collagen I, III, and fibronectin. Taken together, DK223 potentially aids wound healing and attenuates keloid scar development.

Acknowledgments

This work was supported by a grant from the Next Generation BioGreen 21 Program (No. PJ009045) funded by the Rural Development Administration, Korea.

Author Contributions

Manh Tin Ho and Hyun Sik Kang designed and carried out the experiments. Jung Sik Huh prepared and supplied primary human dermal fibroblast. Young Mee Kim planned and discussed in results analysis and arrangement. Youngho Lim synthesized and supplied the novel compound DK223. Moonjae Cho wrote the manuscript and supervised all the process.

References

1. Reinke, J.M.; Sorg, H. Wound repair and regeneration. *Eur. Surg. Res. Eur. Chir. Forsch. Rech. Chir. Eur.* **2012**, *49*, 35–43.
2. Gurtner, G.C.; Werner, S.; Barrandon, Y.; Longaker, M.T. Wound repair and regeneration. *Nature* **2008**, *453*, 314–321.
3. Cowan, M.M. Plant products as antimicrobial agents. *Clin. Microbiol. Rev.* **1999**, *12*, 564–582.
4. Lopez-Jornet, P.; Camacho-Alonso, F.; Gomez-Garcia, F.; Molina Minano, F.; Canas, X.; Serafin, A.; Castillo, J.; Vicente-Ortega, V. Effects of potassium apigenin and verbena extract on the wound healing process of SKH-1 mouse skin. *Int. Wound J.* **2012**, doi:10.1111/j.1742-481X.2012.01114.x.
5. Duarte, C.M.; Quirino, M.R.; Patrocinio, M.C.; Anbinder, A.L. Effects of *Chamomilla recutita* (L.) on oral wound healing in rats. *Med. Oral Patol. Oral Y Cir. Bucal* **2011**, *16*, e716–e721.
6. Philips, N.; Samuel, M.; Arena, R.; Chen, Y.J.; Conte, J.; Natarajan, P.; Haas, G.; Gonzalez, S. Direct inhibition of elastase and matrixmetalloproteinases and stimulation of biosynthesis of fibrillar collagens, elastin, and fibrillins by xanthohumol. *J. Cosmet. Sci.* **2010**, *61*, 125–132.
7. Galicka, A.; Nazaruk, J. Stimulation of collagen biosynthesis by flavonoid glycosides in skin fibroblasts of osteogenesis imperfecta type I and the potential mechanism of their action. *Int. J. Mol. Med.* **2007**, *20*, 889–895.
8. Johnson, L.L.; Dyer, R.; Hupe, D.J. Matrix metalloproteinases. *Curr. Opin. Chem. Biol.* **1998**, *2*, 466–471.
9. Dang, C.M.; Beanes, S.R.; Lee, H.; Zhang, X.; Soo, C.; Ting, K. Scarless fetal wounds are associated with an increased matrix metalloproteinase-to-tissue-derived inhibitor of metalloproteinase ratio. *Plast. Reconstr. Surg.* **2003**, *111*, 2273–2285.
10. Kahari, V.M.; Saarialho-Kere, U. Matrix metalloproteinases in skin. *Exp. Dermatol.* **1997**, *6*, 199–213.
11. Catanzaro, R.; Marotta, F.; Jain, S.; Rastmanesh, R.; Allegri, F.; Celep, G.; Lorenzetti, A.; Polimeni, A.; Yadav, H. Beneficial effect of a sturgeon-based bioactive compound on gene expression of tumor necrosis factor-alpha, matrix metalloproteinases and type-10 collagen in human chondrocytes. *J. Biol. Regul. Homeost. Agents* **2012**, *26*, 337–345.
12. Lee, K.H. Discovery and development of natural product-derived chemotherapeutic agents based on a medicinal chemistry approach. *J. Nat. Prod.* **2010**, *73*, 500–516.
13. Rasanen, K.; Vaheri, A. TGF-beta1 causes epithelial-mesenchymal transition in HaCaT derivatives, but induces expression of COX-2 and migration only in benign, not in malignant keratinocytes. *J. Dermatol. Sci.* **2010**, *58*, 97–104.
14. Barrientos, S.; Stojadinovic, O.; Golinko, M.S.; Brem, H.; Tomic-Canic, M. Growth factors and cytokines in wound healing. *Wound Repair Regen.* **2008**, *16*, 585–601.
15. Visse, R.; Nagase, H. Matrix metalloproteinases and tissue inhibitors of metalloproteinases: Structure, function, and biochemistry. *Circ. Res.* **2003**, *92*, 827–839.
16. McDougall, S.; Dallon, J.; Sherratt, J.; Maini, P. Fibroblast migration and collagen deposition during dermal wound healing: Mathematical modelling and clinical implications. *Philos. Trans. Ser. A Math. Phys. Eng. Sci.* **2006**, *364*, 1385–1405.
17. Wick, G.; Backovic, A.; Rabensteiner, E.; Plank, N.; Schwentner, C.; Sgonc, R. The immunology of fibrosis: Innate and adaptive responses. *Trends Immunol.* **2010** *31*, 110–119.

18. Leask, A.; Abraham, D.J. TGF-beta signaling and the fibrotic response. *FASEB J.* **2004**, *18*, 816–827.
19. Steelman, L.S.; Chappell, W.H.; Abrams, S.L.; Kempf, R.C.; Long, J.; Laidler, P.; Mijatovic, S.; Maksimovic-Ivanic, D.; Stivala, F.; Mazzarino, M.C.; *et al.* Roles of the Raf/MEK/ERK and PI3K/PTEN/Akt/mTOR pathways in controlling growth and sensitivity to therapy-implications for cancer and aging. *Aging* **2011**, *3*, 192–222.
20. Chang, F.; Steelman, L.S.; Lee, J.T.; Shelton, J.G.; Navolanic, P.M.; Blalock, W.L.; Franklin, R.A.; McCubrey, J.A. Signal transduction mediated by the Ras/Raf/MEK/ERK pathway from cytokine receptors to transcription factors: Potential targeting for therapeutic intervention. *Leukemia* **2003**, *17*, 1263–1293.
21. Murawala, P.; Tanaka, E.M.; Currie, J.D. Regeneration: The ultimate example of wound healing. *Semin. Cell Dev. Biol.* **2012**, *23*, 954–962.
22. Bui, N.T.; Ho, M.T.; Kim, Y.M.; Lim, Y.; Cho, M. Flavonoids promoting HaCaT migration: II. Molecular mechanism of 4',6,7-trimethoxyisoflavone via NOX2 activation. *Phytomedicine* **2014**, *21*, 570–577.
23. Li, L.; Hartley, R.; Reiss, B.; Sun, Y.; Pu, J.; Wu, D.; Lin, F.; Hoang, T.; Yamada, S.; Jiang, J.; *et al.* E-cadherin plays an essential role in collective directional migration of large epithelial sheets. *Cell Mol. Life Sci.* **2012**, *69*, 2779–2789.
24. Kim, J.S.; Bak, E.J.; Lee, B.C.; Kim, Y.S.; Park, J.B.; Choi, I.G. Neuregulin induces HaCaT keratinocyte migration via Rac1-mediated NADPH-oxidase activation. *J. Cell. Physiol.* **2011**, *226*, 3014–3021.
25. Irie, H.Y.; Pearline, R.V.; Grueneberg, D.; Hsia, M.; Ravichandran, P.; Kothari, N.; Natesan, S.; Brugge, J.S. Distinct roles of Akt1 and Akt2 in regulating cell migration and epithelial-mesenchymal transition. *J. Cell Biol.* **2005**, *171*, 1023–1034.
26. Thannickal, V.J.; Fanburg, B.L. Reactive oxygen species in cell signaling. *Am. J. Physiol. Lung Cell Mol. Physiol.* **2000**, *279*, L1005–L1028.
27. Jiang, F.; Zhang, Y.; Dusting, G.J. NADPH oxidase-mediated redox signaling: Roles in cellular stress response, stress tolerance, and tissue repair. *Pharmacol. Rev.* **2011**, *63*, 218–242.
28. Huang, C.; Jacobson, K.; Schaller, M.D. MAP kinases and cell migration. *J. Cell Sci.* **2004**, *117*, 4619–4628.
29. Roh, S.S.; Lee, M.H.; Hwang, Y.L.; Song, H.H.; Jin, M.H.; Park, S.G.; Lee, C.K.; Kim, C.D.; Yoon, T.J.; Lee, J.H. Stimulation of the extracellular matrix production in dermal fibroblasts by velvet antler extract. *Ann. Dermatol.* **2010**, *22*, 173–179.
30. Van de Water, L.; Varney, S.; Tomasek, J.J. Mechanoregulation of the myofibroblast in wound contraction, scarring, and fibrosis: Opportunities for new therapeutic intervention. *Adv. Wound Care* **2013**, *2*, 122–141.
31. Kischer, C.W.; Hendrix, M.J. Fibronectin (FN) in hypertrophic scars and keloids. *Cell Tissue Res.* **1983**, *231*, 29–37.
32. Spyrou, G.E.; Naylor, I.L. The effect of basic fibroblast growth factor on scarring. *Br. J. Plast. Surg.* **2002**, *55*, 275–282.
33. Xie, J.; Bian, H.; Qi, S.; Xu, Y.; Tang, J.; Li, T.; Liu, X. Effects of basic fibroblast growth factor on the expression of extracellular matrix and matrix metalloproteinase-1 in wound healing. *Clin. Exp. Dermatol.* **2008**, *33*, 176–182.

34. Lee, H.; Lee, J.Y.; Song, K.C.; Kim, J.; Park, J.H.; Chun, K.H.; Hwang, G.S. Protective effect of processed panax ginseng, sun ginseng on UVB-irradiated human skin keratinocyte and human dermal fibroblast. *J. Ginseng Res.* **2012**, *36*, 68–77.
35. Werner, S.; Krieg, T.; Smola, H. Keratinocyte-fibroblast interactions in wound healing. *J. Investig. Dermatol.* **2007**, *127*, 998–1008.
36. Singh, D.; Choi, S.M.; Zo, S.M.; Painuli, R.M.; Kwon, S.W.; Han, S.S. Effect of extracts of terminalia chebula on proliferation of keratinocytes and fibroblasts cells: An alternative approach for wound healing. *Evid. Based Complement. Altern. Med.* **2014**, *2014*, 701656.
37. Werner, S.; Grose, R. Regulation of wound healing by growth factors and cytokines. *Physiol. Rev.* **2003**, *83*, 835–870.
38. Werb, Z.; Tremble, P.; Damsky, C.H. Regulation of extracellular matrix degradation by cell extracellular matrix interations. *Cell Differ. Dev.* **1990**, *32*, 299–306.
39. Lin, R.Y.; Sullivan, K.M.; Argenta, P.A.; Meuli, M.; Lorenz, H.P.; Adzick, N.S. Exogenous transforming growth factor-beta amplifies its own expression and induces scar formation in a model of human fetal skin repair. *Ann. Surg.* **1995**, *222*, 146–154.
40. Ghahary, A.; Shen, Y.J.; Scott, P.G.; Gong, Y.; Tredget, E.E. Enhanced expression of mRNA for transforming growth factor-beta, type I and type III procollagen in human post-burn hypertrophic scar tissues. *J. Lab. Clin. Med.* **1993**, *122*, 465–473.
41. Rando, D.G.; Doriguetto, A.C.; Tomich de Paula da Silva, C.H.; Ellena, J.; Sato, D.N.; Leite, C.Q.; Varanda, E.A.; Ferreira, E.I. A duplicated nitrotienyl derivative with antimycobacterial activity: Synthesis, X-ray crystallography, biological and mutagenic activity tests. *Eur. J. Med. Chem.* **2006**, *41*, 1196–200.
42. Park, S.-Y.; Lim, H.K.; Lee, S.; Hwang, H.C.; Cho, S.K.; Cho, M. Pepsin-solubilised collagen (PSC) from Red Sea cucumber (Stichopus japonicas) regulates cell cycle and the fibronectin synthesis in HaCaT cell migration. *Food Chem.* **2012**, *132*, 487–492.
43. Gogly, B.; Groult, N.; Hornebeck, W.; Godeau, G.; Pellat, B. Collagen zymography as a sensitive and specific technique for the determination of subpicogram levels of interstitial collagenase. *Anal. Biochem.* **1998**, *255*, 211–216.
44. Wang, H.; Joseph, J.A. Quantifying cellular oxidative stress by dichlorofluorescein assay using microplate reader. *Free Radic. Biol. Med.* **1999**, *27*, 612–616.

12

Colonization and Infection of the Skin by *S. aureus*: Immune System Evasion and the Response to Cationic Antimicrobial Peptides

Sunhyo Ryu [1], Peter I. Song [2], Chang Ho Seo [3], Hyeonsook Cheong [1] and Yoonkyung Park [1,*]

1 Department of Biotechnology, Chosun University, Gwangju 501-759, Korea; E-Mails: bktsh0328@gmail.com (S.R.); hscheong@chosun.ac.kr (H.C.)

2 Department of Dermatology, University of Arkansas for Medical Sciences, Little Rock, AR 72205, USA; E-Mail: psong@uams.edu

3 Department of Bioinformatics, Kongju National University, Kongju 314-701, Korea; E-Mail: chseo@kongju.ac.kr

* Author to whom correspondence should be addressed; E-Mail: y_k_park@chosun.ac.kr

---

Abstract: *Staphylococcus aureus* (*S. aureus*) is a widespread cutaneous pathogen responsible for the great majority of bacterial skin infections in humans. The incidence of skin infections by *S. aureus* reflects in part the competition between host cutaneous immune defenses and *S. aureus* virulence factors. As part of the innate immune system in the skin, cationic antimicrobial peptides (CAMPs) such as the β-defensins and cathelicidin contribute to host cutaneous defense, which prevents harmful microorganisms, like *S. aureus*, from crossing epithelial barriers. Conversely, *S. aureus* utilizes evasive mechanisms against host defenses to promote its colonization and infection of the skin. In this review, we focus on host-pathogen interactions during colonization and infection of the skin by *S. aureus* and methicillin-resistant *Staphylococcus aureus* (MRSA). We will discuss the peptides (defensins, cathelicidins, RNase7, dermcidin) and other mediators (toll-like receptor, IL-1 and IL-17) that comprise the host defense against *S. aureus* skin infection, as well as the various mechanisms by which *S. aureus* evades host defenses. It is anticipated that greater understanding of these mechanisms will enable development of more sustainable antimicrobial compounds and new therapeutic approaches to the treatment of *S. aureus* skin infection and colonization.

Keywords: *Staphylococcus aureus*; skin colonization; skin infection; immune system evasion; cationic antimicrobial peptides (CAMPs)

1. Introduction

Staphylococcus aureus (*S. aureus*) is a Gram-positive bacterium that can live as a commensal organism on the skin and in the nose and throat. Approximately 30% of healthy people are asymptomatically colonized by *S. aureus*, which permanently colonizes the anterior nares in 10%–20% of the population and intermittently colonizes 30%–50%; the rest of the population never becomes colonized [1,2]. Importantly, this colonization is a known risk factor for infection [3–7], and *S. aureus* causes a range of infections, from minor skin infections to abscesses, endocarditis and sepsis. *S. aureus* is also a major cause of food poising induced by heat resistant enterotoxin A and is a leading cause of nosocomial infections [2], as colonized healthcare workers can transmit the pathogen to immunosuppressed patients. In addition, several cases of community-acquired methicillin-resistant *S. aureus* (CA-MRSA) infections have been recently reported [8–10]. Notably, these reports describe severe and even lethal infections by highly virulent strains of *S. aureus* in immunocompetent individuals.

S. aureus is exposed to a large arsenal of highly efficient antimicrobial host factors during skin colonization and infection. However, a growing number of dedicated resistance mechanisms now contribute to the ability of *S. aureus* to evade host cutaneous defenses and survive during colonization [11,12]. Furthermore, Glaser *et al.* recently reported that *S. aureus* small colony variants (SCVs) are less susceptible to the bactericidal activity of different human skin-derived AMP, which are associated with a higher resistance to the killing activity of human stratum corneum [13]. Both host cutaneous defense mechanisms and *S. aureus* virulence factors appear to be the focus of actively ongoing co-evolution, leading to major variations between different host species and bacterial strains, respectively [14,15]. Understanding how ones immune system combats the evasion strategies of *S. aureus* could be useful for the development of novel and more sustainable antimicrobial agents that are not subject to the evolution of microbial resistance.

While bacterial resistance to most available antibiotics is increasing and our knowledge about the arsenal of host cutaneous defense strategies is growing, it is becoming increasingly attractive to consider endogenous antimicrobial peptides (AMPs) as sources for more sustainable antimicrobial agents. Of the variety of host defense molecules expressed by organisms, cationic AMPs (CAMPs) have proven to be particularly promising for future development as new antimicrobials. This review focuses on the role of host CAMPs in staphylococcal skin infections, and on the mechanisms underlying *S. aureus* resistance to CAMPs.

2. Host-Pathogen Interactions during *S. aureus* Skin Colonization and Infection

The epidermis is composed of proliferating basal and differentiated suprabasal keratinocytes, within which sweat glands, sebaceous glands and hair follicles are sparsely distributed. Langerhans cells in the epidermis as well as dendritic cells, macrophages, mast cells, T and B cells, plasma cells and natural killer cells in the dermis participate in immune responses within the skin. As mentioned, approximately 30% of healthy individuals are colonized by *S. aureus* [16] through a process that reflects the competition between host factors and commensal organisms that resist colonization and *S. aureus* virulence factors that facilitate colonization and, possibly, subsequent infection [17]. Among the constitutive properties of skin that help to prevent colonization and infection by *S. aureus* are its low temperature and acidic pH [18,19]. For instance, an epidermal structural component, filaggrin, is broken down during epidermal differentiation into urocanic acid and pyrrolidone carboxylic acid [20]. These acidic breakdown products then not only contribute to the low pH of the skin surface but also inhibit the growth of *S. aureus* and the expression of at least two factors involved in *S. aureus* colonization, clumping factor B (ClfB) and fibronectin binding protein A (FnbpA) [20]. In addition, commensal organisms such as *S. epidermidis*, *P. acnes* and the *Malassezia* species are normally present on the skin surface occupying microbial niches and thus preventing colonization and invasion by *S. aureus* and other pathogens [18,19]. Skin commensals have also been shown to directly inhibit *S. aureus* colonization of skin and nasal mucosa. For example, *S. epidermidis* secretes a serine protease, Esp, which inhibits *S. aureus* colonization by destroying its biofilms [21]. *S. epidermidis* also produces phenol-soluble modulins (PSMγ and PSMδ), which have direct antimicrobial activity against *S. aureus* [22] and activate toll-like receptor 2 (TLR2) on keratinocytes, leading to production of CAMPs (e.g., human β-defensin 2 [hBD2], hBD3 and RNase 7), which amplify the immune response and promote killing of *S. aureus* [23,24]. CAMPs such as hBD2, hBD3, LL-37 (cathelicidin) and RNase 7, which are produced by keratinocytes in the skin and corneal layer, have bacteriostatic or bactericidal activity against *S. aureus* [25–28], as evidenced by the observation that *S. aureus* colonization is increased in skin lesions caused by atopic dermatitis due to reductions in the levels of β-defensins and cathelicidin [29].

To promote colonization of human nasal mucosa and skin, *S. aureus* expresses various factors that facilitate skin surface binding and survival. To bind to host surface components such as fibrinogen, fibronectin and cytokeratins, which are derived from epidermal keratinocytes or nasal epithelium, *S. aureus* utilizes microbial surface components recognizing adhesive matrix molecules (MSCRAMMs), which include fibronectin-binding protein A (Fnbp A) and Fnbp B, fibrinogen-binding proteins (ClfA and ClfB), iron-regulated surface determinant A (IsdA) and wall teichoic acid [30–33]. *S. aureus*-mediated fibronectin and fibrinogen binding is also enhanced by elevated levels of Th2 cytokines. For example, interleukin (IL)-4 is elevated in the skin lesions of atopic dermatitis patients, which are highly susceptible to *S. aureus* colonization [31]. *S. aureus* also produces superantigens such as staphylococcal enterotoxins A and B (SEA and SEB) and toxic shock syndrome toxin-1 (TSST-1), which skew the cutaneous immune response towards the Th2 cytokines and thus contribute to the increased colonization of *S. aureus* in atopic dermatitis patients [34]. In addition, *S. aureus* expresses factors that enable it to directly counter host CAMP responses. For example, IsdA enhances bacterial cellular hydrophobicity, which renders *S. aureus* resistant to bactericidal fatty acids in sebum and to β-defensins and cathelicidin [35]. It also secretes a protein, aureolysin, which is an extracellular metalloproteinase that inhibits cathelicidin antimicrobial activity [36]. Virulence factors from *S. aureus* are also closely related with evasion from human innate immune defenses [37]. In the following section, the mechanisms by which *S. aureus* inhibits the activities of CAMPs will be described in detail.

3. Methicillin-Resistant *S. aureus* (MRSA) Infection

Antibiotic resistance is now recognized to be a serious hindrance to the management of *S. aureus*. For instance, β-lactam antibiotics (e.g., methicillin) have proven unfavorable for the management of toxic *S. aureus* infections, because even subinhibitory concentrations lead to increased expression of α-toxin through a stimulatory effect on exoprotein synthesis [38–40]. Instead, protein-synthesis-suppressing antibiotics such as clindamycin and linezolid are recommended for the treatment of *S. aureus*-induced toxicity syndromes, as concentrations below the MIC impair expression of *S. aureus* virulence factors [41,42]. Clindamycin at a concentration of 1/8 MIC inhibits the expression of α- and δ-haemolysin as well as coagulase [43]. In addition, the expression of protein A is reduced when *S. aureus* is exposed to clindamycin at concentrations below the MIC, leading to increased bacterial susceptibility to phagocytosis and suggesting additional therapeutic efficacy [44]. However, clindamycin cannot be used to treat toxic MRSA infections because MRSA is largely resistant to clindamycin.

MRSA infections are caused by strains of *S. aureus* that have become resistant to the antibiotics commonly used to treat ordinary infections. Most MRSA infections occur in people who have been in hospitals or other health care settings, such as nursing homes and dialysis centers. When it occurs in these settings, it is known as health care-associated MRSA (HA-MRSA). HA-MRSA infections are typically associated with invasive procedures or devices, such as surgeries, intravenous tubing or artificial joints. However, another type of MRSA infection occurs in the wider community, among otherwise healthy individuals. This form, community-associated MRSA (CA-MRSA) is spread by skin-to-skin contact. It often begins as a painful skin boil and generally causes skin and soft tissue infections, but it is also capable of causing invasive disease such as endocarditis, necrotizing pneumonia and sepsis [45–50]. HA-MRSA, by contrast, is considered a nosocomial pathogen typically associated with invasive disease, such as bloodstream infections, pneumonia, surgical site infections and urinary tract infections [45,51–53]. It is now recognized that these two entities are genetically distinct. Isolates of HA-MRSA are likely to be resistant to three or more antibiotic classes, whereas CA-MRSA is usually resistant only to β-lactams and macrolides [47,51,53,54].

Resistance to methicillin is mediated in *S. aureus* by PBP2a, a penicillin-binding protein with a low affinity for β-lactams. PBPs are membrane-bound enzymes that catalyze the transpeptidation reaction, which is necessary for cross-linkage of peptidoglycan chains [55]. PBP2a substitutes for the other PBPs and, because of its low affinity for all β-lactam antibiotics, enables staphylococci to survive exposure to high concentrations of these agents. Thus, resistance to methicillin confers resistance to all β-lactam agents, including cephalosporins. Expression of resistance in some MRSA strains is regulated by homologues of the regulatory genes for *blaZ*. These genes, *mecI* and *mecR1*, regulate the *mecA* response to β-lactam antibiotics in a fashion similar to the regulation of the *blaZ* response to penicillin by *blaR1* and *blaI*. Katayama *et al.* demonstrated that *mecA* is carried on a mobile genetic element and is part of a genomic island designated staphylococcal cassette chromosome *mec* (SCC*mec*) [56]. To date, four different SCC*mec* elements varying in size from 21 to 67 kb have been characterized [57]. Such islands may also contain additional genes for antimicrobial resistance and insertion sequences, as well as genes whose function is uncertain.

As *S. aureus* isolates from intensive care units and blood cultures have become increasingly resistant to greater numbers of antimicrobial agents [2,58], this has inevitably diminished the number of effective bactericidal antibiotics available to treat these often life-threatening infections. As rapidly as new antibiotics are introduced, staphylococci are developing efficient mechanisms to neutralize them. Recent reports of *S. aureus* isolates with intermediate or complete resistance to vancomycin portend a chemotherapeutic era in which effective bactericidal antibiotics against this organism may no longer be readily available [59,60]. Consequently the need to identify new alternative therapeutic targets and to develop novel drugs that can be used against these targets is increasing.

4. Human AMPs Effective against *S. aureus*

AMPs are a diverse group of polypeptides that are typically less than 50 amino acids in length and exhibit bactericidal activity under physiologic conditions [61–63]. Most AMPs are cationic and interact with the anionic microbial membrane leading to osmotic lysis [61–63]. Autolytic enzymes induced by AMPs may also be associated with bacterial cell death [64]. Whereas some AMPs are produced by keratinocytes and are normally present in the skin, others are induced during infection and inflammation/wounding [65,66]. In this section, we will focus on the specific bacteriostatic or bactericidal AMPs expressed by keratinocytes and by immune cells thought to contribute to host defense against *S. aureus* (Table 1).

Table 1. Cationic antimicrobial peptides (CAMPs) that contribute to human cutaneous immune defenses against *S. aureus*.

Peptides	Cellular source in the skin	Mechanism of *S. aureus* evasion	References
α-Defensins	Neutrophils	Staphylokinase, MprF, *dlt*ABCD operon	[67–73]
hBD2	Keratinocytes, macrophages, and dendritic cells	IsdA, *dlt*ABCD	[26,29,35,74–76]
hBD3	Keratinocytes	*dlt*ABCD operon	[23,24,27,75–80]
hBD4	Keratinocytes	Please check	[81]
LL-37	Keratinocytes, macrophages, and neutrophils	IsdA, Aureolysin, MprF, *dlt*ABCD	[25,29,35,36,69,71–73,75]
Dermcidin	Sweat glands	Extracellular proteases, *dlt*ABCD operon	[82–84]
RNase 7	Keratinocytes	*dlt*ABCD operon	[24,28,61,76]

These include α-defensins (also called human neutrophil peptides [HNPs]), β-defensins (hBD1-4) cathelicidin (LL-37), RNase7 and dermcidin [61–63]. These AMPs not only have bactericidal activity against *S. aureus*, they also promote the recruitment of immune cells to sites of infection. For example, HNPs promote recruitment of macrophages, T cells and mast cells through a PKC-dependent mechanism [85], while hBD2 and hBD3 promote CCR6-mediated chemotaxis of immature dendritic cells and memory CD4+ T cells and CCR2-mediated chemotaxis of monocytes/macrophages [86,87]. In addition, LL-37 promotes chemotaxis of neutrophils, monocytes and T cells by activating formyl peptide receptor-like 1 [88,89]. Through these various mechanisms, AMPs enhance host defenses against *S. aureus*.

4.1. Defensins

Neutrophils express high levels of HNP1-3 and lower levels of HNP4, which together constitute nearly 50% of the peptides within neutrophil granules [67]. HNP2 has the highest degree of bactericidal activity against *S. aureus*, though HNP1, 3 and 4 also exhibit some activity against *S. aureus* [68].

Most AMPs expressed in humans belong to the β-defensin family. These amphipathic peptides have a β-sheet structure and are subcategorized according to the number and location of their disulfide bridges [90]. Four well-characterized human β-defensins (hBD1-4) are expressed by epithelial cells, including keratinocytes, as well as by activated monocytes/macrophages and dendritic cells [62,63]. *hBD1* is constitutively expressed, while *hBD2* and *hBD3* are inducible by bacterial infection or cytokines [91]. hBD1 has no antimicrobial activity against *S. aureus*, while hBD2 and hBD4 show weak bacteriostatic activity against *S. aureus in vitro* [26,81]. By contrast, hBD3 exhibits strong bactericidal activity against *S. aureus in vitro* and in skin explants *ex vivo* [27,77]. In keratinocytes, production of hBD2, hBD3 and LL-37 can be induced by live or heat-killed *S. aureus* or by bacterial components such as lipopeptides and lipoteichoic acid [74,75,78–80]. Activation of the epidermal growth factor receptor through wounding of human skin also leads to increased hBD3 production, providing another mechanism for enhancing antimicrobial activity against *S. aureus* [66,92]. Finally, defensins induce production of cytokines, including IL-8, and have chemotactic activity [93].

4.2. Cathelicidins

Cathelicidins are a family of AMPs whose named reflects their resemblance to the precursor forms of the protein cathelin [94]. The *N*-terminal cathelin domain keeps the AMP precursor inactive until proteolytic cleavage releases the active *C*-terminal peptide. Although they may vary in structure, most mature cathelicidins are α-helical, amphipathic and cationic. Cathelicidin is constitutively expressed in neutrophils and has potent bactericidal activity against *S. aureus*. It is also called LL-37, referring its first two amino acids and total length of 37 amino acids [25,62,63]. Two other forms, RK-31 and KS-30, may be produced through alternative cleavage, especially on the skin [95]. Both KS-30 and RK-31 show greater antimicrobial activity than LL-37 and also differ from LL-37 in their ability to elicit cytokine release. Like defensins, LL-37 can induce both chemotaxis and cytokine release [93].

Vitamin D may also play a role in host defense against *S. aureus* skin infections, since it induces production of LL-37 in keratinocytes, neutrophils and monocytes/macrophages. However, the link between vitamin D and host defense against *S. aureus* has yet to be demonstrated in the skin [96–98].

4.3. RNase7

The cationic peptide RNase 7 is produced by many cell types, including keratinocytes, and has bactericidal activity against a broad range of bacteria, including *S. aureus* [61,99]. The high levels of RNase 7 present in the stratum corneum prevents *S. aureus* colonization of skin explants [28].

4.4. Dermcidin

Dermcidin is produced by human eccrine sweat glands and its processed forms have activity against numerous bacteria, including *S. aureus* [82,83,100,101]. While the DCD-1L and DCD-1 processed forms of dermcidin are negatively charged [69], a further processed cationic form (SSl-25) also shows antimicrobial activity, suggesting that charge is of no importance to the mode of action of dermcidin-derived peptides [83].

Figure 1. Toll-like receptor-mediated cutaneous immune response against *S. aureus*. Toll-like receptor 2 (TLR2) and nucleotide-binding oligomerization domain containing 2 (NOD2), which are expressed by keratinocytes, respectively recognize *S. aureus* lipopeptides/lipoteichoic acid and muramyl dipeptide. Both TLR2 and NOD2 signaling triggers the activation of nuclear factor-κB (NF-κB), which leads to the production of AMPs, cytokines, chemokines, adhesion molecules and granulopoesis factors, all of which contribute to the cutaneous host defense against *S. aureus*.

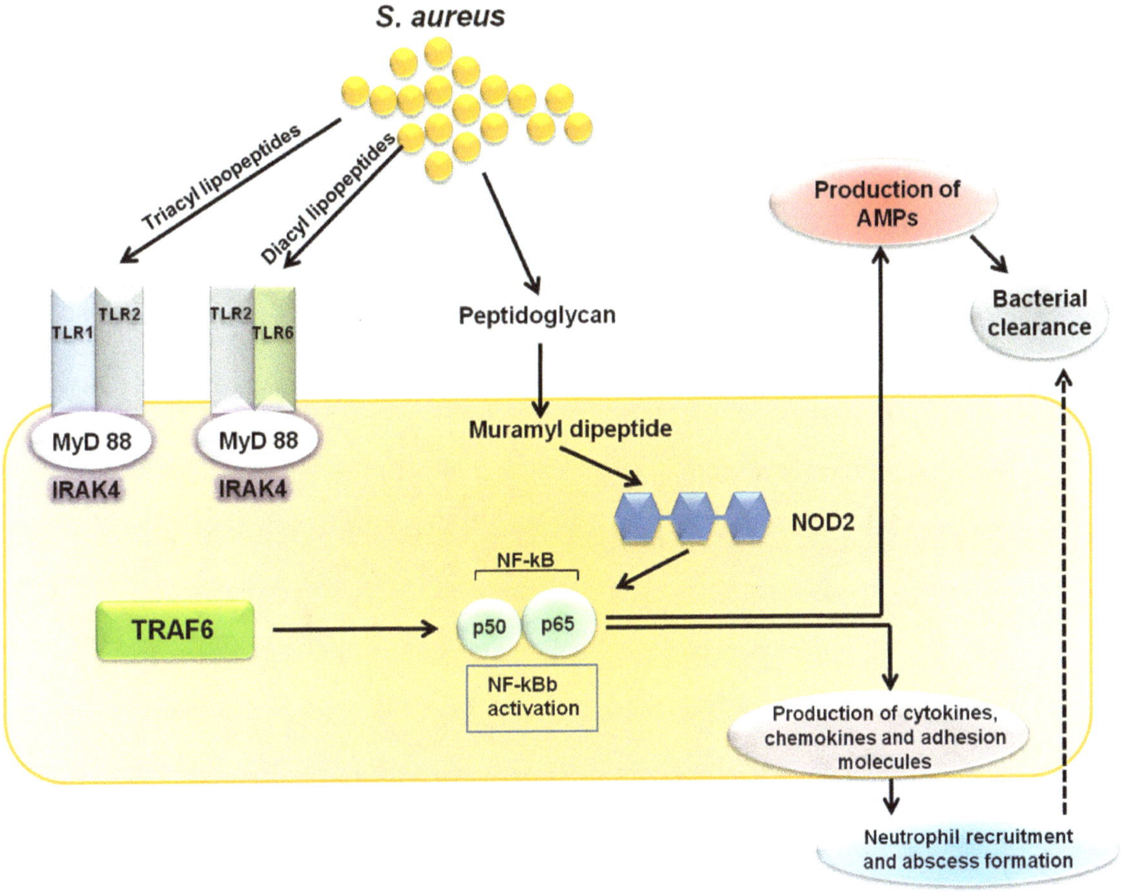

5. Cutaneous Host Defense Involving TLR-Mediated AMP Activity against *S. aureus*

Keratinocytes express pattern recognition receptors such as TLR2, which recognizes *S. aureus* lipopeptides and lipoteichoic acid, and nucleotide-binding oligomerization domain containing 2 (NOD2), which recognizes the *S. aureus* peptidoglycan breakdown product muramyl dipeptide. Both the TLR2 and NOD2 signals lead to activation of nuclear factor-κB (NF-κB) and other transcription factors that induce transcription of the proinflammatory mediators (cytokines, chemokines, adhesion molecules and AMPs) involved in cutaneous host defense against *S. aureus* (Figure 1) [102,103]. Upon cutaneous *S. aureus* infection, the epidermal barrier is breached and keratinocytes and resident skin immune cells (e.g., Langerhans cells and γδ T cells in the epidermis, as well as dendritic cells, macrophages, fibroblasts, mast cells, B and T cells, plasma cells and natural killer cells in the dermis) produce pro-inflammatory cytokines, chemokines and adhesion molecules. These molecules promote the recruitment of neutrophils from the bloodstream, which help to control the infection by forming an abscess. Neutrophilic abscess formation is a hallmark of *S. aureus* infections, which are typically pyogenic, and is required for bacterial clearance. Pro-inflammatory cytokines also induce the production of AMPs (e.g., β-defensins and cathelicidins) with bacteriostatic or bactericidal activity against *S. aureus* [104,105].

Figure 2. IL-1- and IL-17-mediated cutaneous immune response against *S. aureus*. Infection of the skin by *S. aureus* leads to the production of IL-1α, IL-1β and IL-17, which in turn triggers activation of nuclear factor-κB (NF-κB). These signaling pathways lead to the production of AMPs, cytokines, chemokines, adhesion molecules and granulopoesis factors, which recruit neutrophils from the circulation to the site of *S. aureus* infection in the skin. The recruited neutrophils form an abscess that helps control and limit the spread of the infection, and is ultimately required for bacterial clearance. IL-1R1, interleukin-1 receptor 1; IL-17R, interleukin-17 receptor.

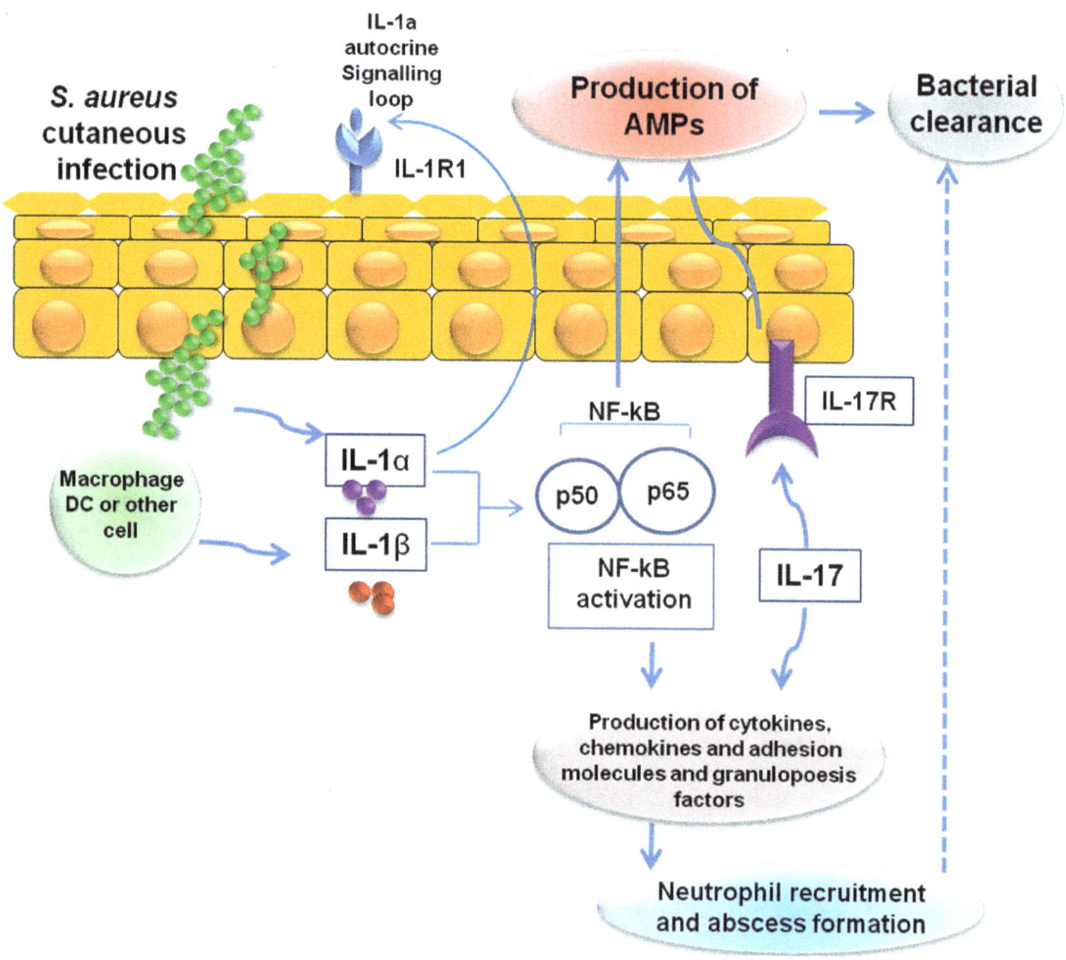

6. Cutaneous Host Defense Involving IL-1- and IL-17-Mediated AMP Activity against *S. aureus*

IL-1α, which is produced and released by keratinocytes, and IL-1β, which is produced by resident and recruited immune cells (e.g., macrophages and dendritic cells), trigger activation of NF-κB. These signaling pathways lead to the production of β-defensins 2 and 3, cathelicidins and RNase 7. IL-1-mediated responses also result in the production of pro-inflammatory cytokines, chemokines and adhesion molecules that promote the recruitment of neutrophils from the circulation to sites of *S. aureus* infection in the skin and abscess formation (Figure 2) [106]. In addition to IL-1, recent studies have uncovered the critical role played by IL-17, which is predominantly expressed by recruited T cell subsets (Th17 cells, NKT cells and γδ T cells) and natural killer cells in response to TLR2 activation. The IL-17 produced stimulates production of β-defensins 2 and 3 and cathelicidins by keratinocytes and induces neutrophil recruitment via induction of various chemokines (CXCL1, CXCL2 and IL-8) and granulopoesis factors (G-CSF and GM-CSF) [107].

7. Mechanisms by Which *S. aureus* Evades Skin-Derived CAMPs

The importance of CAMPs in host cutaneous defense against *S. aureus* is evidenced by the mechanisms that have evolved in *S. aureus* to resist and evade these peptides. As shown in Figure 3, *S. aureus* counteracts CAMPs and antimicrobial fatty acids through at least four mechanisms: (i) production of CAMP-binding molecules, like the fibrinolytic enzyme staphylokinase (SAK), which binds to and inhibits α-defensins; (ii) proteolytic degradation of CAMPs by secreted proteases such as aureolysin, which cleaves and inactivates LL-37; (iii) reduction of the bacterial cell surface net negative charge by modification of teichoic acids using D-alanine or phospholipids with L-lysine; and (iv) alteration of bacterial cell surface hydrophobicity [11,108]. In the following sections, these mechanisms will be discussed in additional detail.

Figure 3. Strategies by which *S. aureus* evades CAMPs. *S. aureus* counteracts CAMPs by secreting trapping molecules and proteases that inactivate CAMPs and by modifying the cell membrane hydrophobicity or net charge [108].

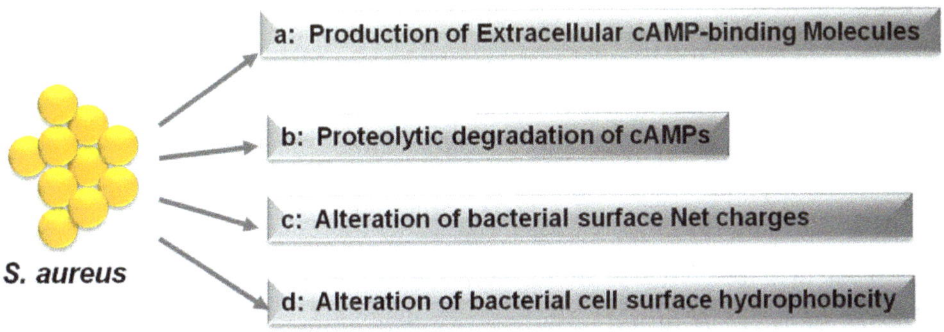

7.1. *Secretion of Extracellular CAMP-Binding Molecules*

S. aureus resists α-defensins through the production of SAK, which binds human α-defensins with high affinity, thereby mediating significant α-defensin resistance. *In vitro*, SAK levels correlate inversely with the susceptibility of *S. aureus* isolates to α-defensins (Figure 3a) [70].

7.2. *Proteolytic Degradation of CAMPs by Secreted Proteases*

S. aureus and many other bacterial species produce peptidases and proteases capable of cleaving CAMPs. *In vitro*, production of *S. aureus* protease correlates with staphylococcal resistance to

CAMPs [36]. For example, *S. aureus* produces a metalloproteinase, aureolysin, which cleaves and inactivates LL-37 [36]. *S. aureus* also secretes extracellular proteases that degrade dermcidin, neutralizing its antimicrobial activity [84], and similar observations have been made with the *S. epidermidis* protease SepA (Figure 3b) [84].

7.3. Resistance to CAMPs through Reduction of Bacterial Surface Net Negative Charges

CAMPs and most other antimicrobial molecules, including lysozyme, phospholipase A2 and RNase5, have net positive charges. The surface of human cells is normally composed mainly of uncharged or zwitterionic lipids, whereas bacterial surfaces are composed of various anionic components, including as peptidoglycan, the phospholipids phosphatidylglycerol and cardiolipin, lipid A, and teichoic acids, which give it an anionic net charge [109]. Presumably, antimicrobial host factors have evolved to be cationic to achieve strong, selective affinity for the anionic surfaces of bacteria. However, some bacterial species, like *S. aureus*, are able to reduce the negative charge of their cell envelope, thereby becoming resistant to inactivation by many CAMPs (Figure 3c) [69,71–73,110–112].

7.3.1. Modification of Phospholipids with L-lysine

To reduce anionic charge, *S. aureus* and other bacteria are able to modify most of their phosphatidylglycerol with L-lysine [113]. The lysinylation of phosphatidylglycerol is mediated by a membrane protein, multiple peptide resistance factor protein (MprF) [112,114], which neutralizes the bacterial cell envelope and thus reduces susceptibility to many CAMPs, including α-defensins, LL-37 and Group IIA-phospholipase A_2 [69,71,110,111].

7.3.2. Modification of Teichoic Acids with D-alanine

Products of the *dlt*ABCD operon attach positively charged D-alanine residues to negatively charged phosphate groups in the backbone of teichoic acids, rendering bacteria less susceptible to α-defensins and LL-37 [72,73]. Teichoic acids in *S. aureus* and other Gram-positive bacteria consist of alternating glycerolphosphate or ribitolphosphate units, which are substituted with *N*-acetyl-glucosamine or D-alanine [113]. These polymers are either anchored to the cytoplasmic membrane (lipoteichoic acid) or to the peptidoglycan cell wall (wall teichoic acid) and are anionic due to the presence of negatively charged phosphate groups. In a fashion similar to lysinylation of phospholipids, modification of teichoic acids with D-alanine leads to a partial neutralization of the polymer [73], which reduces the interaction of CAMPs with the bacterial surface, in turn reducing the susceptibility to cationic host defense molecules, including α-defensins and LL-37 [73]. Consistent with this scenario, an *S. aureus* mutant lacking D-alanine in its teichoic acids (*dlt*A mutant) as well as clinical isolates expressing lower levels of *dlt*A showed greater susceptibility to CAMPs, including dermcidin, RNase 7, hBD2 and hBD3 [76]. With dermcidin, cationic structures in the *N*-terminal part of the peptide appear crucial for interaction with the negative bacterial cell surface, which likely explains why D-alanylation influences its efficacy [83]. Also, several studies in animal models have demonstrated that alanylated teichoic acids contribute to an increased virulence of *S. aureus* [115–117].

7.4. Resistance to CAMPs through Alteration of Bacterial Cell Surface Hydrophobicity

Human skin is rich in antimicrobial fatty acids produced by sebaceous glands. *S. aureus* produces IsdA, which alters its surface hydrophobicity, thereby reducing the efficiency with which fatty acids gain access to the cells [35]. Indeed, by decreasing cellular hydrophobicity, IsdA renders *S. aureus* resistant to hBD2 and LL-37 on human skin (Figure 3d) [35].

8. Conclusions

S. aureus is a frequent component of human skin and nose microbiota. However, it can also cause various skin diseases, sometimes leading to systemic infections. The ability of *S. aureus* to colonize and infect the skin is apparently dependent on specific mechanisms that subvert host cutaneous defenses. The existence of these multiple resistance mechanisms makes it clear that CAMPs play a key role in the host cutaneous defense against *S. aureus*. Peschel *et al.* proposed the coevolution of CAMP structures and bacterial resistance mechanisms, which has led to the existence of the currently observed CAMPs [118]. One mechanism that renders CAMPs resistant to degradation by proteases is stabilization through disulphide bridges [118]. Other modifications that increase the efficacy of CAMPs include variation in the amino acid sequence, increases in the net positive charge through incorporation of larger numbers of cationic amino acids, and combining multiple antimicrobial mechanisms in a single molecule. These potential modifications of CAMPs are reviewed in detail by Peschel and Sahl [118].

Ouhara *et al.* showed that several clinical isolates of MRSA strains exhibited reduced susceptibility to the human LL-37 but not to the hBD3 [119]. The greater resistance to LL-37 is based on the more positive net cell-surface charge in MRSA strains than methicillin-susceptible *S. aureus* strains (MSSA). The fact that the efficacy of hBD3 appears unaffected may be due to its more positive net charge, as compared to LL-37 (+11 *vs.* +6), which would favor stronger interaction with the bacterial cell surface [119]. This suggests targeting highly conserved bacterial CAMP resistance mechanisms such as lysinylation of phospholipids by MprF or the alanylation of teichoic acids by *dlt*ABCD could be an effective treatment strategy. Moreover, in addition to its essential role in mediating resistance to CAMPs [69,111], it appears MprF may dramatically reduce the susceptibility of *S. aureus* to the novel lipopeptide antibiotic daptomycin [120,121]. Thus, new therapeutics targeting CAMP resistance factors, like MprF, could not only render a pathogen susceptible to host antimicrobial defense, but might also act synergistically to combat infections in combination with currently available antibiotics. Although targeting resistance factors would not directly inactivate *S. aureus*, it would render it more susceptible to CAMPs, thus assisting host cutaneous defenses to successfully combat skin infections.

The increasing numbers of reports of virulent and drug-resistant strains of *S. aureus* prompt further investigation into the mechanisms that enable this pathogen to cause infection and overcome the broad spectrum of human cutaneous antimicrobial defenses. We anticipate that future studies will provide further information about the host and bacterial determinants involved in skin colonization and infection by *S. aureus*. Targeted drug development around highly conserved bacterial resistance mechanisms against host CAMPs is a promising pharmacologic approach in this era of highly virulent and drug-resistant strains of *S. aureus*.

Acknowledgments

This work was supported by the IPET (Korea Institute of Planning and Evaluation for Technology in Food, Agriculture, Forestry and Fisheries), Ministry for Food, Agriculture, Forestry and Fisheries, Republic of Korea and the Human Resource Training Project for Regional Innovation (NRF-2013H1B8A2032054).

References

1. Chambers, H.F. The changing epidemiology of *Staphylococcus aureus*? *Emerg. Infect. Dis.* **2001**, *7*, 178–182.
2. Lowy, F.D. *Staphylococcus aureus* infections. *N. Engl. J. Med.* **1998**, *339*, 520–532.
3. Graham, P.L., 3rd; Lin, S. X.; Larson, E.L. A U.S. population-based survey of *Staphylococcus aureus* colonization. *Ann. Intern. Med.* **2006**, *144*, 318–325.
4. Kuehnert, M.J.; Kruszon-Moran, D.; Hill, H.A.; McQuillan, G.; McAllister, S.K.; Fosheim, G.; McDougal, L.K.; Chaitram, J.; Jensen, B.; Fridkin, S.K.; *et al.* Prevalence of *Staphylococcus aureus* nasal colonization in the United States, 2001–2002. *J. Infect. Dis.* **2006**, *193*, 172–179.
5. Perl, T.M.; Cullen, J.J.; Wenzel, R.P.; Zimmerman, M.B.; Pfaller, M.A.; Sheppard, D.; Twombley, J.; French, P.P.; Herwaldt, L.A.; *et al.* Intranasal mupirocin to prevent postoperative *Staphylococcus aureus* infections. *N. Engl. J. Med.* **2002**, *346*, 1871–1877.
6. Shopsin, B.; Mathema, B.; Martinez, J.; Ha, E.; Campo, M.L.; Fierman, A.; Krasinski, K.; Kornblum, J.; Alcabes, P.; Waddington, M.; Riehman, M.; *et al.* Prevalence of methicillin-resistant and methicillin-susceptible *Staphylococcus aureus* in the community. *J. Infect. Dis.* **2000**, *182*, 359–362.
7. Von Eiff, C.; Becker, K.; Machka, K.; Stammer, H.; Peters, G. Nasal carriage as a source of *Staphylococcus aureus* bacteremia. *N. Engl. J. Med.* **2001**, *344*, 11–16.
8. Herwaldt, L.A. *Staphylococcus aureus* nasal carriage and surgical-site infections. *Surgery* **2003**, *134*, S2–S9.
9. Lin, Y.C.; Lauderdale, T.L.; Lin, H.M.; Chen, P.C.; Cheng, M.F.; Hsieh, K.S.; Liu, Y.C. An outbreak of methicillin-resistant *Staphylococcus aureus* infection in patients of a pediatric intensive care unit and high carriage rate among health care workers. *J. Microbiol. Immunol. Infect.* **2007**, *40*, 325–334.
10. Elston, D.M. Community-acquired methicillin-resistant *Staphylococcus aureus*. *J. Am. Acad. Dermatol.* **2007**, *56*, 1–16.
11. Foster, T.J. Immune evasion by staphylococci. *Nat. Rev. Microbiol.* **2005**, *3*, 948–958.
12. Kraus, D.; Peschel, A. Molecular mechanisms of bacterial resistance to antimicrobial peptides. *Curr. Top. Microbiol. Immunol.* **2006**, *306*, 231–250.
13. Glaser, R.; Becker, K.; von Eiff, C.; Meyer-Hoffert, U.; Harder, J. Decreased susceptibility of Staphylococcus aureus small colony variants (SCVs) towards human antimicrobial peptides. *J. Invest. Dermatol.* **2014**, doi:10.1038/jid.2014.176.
14. Grenfell, B.T.; Pybus, O.G.; Gog, J.R.; Wood, J.L.; Daly, J.M.; Mumford, J.A.; Holmes, E.C. Unifying the epidemiological and evolutionary dynamics of pathogens. *Science* **2004**, *303*, 327–332.
15. Woolhouse, M.E.; Webster, J.P.; Domingo, E.; Charlesworth, B.; Levin, B.R. Biological and

biomedical implications of the co-evolution of pathogens and their hosts. *Nat. Genet.* **2002**, *32*, 569–577.

16. Gorwitz, R.J.; Kruszon-Moran, D.; McAllister, S.K.; McQuillan, G.; McDougal, L.K.; Fosheim, G.E.; Jensen, B.J.; Killgore, G.; Tenover, F.C.; Kuehnert, M.J. Changes in the prevalence of nasal colonization with *Staphylococcus aureus* in the United States, 2001–2004. *J. Infect. Dis.* **2008**, *197*, 1226–1234.
17. Miller, L.G.; Diep, B.A. Clinical practice: Colonization, fomites, and virulence: Rethinking the pathogenesis of community-associated methicillin-resistant *Staphylococcus aureus* infection. *Clin. Infect. Dis.* **2008**, *46*, 752–760.
18. Grice, E.A.; Kong, H.H.; Conlan, S.; Deming, C.B.; Davis, J.; Young, A.C.; Program, N.C.S.; Bouffard, G.G.; Blakesley, R.W.; Murray, P.R.; *et al.* Topographical and temporal diversity of the human skin microbiome. *Science* **2009**, *324*, 1190–1192.
19. Grice, E.A.; Segre, J.A. The skin microbiome. *Nat. Rev. Microbiol.* **2011**, *9*, 244–253.
20. Miajlovic, H.; Fallon, P.G.; Irvine, A.D.; Foster, T.J. Effect of filaggrin breakdown products on growth of and protein expression by *Staphylococcus aureus*. *J. Allergy. Clin. Immunol.* **2010**, *126*, 1184–1190.
21. Iwase, T.; Uehara, Y.; Shinji, H.; Tajima, A.; Seo, H.; Takada, K.; Agata, T.; Mizunoe, Y. *Staphylococcus epidermidis* Esp inhibits *Staphylococcus aureus* biofilm formation and nasal colonization. *Nature* **2010**, *465*, 346–349.
22. Cogen, A.L.; Yamasaki, K.; Sanchez, K.M.; Dorschner, R.A.; Lai, Y.; MacLeod, D.T.; Torpey, J.W.; Otto, M.; Nizet, V.; Kim, J.E.; *et al.* Selective antimicrobial action is provided by phenol-soluble modulins derived from *Staphylococcus epidermidis*, a normal resident of the skin. *J. Invest. Dermatol.* **2010**, *130*, 192–200.
23. Lai, Y.; Cogen, A.L.; Radek, K.A.; Park, H.J.; Macleod, D.T.; Leichtle, A.; Ryan, A.F.; Di Nardo, A.; Gallo, R.L. Activation of TLR2 by a small molecule produced by *Staphylococcus epidermidis* increases antimicrobial defense against bacterial skin infections. *J. Invest. Dermatol.* **2010**, *130*, 2211–2221.
24. Wanke, I.; Steffen, H.; Christ, C.; Krismer, B.; Gotz, F.; Peschel, A.; Schaller, M.; Schittek, B. Skin commensals amplify the innate immune response to pathogens by activation of distinct signaling pathways. *J. Invest. Dermatol.* **2011**, *131*, 382–390.
25. Braff, M.H.; Zaiou, M.; Fierer, J.; Nizet, V.; Gallo, R.L. Keratinocyte production of cathelicidin provides direct activity against bacterial skin pathogens. *Infect. Immun.* **2005**, *73*, 6771–6781.
26. Harder, J.; Bartels, J.; Christophers, E.; Schroder, J.M. A peptide antibiotic from human skin. *Nature* **1997**, *387*, 861.
27. Kisich, K.O.; Howell, M.D.; Boguniewicz, M.; Heizer, H.R.; Watson, N.U.; Leung, D.Y. The constitutive capacity of human keratinocytes to kill *Staphylococcus aureus* is dependent on β-defensin 3. *J. Invest. Dermatol.* **2007**, *127*, 2368–2380.
28. Simanski, M.; Dressel, S.; Glaser, R.; Harder, J. RNase 7 protects healthy skin from *Staphylococcus aureus* colonization. *J. Invest. Dermatol.* **2010**, *130*, 2836–2838.
29. Ong, P.Y.; Ohtake, T.; Brandt, C.; Strickland, I.; Boguniewicz, M.; Ganz, T.; Gallo, R.L.; Leung, D.Y. Endogenous antimicrobial peptides and skin infections in atopic dermatitis. *N. Engl. J. Med.* **2002**, *347*, 1151–1160.

30. Burian, M.; Rautenberg, M.; Kohler, T.; Fritz, M.; Krismer, B.; Unger, C.; Hoffmann, W.H.; Peschel, A.; Wolz, C.; Goerke, C. Temporal expression of adhesion factors and activity of global regulators during establishment of *Staphylococcus aureus* nasal colonization. *J. Infect. Dis.* **2010**, *201*, 1414–1421.
31. Cho, S.H.; Strickland, I.; Tomkinson, A.; Fehringer, A.P.; Gelfand, E.W.; Leung, D.Y. Preferential binding of *Staphylococcus aureus* to skin sites of Th2-mediated inflammation in a murine model. *J. Invest. Dermatol.* **2001**, *116*, 658–663.
32. Clarke, S.R.; Brummell, K.J.; Horsburgh, M.J.; McDowell, P.W.; Mohamad, S.A.; Stapleton, M.R.; Acevedo, J.; Read, R.C.; Day, N.P.; Peacock, S.J.; *et al.* Identification of *in vivo*-expressed antigens of *Staphylococcus aureus* and their use in vaccinations for protection against nasal carriage. *J. Infect. Dis.* **2006**, *193*, 1098–1108.
33. Weidenmaier, C.; Kokai-Kun, J.F.; Kristian, S.A.; Chanturiya, T.; Kalbacher, H.; Gross, M.; Nicholson, G.; Neumeister, B.; Mond, J.J.; Peschel, A. Role of teichoic acids in *Staphylococcus aureus* nasal colonization, a major risk factor in nosocomial infections. *Nat. Med.* **2004**, *10*, 243–245.
34. Laouini, D.; Kawamoto, S.; Yalcindag, A.; Bryce, P.; Mizoguchi, E.; Oettgen, H.; Geha, R.S. Epicutaneous sensitization with superantigen induces allergic skin inflammation. *J. Allergy. Clin. Immunol.* **2003**, *112*, 981–987.
35. Clarke, S.R.; Mohamed, R.; Bian, L.; Routh, A.F.; Kokai-Kun, J.F.; Mond, J.J.; Tarkowski, A.; Foster, S.J. The *Staphylococcus aureus* surface protein IsdA mediates resistance to innate defenses of human skin. *Cell Host Microbe* **2007**, *1*, 199–212.
36. Sieprawska-Lupa, M.; Mydel, P.; Krawczyk, K.; Wojcik, K.; Puklo, M.; Lupa, B.; Suder, P.; Silberring, J.; Reed, M.; Pohl, J.; *et al.* Degradation of human antimicrobial peptide LL-37 by *Staphylococcus aureus*-derived proteinases. *Antimicrob. Agents Chemother.* **2004**, *48*, 4673–4679.
37. Zecconi, A.; Scali, F. *Staphylococcus aureus* virulence factors in evasion from innate immune defenses in human and animal diseases. *Immunol. Lett.* **2013**, *150*, 12–22.
38. Hallander, H.O.; Laurell, G.; Lofstrom, G. Enhancement of staphylococcal pathogenicity in the presence of penicillin. *Acta Pathol. Microbiol. Scand.* **1966**, *68*, 463–464.
39. Ohlsen, K.; Ziebuhr, W.; Koller, K.P.; Hell, W.; Wichelhaus, T.A.; Hacker, J. Effects of subinhibitory concentrations of antibiotics on α-toxin (*hla*) gene expression of methicillin-sensitive and methicillin-resistant *Staphylococcus aureus* isolates. *Antimicrob. Agents Chemother.* **1998**, *42*, 2817–2823.
40. Shibl, A.M. Effect of antibiotics on production of enzymes and toxins by microorganisms. *Rev. Infect. Dis.* **1983**, *5*, 865–875.
41. Bernardo, K.; Pakulat, N.; Fleer, S.; Schnaith, A.; Utermohlen, O.; Krut, O.; Muller, S.; Kronke, M. Subinhibitory concentrations of linezolid reduce *Staphylococcus aureus* virulence factor expression. *Antimicrob. Agents Chemother.* **2004**, *48*, 546–555.
42. Schlievert, P.M.; Kelly, J.A. Clindamycin-induced suppression of toxic-shock syndrome—Associated exotoxin production. *J. Infect. Dis.* **1984**, *149*, 471.
43. Shibl, A.M. Role of *Staphylococcus aureus* exfoliatin toxin in staphylococcal infections in mice. *Chemotherapy* **1981**, *27*, 224–227.
44. Veringa, E. M.; Verhoef, J. Influence of subinhibitory concentrations of clindamycin on

opsonophagocytosis of *Staphylococcus aureus*, a protein-A-dependent process. *Antimicrob. Agents Chemother.* **1986**, *30*, 796–797.

45. Beilman, G.J.; Sandifer, G.; Skarda, D.; Jensen, B.; McAllister, S.; Killgore, G.; Srinivasan, A. Emerging infections with community-associated methicillin-resistant *Staphylococcus aureus* in outpatients at an Army Community Hospital. *Surg. Infect. (Larchmt)* **2005**, *6*, 87–92.
46. Daum, R.S. Clinical practice: Skin and soft-tissue infections caused by methicillin-resistant *Staphylococcus aureus*. *N. Engl. J. Med.* **2007**, *357*, 380–390.
47. David, M.Z.; Daum, R.S. Community-associated methicillin-resistant *Staphylococcus aureus*: Epidemiology and clinical consequences of an emerging epidemic. *Clin. Microbiol. Rev.* **2010**, *23*, 616–687.
48. DeLeo, F.R.; Otto, M.; Kreiswirth, B.N.; Chambers, H.F. Community-associated meticillin-resistant *Staphylococcus aureus*. *Lancet* **2010**, *375*, 1557–1568.
49. Deurenberg, R.H.; Stobberingh, E.E. The evolution of *Staphylococcus aureus*. *Infect. Genet. Evol.* **2008**, *8*, 747–763.
50. Mediavilla, J.R.; Chen, L.; Mathema, B.; Kreiswirth, B.N. Global epidemiology of community-associated methicillin resistant *Staphylococcus aureus* (CA-MRSA). *Curr. Opin. Microbiol.* **2012**, *15*, 588–595.
51. Chavez, T.T.; Decker, C.F. Health care-associated MRSA *versus* community-associated MRSA. *Dis. Mon.* **2008**, *54*, 763–768.
52. Enright, M.C. The evolution of a resistant pathogen—The case of MRSA. *Curr. Opin. Pharmacol.* **2003**, *3*, 474–479.
53. Naimi, T.S.; LeDell, K.H.; Como-Sabetti, K.; Borchardt, S.M.; Boxrud, D.J.; Etienne, J.; Johnson, S.K.; Vandenesch, F.; Fridkin, S.; O'Boyle, C.; *et al.* Comparison of community- and health care-associated methicillin-resistant *Staphylococcus aureus* infection. *J. Am. Med. Assoc.* **2003**, *290*, 2976–2984.
54. Klein, E.; Smith, D.L.; Laxminarayan, R. Community-associated methicillin-resistant *Staphylococcus aureus* in outpatients, United States, 1999–2006. *Emerg. Infect. Dis.* **2009**, *15*, 1925–1930.
55. Ghuysen, J.M. Molecular structures of penicillin-binding proteins and β-lactamases. *Trends. Microbiol.* **1994**, *2*, 372–380.
56. Katayama, Y.; Ito, T.; Hiramatsu, K. A new class of genetic element, staphylococcus cassette chromosome *mec*, encodes methicillin resistance in *Staphylococcus aureus*. *Antimicrob. Agents Chemother.* **2000**, *44*, 1549–1555.
57. Hiramatsu, K.; Cui, L.; Kuroda, M.; Ito, T. The emergence and evolution of methicillin-resistant *Staphylococcus aureus*. *Trends. Microbiol.* **2001**, *9*, 486–493.
58. Diekema, D.J.; Pfaller, M.A.; Schmitz, F.J.; Smayevsky, J.; Bell, J.; Jones, R.N.; Beach, M.; Group, S.P. Survey of infections due to *Staphylococcus* species: Frequency of occurrence and antimicrobial susceptibility of isolates collected in the United States, Canada, Latin America, Europe, and the Western Pacific region for the SENTRY Antimicrobial Surveillance Program, 1997–1999. *Clin. Infect. Dis.* **2001**, *32*, S114–S132.
59. Centers for Disease Control and Prevention. *Staphylococcus aureus* resistant to vancomycin—United States, 2002. *MMWR Morb. Mortal. Wkly. Rep.* **2002**, *51*, 565–567.
60. Hiramatsu, K.; Hanaki, H.; Ino, T.; Yabuta, K.; Oguri, T.; Tenover, F.C. Methicillin-resistant

Staphylococcus aureus clinical strain with reduced vancomycin susceptibility. *J. Antimicrob. Chemother.* **1997**, *40*, 135–136.

61. Cho, J.S.; Xuan, C.; Miller, L.S. Lucky number seven: RNase 7 can prevent *Staphylococcus aureus* skin colonization. *J. Invest. Dermatol.* **2010**, *130*, 2703–2706.
62. Otto, M. Staphylococcus colonization of the skin and antimicrobial peptides. *Expert. Rev. Dermatol.* **2010**, *5*, 183–195.
63. Schauber, J.; Gallo, R.L. Antimicrobial peptides and the skin immune defense system. *J. Allergy. Clin. Immunol.* **2009**, *124*, R13–R18.
64. Sahl, H.G.; Pag, U.; Bonness, S.; Wagner, S.; Antcheva, N.; Tossi, A. Mammalian defensins: Structures and mechanism of antibiotic activity. *J. Leukoc. Biol.* **2005**, *77*, 466–475.
65. Miller, L.S.; Sorensen, O.E.; Liu, P.T.; Jalian, H.R.; Eshtiaghpour, D.; Behmanesh, B.E.; Chung, W.; Starner, T.D.; Kim, J.; Sieling, P.A.; *et al.* TGF-α regulates TLR expression and function on epidermal keratinocytes. *J. Immunol.* **2005**, *174*, 6137–6143.
66. Sorensen, O.E.; Thapa, D.R.; Roupe, K.M.; Valore, E.V.; Sjobring, U.; Roberts, A.A.; Schmidtchen, A.; Ganz, T. Injury-induced innate immune response in human skin mediated by transactivation of the epidermal growth factor receptor. *J. Clin. Invest.* **2006**, *116*, 1878–1885.
67. Lehrer, R.I. Multispecific myeloid defensins. *Curr. Opin. Hematol.* **2007**, *14*, 16–21.
68. Ericksen, B.; Wu, Z.; Lu, W.; Lehrer, R.I. Antibacterial activity and specificity of the six human α-defensins. *Antimicrob. Agents Chemother.* **2005**, *49*, 269–275.
69. Peschel, A.; Jack, R.W.; Otto, M.; Collins, L.V.; Staubitz, P.; Nicholson, G.; Kalbacher, H.; Nieuwenhuizen, W.F.; Jung, G.; Tarkowski, A.; *et al. Staphylococcus aureus* resistance to human defensins and evasion of neutrophil killing via the novel virulence factor MprF is based on modification of membrane lipids with L-lysine. *J. Exp. Med.* **2001**, *193*, 1067–1076.
70. Jin, T.; Bokarewa, M.; Foster, T.; Mitchell, J.; Higgins, J.; Tarkowski, A. *Staphylococcus aureus* resists human defensins by production of staphylokinase, a novel bacterial evasion mechanism. *J. Immunol.* **2004**, *172*, 1169–1176.
71. Ernst, C.M.; Staubitz, P.; Mishra, N.N.; Yang, S.J.; Hornig, G.; Kalbacher, H.; Bayer, A.S.; Kraus, D.; Peschel, A. The bacterial defensin resistance protein MprF consists of separable domains for lipid lysinylation and antimicrobial peptide repulsion. *PLoS Pathog.* **2009**, *5*, e1000660.
72. Jann, N.J.; Schmaler, M.; Kristian, S.A.; Radek, K.A.; Gallo, R.L.; Nizet, V.; Peschel, A.; Landmann, R. Neutrophil antimicrobial defense against *Staphylococcus aureus* is mediated by phagolysosomal but not extracellular trap-associated cathelicidin. *J. Leukoc. Biol.* **2009**, *86*, 1159–1169.
73. Peschel, A.; Otto, M.; Jack, R.W.; Kalbacher, H.; Jung, G.; Gotz, F. Inactivation of the dlt operon in *Staphylococcus aureus* confers sensitivity to defensins, protegrins, and other antimicrobial peptides. *J. Biol. Chem.* **1999**, *274*, 8405–8410.
74. Dinulos, J.G.; Mentele, L.; Fredericks, L.P.; Dale, B.A.; Darmstadt, G.L. Keratinocyte expression of human β-defensin 2 following bacterial infection: Role in cutaneous host defense. *Clin. Diagn. Lab. Immunol.* **2003**, *10*, 161–166.
75. Sayama, K.; Komatsuzawa, H.; Yamasaki, K.; Shirakata, Y.; Hanakawa, Y.; Ouhara, K.; Tokumaru, S.; Dai, X.; Tohyama, M.; Ten Dijke, P.; *et al.* New mechanisms of skin innate immunity: ASK1-mediated keratinocyte differentiation regulates the expression of β-defensins, LL37, and TLR2. *Eur. J. Immunol.* **2005**, *35*, 1886–1895.

76. Simanski, M.; Glaser, R.; Koten, B.; Meyer-Hoffert, U.; Wanner, S.; Weidenmaier, C.; Peschel, A.; Harder, J. *Staphylococcus aureus* subverts cutaneous defense by D-alanylation of teichoic acids. *Exp. Dermatol.* **2013**, *22*, 294–296.
77. Harder, J.; Bartels, J.; Christophers, E.; Schroder, J.M. Isolation and characterization of human β-defensin 3, a novel human inducible peptide antibiotic. *J. Biol. Chem.* **2001**, *276*, 5707–5713.
78. Menzies, B.E.; Kenoyer, A. Signal transduction and nuclear responses in *Staphylococcus aureus*-induced expression of human β-defensin 3 in skin keratinocytes. *Infect. Immun.* **2006**, *74*, 6847–6854.
79. Sumikawa, Y.; Asada, H.; Hoshino, K.; Azukizawa, H.; Katayama, I.; Akira, S.; Itami, S. Induction of β-defensin 3 in keratinocytes stimulated by bacterial lipopeptides through Toll-like receptor 2. *Microbes. Infect.* **2006**, *8*, 1513–1521.
80. Zanger, P.; Holzer, J.; Schleucher, R.; Scherbaum, H.; Schittek, B.; Gabrysch, S. Severity of *Staphylococcus aureus* infection of the skin is associated with inducibility of human β-defensin 3 but not human β-defensin 2. *Infect. Immun.* **2010**, *78*, 3112–3117.
81. Garcia, J.R.; Krause, A.; Schulz, S.; Rodriguez-Jimenez, F.J.; Kluver, E.; Adermann, K.; Forssmann, U.; Frimpong-Boateng, A.; Bals, R.; Forssmann, W.G. Human β-defensin 4: A novel inducible peptide with a specific salt-sensitive spectrum of antimicrobial activity. *FASEB J.* **2001**, *15*, 1819–1821.
82. Rieg, S.; Steffen, H.; Seeber, S.; Humeny, A.; Kalbacher, H.; Dietz, K.; Garbe, C.; Schittek, B. Deficiency of dermcidin-derived antimicrobial peptides in sweat of patients with atopic dermatitis correlates with an impaired innate defense of human skin *in vivo*. *J. Immunol.* **2005**, *174*, 8003–8010.
83. Steffen, H.; Rieg, S.; Wiedemann, I.; Kalbacher, H.; Deeg, M.; Sahl, H.G.; Peschel, A.; Gotz, F.; Garbe, C.; Schittek, B. Naturally processed dermcidin-derived peptides do not permeabilize bacterial membranes and kill microorganisms irrespective of their charge. *Antimicrob. Agents Chemother.* **2006**, *50*, 2608–2620.
84. Lai, Y.; Villaruz, A.E.; Li, M.; Cha, D.J.; Sturdevant, D.E.; Otto, M. The human anionic antimicrobial peptide dermcidin induces proteolytic defence mechanisms in staphylococci. *Mol. Microbiol.* **2007**, *63*, 497–506.
85. Grigat, J.; Soruri, A.; Forssmann, U.; Riggert, J.; Zwirner, J. Chemoattraction of macrophages, T lymphocytes, and mast cells is evolutionarily conserved within the human α-defensin family. *J. Immunol.* **2007**, *179*, 3958–3965.
86. Rohrl, J.; Yang, D.; Oppenheim, J.J.; Hehlgans, T. Human β -defensin 2 and 3 and their mouse orthologs induce chemotaxis through interaction with CCR2. *J. Immunol.* **2010**, *184*, 6688–6694.
87. Yang, D.; Chertov, O.; Bykovskaia, S.N.; Chen, Q.; Buffo, M.J.; Shogan, J.; Anderson, M.; Schroder, J.M.; Wang, J.M.; Howard, O.M.; *et al.* β-Defensins: Linking innate and adaptive immunity through dendritic and T cell CCR6. *Science* **1999**, *286*, 525–528.
88. De, Y.; Chen, Q.; Schmidt, A.P.; Anderson, G.M.; Wang, J.M.; Wooters, J.; Oppenheim, J.J.; Chertov, O. LL-37, the neutrophil granule- and epithelial cell-derived cathelicidin, utilizes formyl peptide receptor-like 1 (FPRL1) as a receptor to chemoattract human peripheral blood neutrophils, monocytes, and T cells. *J. Exp. Med.* **2000**, *192*, 1069–1074.

89. Tjabringa, G.S.; Ninaber, D.K.; Drijfhout, J.W.; Rabe, K.F.; Hiemstra, P.S. Human cathelicidin LL-37 is a chemoattractant for eosinophils and neutrophils that acts via formyl-peptide receptors. *Int. Arch. Allergy. Immunol.* **2006**, *140*, 103–112.
90. Ganz, T. Defensins: Antimicrobial peptides of innate immunity. *Nat. Rev. Immunol.* **2003**, *3*, 710–720.
91. Harder, J.; Meyer-Hoffert, U.; Wehkamp, K.; Schwichtenberg, L.; Schroder, J.M. Differential gene induction of human β-defensins (hBD-1, -2, -3, and -4) in keratinocytes is inhibited by retinoic acid. *J. Invest. Dermatol.* **2004**, *123*, 522–529.
92. Miller, L.S.; Modlin, R.L. Human keratinocyte Toll-like receptors promote distinct immune responses. *J. Invest. Dermatol.* **2007**, *127*, 262–263.
93. Yang, D.; Chertov, O.; Oppenheim, J.J. Participation of mammalian defensins and cathelicidins in anti-microbial immunity: Receptors and activities of human defensins and cathelicidin (LL-37). *J. Leukoc. Biol.* **2001**, *69*, 691–697.
94. Zanetti, M. Cathelicidins, multifunctional peptides of the innate immunity. *J. Leukoc. Biol.* **2004**, *75*, 39–48.
95. Murakami, M.; Ohtake, T.; Dorschner, R.A.; Schittek, B.; Garbe, C.; Gallo, R.L. Cathelicidin anti-microbial peptide expression in sweat, an innate defense system for the skin. *J. Invest. Dermatol.* **2002**, *119*, 1090–1095.
96. Liu, P.T.; Stenger, S.; Li, H.; Wenzel, L.; Tan, B.H.; Krutzik, S.R.; Ochoa, M.T.; Schauber, J.; Wu, K.; Meinken, C.; *et al.* Toll-like receptor triggering of a vitamin D-mediated human antimicrobial response. *Science* **2006**, *311*, 1770–1773.
97. Schauber, J.; Dorschner, R.A.; Coda, A.B.; Buchau, A.S.; Liu, P.T.; Kiken, D.; Helfrich, Y.R.; Kang, S.; Elalieh, H.Z.; Steinmeyer, A.; *et al.* Injury enhances TLR2 function and antimicrobial peptide expression through a vitamin D-dependent mechanism. *J. Clin. Invest.* **2007**, *117*, 803–811.
98. Wang, T.T.; Nestel, F.P.; Bourdeau, V.; Nagai, Y.; Wang, Q.; Liao, J.; Tavera-Mendoza, L.; Lin, R.; Hanrahan, J.W.; Mader, S.; *et al.* Cutting edge: 1,25-Dihydroxyvitamin D3 is a direct inducer of antimicrobial peptide gene expression. *J. Immunol.* **2004**, *173*, 2909–2912.
99. Zhang, J.; Dyer, K.D.; Rosenberg, H.F. Human RNase 7: A new cationic ribonuclease of the RNase A superfamily. *Nucleic. Acids. Res.* **2003**, *31*, 602–607.
100. Rieg, S.; Garbe, C.; Sauer, B.; Kalbacher, H.; Schittek, B. Dermcidin is constitutively produced by eccrine sweat glands and is not induced in epidermal cells under inflammatory skin conditions. *Br. J. Dermatol.* **2004**, *151*, 534–539.
101. Schittek, B.; Hipfel, R.; Sauer, B.; Bauer, J.; Kalbacher, H.; Stevanovic, S.; Schirle, M.; Schroeder, K.; Blin, N.; Meier, F.; *et al.* Dermcidin: A novel human antibiotic peptide secreted by sweat glands. *Nat. Immunol.* **2001**, *2*, 1133–1137.
102. Hruz, P.; Zinkernagel, A.S.; Jenikova, G.; Botwin, G.J.; Hugot, J.P.; Karin, M.; Nizet, V.; Eckmann, L. NOD2 contributes to cutaneous defense against *Staphylococcus aureus* through α-toxin-dependent innate immune activation. *Proc. Natl. Acad. Sci. USA* **2009**, *106*, 12873–12878.
103. Takeuchi, O.; Akira, S. Pattern recognition receptors and inflammation. *Cell* **2010**, *140*, 805–820.
104. Kim, M.H.; Granick, J.L.; Kwok, C.; Walker, N.J.; Borjesson, D.L.; Curry, F.R.; Miller, L.S.; Simon, S.I. Neutrophil survival and c-kit$^+$-progenitor proliferation in

Staphylococcus aureus-infected skin wounds promote resolution. *Blood* **2011**, *117*, 3343–3352.

105. Molne, L.; Verdrengh, M.; Tarkowski, A. Role of neutrophil leukocytes in cutaneous infection caused by *Staphylococcus aureus*. *Infect. Immun.* **2000**, *68*, 6162–6167.
106. Miller, L.S.; Cho, J.S. Immunity against *Staphylococcus aureus* cutaneous infections. *Nat. Rev. Immunol.* **2011**, *11*, 505–518.
107. Cua, D.J.; Tato, C.M. Innate IL-17-producing cells: The sentinels of the immune system. *Nat. Rev. Immunol.* **2010**, *10*, 479–489.
108. Kraus, D.; Peschel, A. *Staphylococcus aureus* evasion of innate antimicrobial defense. *Future Microbiol.* **2008**, *3*, 437–451.
109. Huijbregts, R.P.; de Kroon, A.I.; de Kruijff, B. Topology and transport of membrane lipids in bacteria. *Biochim. Biophys. Acta* **2000**, *1469*, 43–61.
110. Koprivnjak, T.; Peschel, A.; Gelb, M.H.; Liang, N.S.; Weiss, J.P. Role of charge properties of bacterial envelope in bactericidal action of human group IIA phospholipase A2 against *Staphylococcus aureus*. *J. Biol. Chem.* **2002**, *277*, 47636–47644.
111. Kristian, S.A.; Durr, M.; van Strijp, J.A.; Neumeister, B.; Peschel, A. MprF-mediated lysinylation of phospholipids in *Staphylococcus aureus* leads to protection against oxygen-independent neutrophil killing. *Infect. Immun.* **2003**, *71*, 546–549.
112. Staubitz, P.; Neumann, H.; Schneider, T.; Wiedemann, I.; Peschel, A. MprF-mediated biosynthesis of lysylphosphatidylglycerol, an important determinant in staphylococcal defensin resistance. *FEMS Microbiol. Lett.* **2004**, *231*, 67–71.
113. Neuhaus, F.C.; Baddiley, J.A continuum of anionic charge: Structures and functions of D-alanyl-teichoic acids in gram-positive bacteria. *Microbiol. Mol. Biol. Rev.* **2003**, *67*, 686–723.
114. Oku, Y.; Kurokawa, K.; Ichihashi, N.; Sekimizu, K. Characterization of the *Staphylococcus aureus mprF* gene, involved in lysinylation of phosphatidylglycerol. *Microbiology* **2004**, *150*, 45–51.
115. Collins, L.V.; Kristian, S.A.; Weidenmaier, C.; Faigle, M.; van Kessel, K.P.; van Strijp, J.A.; Gotz, F.; Neumeister, B.; Peschel, A. *Staphylococcus aureus* strains lacking D-alanine modifications of teichoic acids are highly susceptible to human neutrophil killing and are virulence attenuated in mice. *J. Infect. Dis.* **2002**, *186*, 214–219.
116. Kristian, S.A.; Lauth, X.; Nizet, V.; Goetz, F.; Neumeister, B.; Peschel, A.; Landmann, R. Alanylation of teichoic acids protects *Staphylococcus aureus* against Toll-like receptor 2-dependent host defense in a mouse tissue cage infection model. *J. Infect. Dis.* **2003**, *188*, 414–423.
117. Weidenmaier, C.; Peschel, A.; Kempf, V.A.; Lucindo, N.; Yeaman, M.R.; Bayer, A.S. DltABCD- and MprF-mediated cell envelope modifications of *Staphylococcus aureus* confer resistance to platelet microbicidal proteins and contribute to virulence in a rabbit endocarditis model. *Infect. Immun.* **2005**, *73*, 8033–8038.
118. Peschel, A.; Sahl, H.G. The co-evolution of host cationic antimicrobial peptides and microbial resistance. *Nat. Rev. Microbiol.* **2006**, *4*, 529–536.
119. Ouhara, K.; Komatsuzawa, H.; Kawai, T.; Nishi, H.; Fujiwara, T.; Fujiue, Y.; Kuwabara, M.; Sayama, K.; Hashimoto, K.; Sugai, M. Increased resistance to cationic antimicrobial peptide LL-37 in methicillin-resistant strains of *Staphylococcus aureus*. *J. Antimicrob. Chemother.* **2008**, *61*, 1266–1269.

120. Friedman, L.; Alder, J.D.; Silverman, J.A. Genetic changes that correlate with reduced susceptibility to daptomycin in *Staphylococcus aureus*. *Antimicrob. Agents Chemother.* **2006**, *50*, 2137–2145.

121. Jones, T.; Yeaman, M.R.; Sakoulas, G.; Yang, S.J.; Proctor, R.A.; Sahl, H.G.; Schrenzel, J.; Xiong, Y.Q.; Bayer, A.S. Failures in clinical treatment of *Staphylococcus aureus* Infection with daptomycin are associated with alterations in surface charge, membrane phospholipid asymmetry, and drug binding. *Antimicrob. Agents Chemother.* **2008**, *52*, 269–278.

13

4-Hydroxyphenylacetic Acid Attenuated Inflammation and Edema via Suppressing HIF-1α in Seawater Aspiration-Induced Lung Injury in Rats

Zhongyang Liu [1,2,†], **Ronggang Xi** [1,†], **Zhiran Zhang** [1], **Wangping Li** [2], **Yan Liu** [1], **Faguang Jin** [2,*] **and Xiaobo Wang** [1,*]

[1] Department of Pharmacological and Toxicological Research Centre, No. 210 Hospital of Chinese People's Liberation Army, Dalian 116021, China; E-Mails: lhw@wfmc.edu.cn (Z.L.); yyyes@wfmc.edu.cn (R.X.); wangfei@wfmc.edu.cn (Z.Z.); shifuyan@wfmc.edu.cn (Y.L.)

[2] Department of Respiration, Tangdu Hospital, Fourth Military Medical University, Xi'an 710038, China; E-Mail: wangdongrui@gmail.com

† These authors contributed equally to this work.

* Authors to whom correspondence should be addressed; E-Mails: jinfag@fmmu.edu.cn (F.J.); liwanwei@wfmc.edu.cn (X.W.)

Abstract: 4-Hydroxyphenylacetic acid (4-HPA) is an active component of Chinese herb *Aster tataricus* which had been widely used in China for the treatment of pulmonary diseases. The aim of this study is to investigate the effect of 4-HPA on seawater aspiration-induced lung injury. Pulmonary inflammation and edema were assessed by enzyme-linked immunosorbent assay (ELISA), bronchoalveolar lavage fluid (BALF) white cell count, Evans blue dye analysis, wet to dry weight ratios, and histology study. Hypoxia-inducible factor-1α (HIF-1α) siRNA and permeability assay were used to study the effect of 4-HPA on the production of inflammatory cytokines and monolayer permeability *in vitro*. The results showed that 4-HPA reduced seawater instillation-induced mortality in rats. In lung tissues, 4-HPA attenuated hypoxia, inflammation, vascular leak, and edema, and decreased HIF-1α protein level. In primary rat alveolar epithelial cells (AEC), 4-HPA decreased hypertonicity- and hypoxia-induced HIF-1α protein levels through inhibiting the activations of protein translational regulators and via promoting HIF-1α protein degradation. In addition, 4-HPA lowered inflammatory cytokines levels through suppressing hypertonicity- and hypoxia-induced HIF-1α in NR8383 macrophages. Moreover, 4-HPA decreased monolayer permeability through suppressing hypertonicity and hypoxia-induced HIF-1α, which was mediated by inhibiting vascular endothelial growth factor (*VEGF*) in rat lung microvascular endothelial cell line (RLMVEC). In conclusion, 4-HPA attenuated inflammation and edema through suppressing hypertonic and hypoxic induction of HIF-1α in seawater aspiration-induced lung injury in rats.

Keywords: 4-hydroxyphenylacetic acid; seawater drowning; hypoxia-inducible factor 1α; acute lung injury

1. Introduction

Drowning, one of the three leading causes of unintentional injury death, is a major but often neglected public health problem [1]. The acute lung injury (ALI) is a serious body injuries induced by water aspiration. Some ALI induced by near-drowning would deteriorate into acute respiratory distress syndrome (ARDS) without proper treatments [2–4]. A recent study showed that ALI induced by seawater aspiration is severer than that by freshwater, the reason of which could concern osmotic pressure [5]. Hypoxia and hypertonicity are the two impact factors in seawater aspiration-induced ALI which had an acuter and rapider course than that induced by lipopolysaccharide (LPS) [4,6–8]. Besides mechanical ventilation [9–11], therapies which could attenuate the injuries in lungs at the early stage of seawater aspiration-induced ALI are required to prevent the occurrence of ARDS.

Hypoxia-inducible factor-1 (HIF-1) is a key transcription factor that mediates adaptive responses to changes in tissue oxygenation. It is a basic helix-loop-helix transcription factor that is composed of two subunits, HIF-1α and HIF-1β. HIF-1β is constitutively present, whereas HIF-1α protein is kept at a low or undetectable level by continuous HIF-prolyl hydroxylase domain (PHD) enzyme-mediated degradation which is suppressed by hypoxia [12]. More and more evidences have demonstrated that HIF-1α also responds to nonhypoxic stimuli such as hormones, growth factors, vasoactive peptides, cytokines, heat, LPS, and hypertonicity [13–16]. Furthermore, a previous study reported that LPS-induced lung injury could be inhibited by reducing HIF-1α expression [17]. Since both of the two impact factors, hypoxia and hypertonicity, in seawater aspiration-induced ALI affected HIF-1α which played important roles in inflammation and edema [18,19], HIF-1α could be a potential therapeutic target.

4-Hydroxyphenylacetic acid (4-HPA) is an active component of Chinese herb *Aster tataricus* (fan hun cao) which had been widely used in China for the treatment of pneumonia, HBV, and carcinoma [20–22]. Some previous studies reported that 4-HPA, a metabolite of aromatic amino acid catabolism that is secreted in saliva, controlled the *NadA* gene expression and could become a potential hypopigmenting agent [23–25]. We also found that *Aster tataricus* extract and 4-HPA could inhibit HIF-1α expression in our preliminary experiments. Therefore, we hypothesized that 4-HPA might attenuate ALI induced by seawater aspiration through inhibiting HIF-1α expression. The aim of this study is to investigate the effect of 4-HPA on seawater aspiration-induced lung injury.

2. Results

2.1. 4-Hydroxyphenylacetic Acid (4-HPA) Reduced Seawater Instillation-Induced Mortality in Rats

As shown in Figure 1, treatment with 4-hydroxyphenylacetic acid (4-HPA) significantly reduced seawater instillation-induced death, the accumulative mortalities during 12 h in middle dose (100 mg/kg) and high dose (150 mg/kg) of 4-HPA treatment groups were both significantly lower than that in the seawater instillation group ($p < 0.05$). However, the accumulative mortalities between middle and high does groups had no significant difference and no protection was observed when rats received 4-HPA treatment at dose of 50 mg/kg. Therefore, 100 mg/kg 4-HPA was used in the following studies.

Figure 1. Effects of 4-hydroxyphenylacetic acid (4-HPA) on seawater instillation-induced mortality in rats. Drowning model rats were prepared with or without different does of 4-HPA (50, 100 or 150 mg/kg body weight, i.p.). 4-HPA was administered after seawater instillation for 10 min. The mortality of rats were recorded at 2, 4, 6, 8, 10, and 12 h after seawater instillation in each group ($n = 20$). * $p < 0.05$ *vs.* seawater group, # $p < 0.01$ *vs.* seawater group.

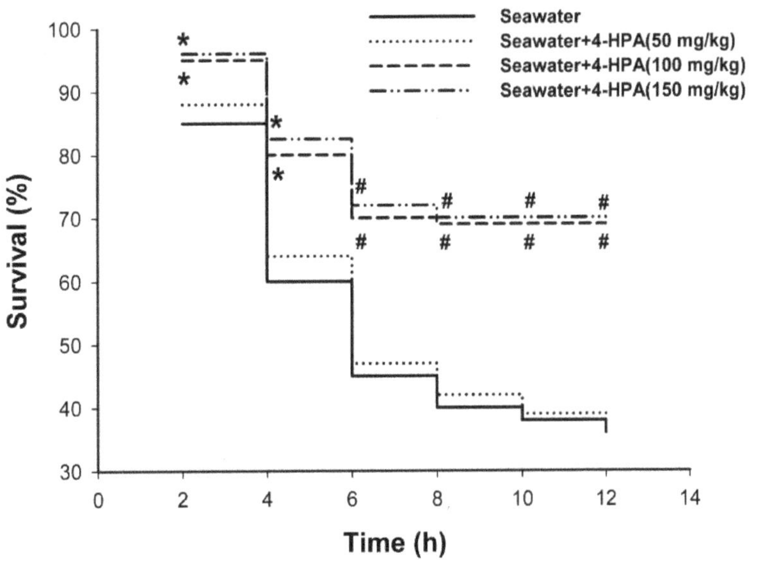

2.2. 4-HPA Increased PaO_2 and Decreased $PaCO_2$ in Seawater Instillation Rats

The response of PaO_2 and $PaCO_2$ after instillation of seawater with or without treatment of 4-HPA at 0.5, 1, 2, 3, and 4 h was observed (Figure 2). The results showed that PaO_2 dropped precipitously to its minimum at 0.5 h after instillation and then recovered gradually. The PaO_2 of rats treated with both seawater instillation and 4-HPA were significantly higher ($p < 0.05$) than that treated with only seawater instillation at 2, 3, and 4 h. Similarly, 4-HPA decreased $PaCO_2$ of rats instilled with seawater at 2, 3, and 4 h.

Figure 2. Effects of 4-HPA on PaO_2 and $PaCO_2$ after seawater instillation in rats. At 0, 0.5, 1, 2, 3, and 4 h after seawater instillation with or without 4-HPA treatment, blood samples were obtained from left carotid artery and then PaO_2 (**A**) and $PaCO_2$ (**B**) were measured by blood gas analyzer. Data are means ± standard deviation (SD) ($n = 10$), * $p < 0.05$ *vs.* seawater group.

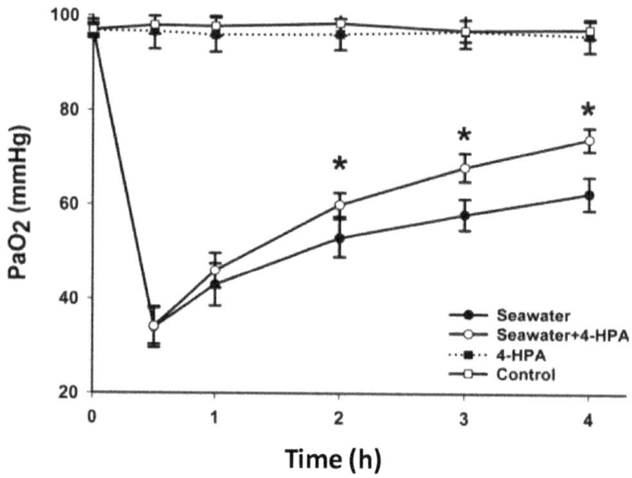

(**A**)

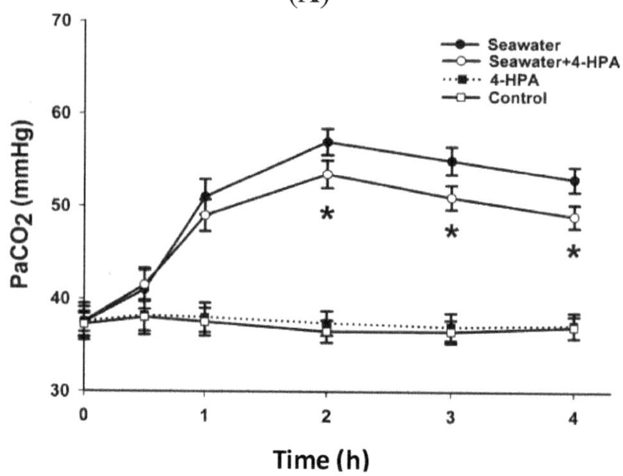

(**B**)

2.3. 4-HPA Attenuated Inflammation, Vascular Leak, and Edema in Seawater Instillation-Induced Lung Injury in Rats

Inflammatory cytokines such as TNF-α, IL-1β, and IL-6 play important roles in the inflammatory response in lungs. Therefore, we detected the TNF-α (Figure 3A), IL-1β (Figure 3B), and IL-6 (Figure 3C) content to study the inflammatory response in lung tissues. After seawater instillation, the contents of TNF-α, IL-1β, and IL-6 increased at 2, 4, and 6 h ($p < 0.05$), and 4-HPA markedly inhibited the expression of these cytokines ($p < 0.05$). Additionally, the degrees of inflammation and vascular leakage in lungs were measured by bronchoalveolar lavage fluid (BALF) white cell count (Figure 3D) and Evans blue dye analysis (Figure 3E), and lung edema was assessed by wet to dry weight ratios (Figure 3F). Seawater instillation caused a significant increase in BALF white cell count, Evans blue dye analysis, and wet to dry weight ratios in seawater group compared with control ($p < 0.05$). However, administration with 4-HPA markedly reduced the three at 2, 4, and 6 h ($p < 0.05$). There was no significant difference in BALF white cell count, Evans blue dye analysis, and wet to dry weight ratios between control and 4-HPA groups in the absence of seawater instillation. The histological results showed that seawater aspiration after 4 h induced pulmonary edema, infiltration of inflammatory cells in the lung tissues and alveoli, and alveolar damage (Figure 3I). However, 4-HPA treatment could improve the lung injury (Figure 3J). There was no obvious change in the lung structure in control and 4-HPA groups (Figure 3G,H).

Figure 3. Effects of 4-HPA on inflammatory cytokines, vascular leakage, and edema after seawater instillation in lungs. After instillation of seawater for 0, 2, 4, and 6 h in the absence or presence of 4-HPA, TNF-α (**A**); IL-1β (**B**); and IL-6 (**C**) contents in lung tissues were assessed by ELISA and white cells in brochoalveolar lavage fluid (BALF) were counted (**D**); Pulmonary vascular leakage was determined by Evans blue dye analysis (**E**); Lung edema was assessed by wet to dry weight ratios (**F**); Lung tissues were stained with hematoxilin and eosin to reveal histopathological changes at 4 h after seawater aspiration. (**G**) Control group; (**H**) 4-HPA group; (**I**) Seawater group; and (**J**) Seawater + 4-HPA group. The data are presented as means ± SD from three independent experiments, * $p < 0.05$ *vs.* control group, # $p < 0.05$ *vs.* seawater group.

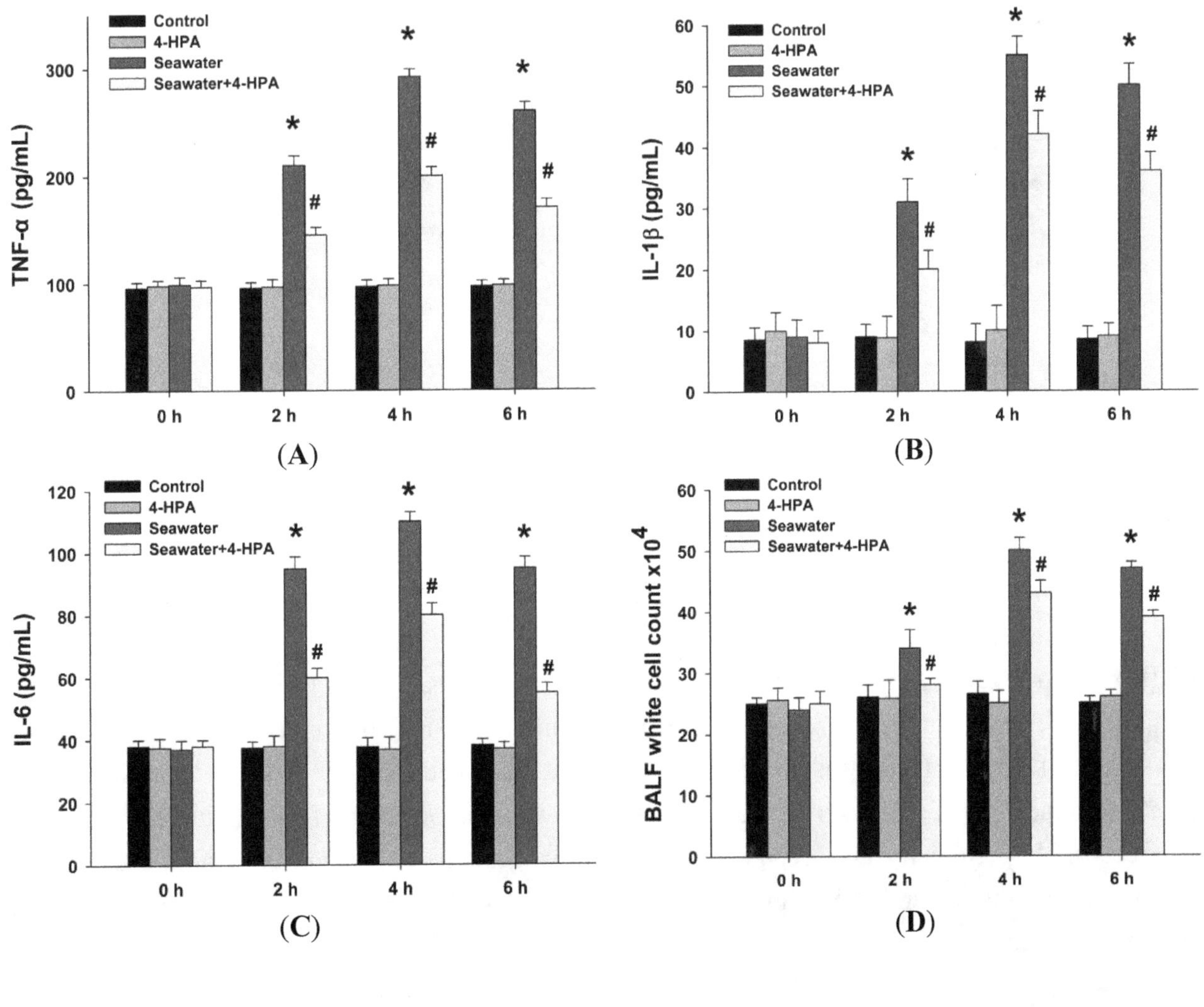

Figure 3. *Cont.*

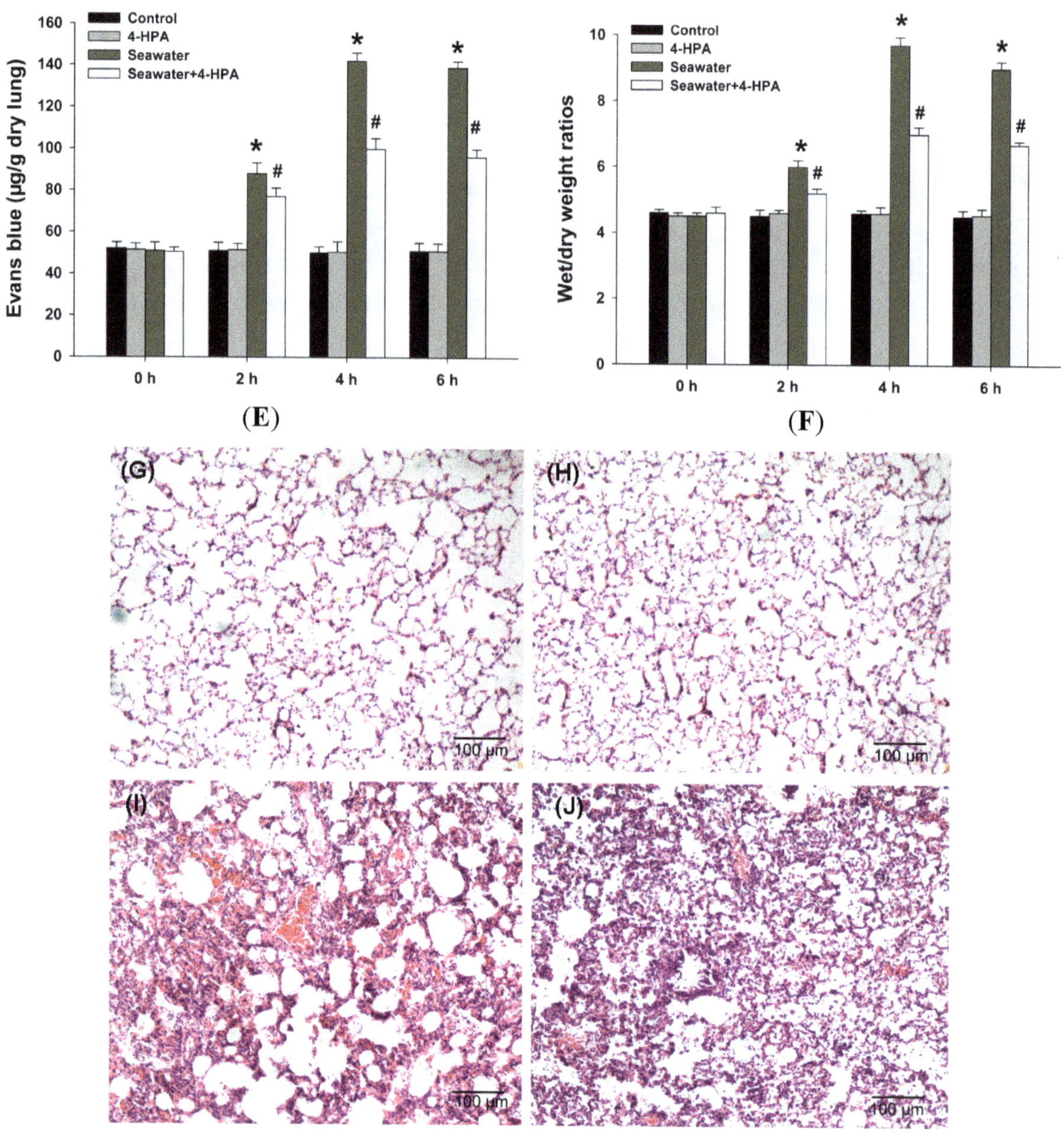

2.4. 4-HPA Decreased Seawater Instillation-Induced HIF-1α Protein Level, but not mRNA Level, in Lung Tissues in Rats

As shown in Figure 4, seawater instillation increased both HIF-1α protein and mRNA levels of lung tissue in rats at 2, 4, and 6 h ($p < 0.05$). However, 4-HPA decreased seawater instillation-induced HIF-1α protein level at each time point ($p < 0.05$), but not mRNA level. In addition, 4-HPA did not affect HIF-1α expression in the absence of seawater instillation. Since hypoxia did not affected *HIF-1α* mRNA level [26–28], there was hypertonicity which promoted *HIF-1α* mRNA level in seawater aspiration-induced lung injury. Therefore, there were two major injury factors and we focused on the effects of hypertonicity and hypoxia in the following studies *in vitro*. To examine that 4-HPA attenuates inflammation and edema in lung through inhibiting HIF-1α, a series of studies *in vitro* were performed as below.

Figure 4. Effects of 4-HPA on seawater instillation-induced HIF-1α protein and mRNA levels in lungs. After instillation of seawater for 0, 2, 4, and 6 h in the absence or presence of 4-HPA, HIF-1α protein (**C**,**D**) and *HIF-1α* mRNA (**A**,**B**) levels of lung tissue were detected by Western blotting and RT-PCR. The ratios of HIF-1α to β-actin in protein and mRNA levels from three independent experiments were obtained by density scanning of the Western blotting and PCR band using an image analysis system. Data are means ± SD, * $p < 0.05$ *vs.* control group, # $p < 0.05$ *vs.* seawater group.

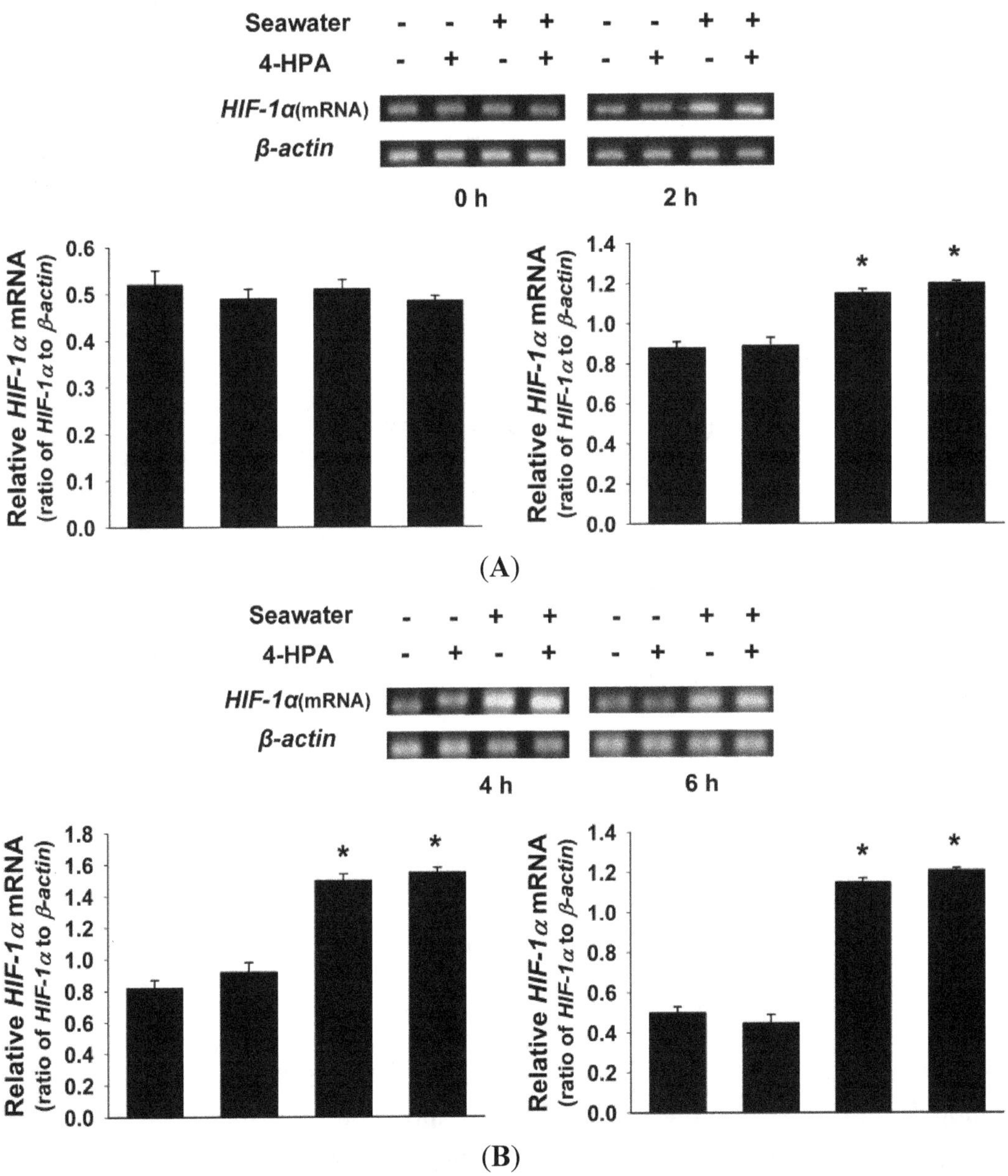

Fgure 4. *Cont.*

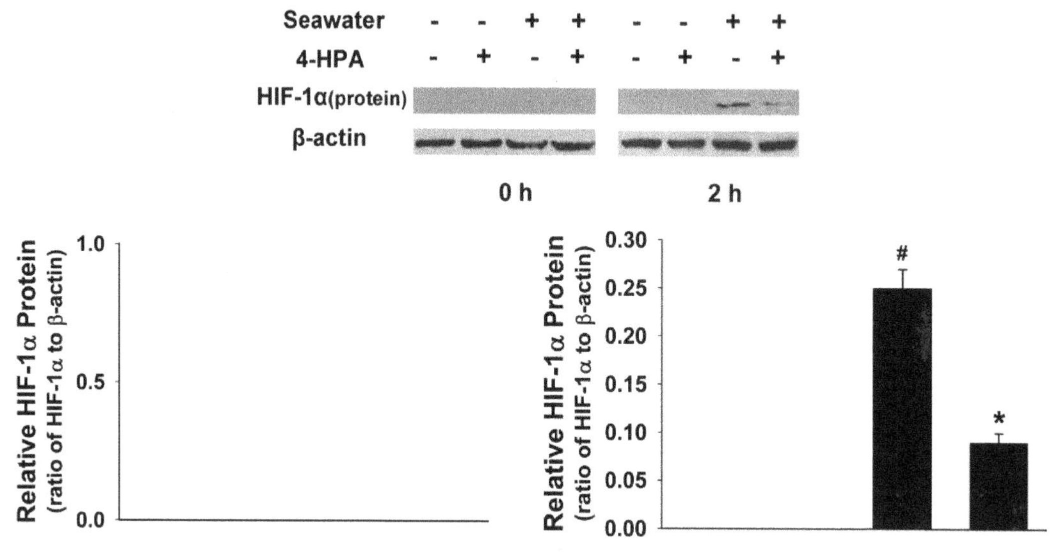

(C)

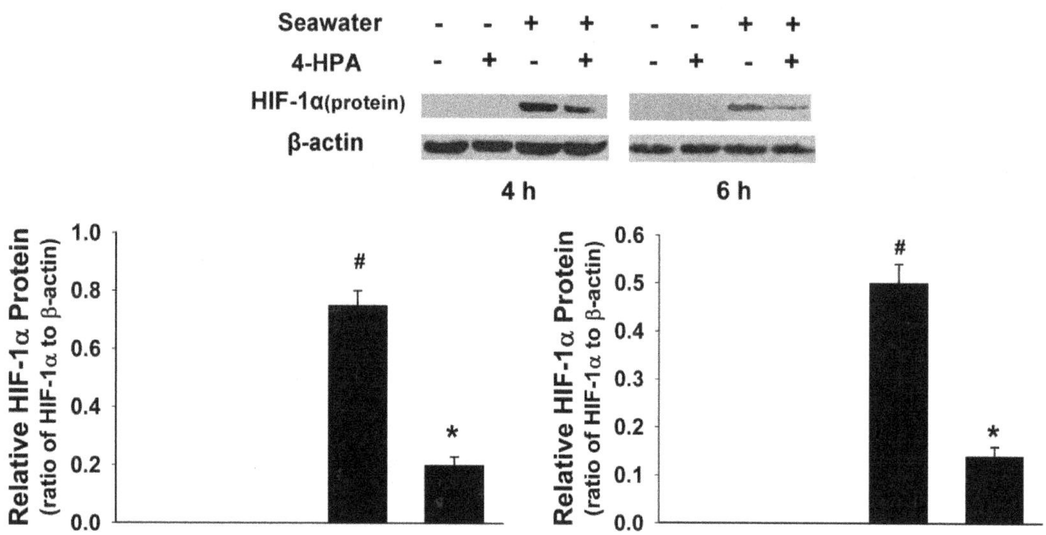

(D)

2.5. 4-HPA Decreased Hypertonicity and Hypoxia-Induced HIF-1α Protein Level, but not mRNA Level, in Primary Rat Alveolar Epithelial Cells (AEC)

As shown in Figure 5, hypertonicity (25% seawater) together with hypoxia (3% O_2) or hypertonicity alone promoted both HIF-1α protein and mRNA expression in primary rat alveolar epithelial cells (AEC) ($p < 0.05$). Moreover, hypertonicity and hypoxia synergistically increased HIF-1α protein level. However, hypoxia alone increased only HIF-1α protein ($p < 0.05$) but not mRNA level. 4-HPA decreased hypertonicity, hypoxia, and both of the two induced HIF-1α protein levels, but not mRNA levels ($p < 0.05$).

Figure 5. Effects of 4-HPA on hypertonicity, hypoxia, and both of the two induced HIF-1α protein and mRNA levels in primary AEC. Treated by hypertonicity, hypoxia, or both of the two with or without 4-HPA treatment for 4 h, primary rat alveolar epithelial cells (AEC) were harvested and HIF-1α protein and mRNA levels were assessed by Western blotting and RT-PCR. The ratios of HIF-1α to β-actin in protein and mRNA levels from three independent experiments were obtained by density scanning of the Western blotting and PCR band using an image analysis system. Data are means ± SD, * $p < 0.05$ *vs.* control group, $^{\#}p < 0.05$ *vs.* the groups with stimuli or stimulus in the absence of 4-HPA treatment.

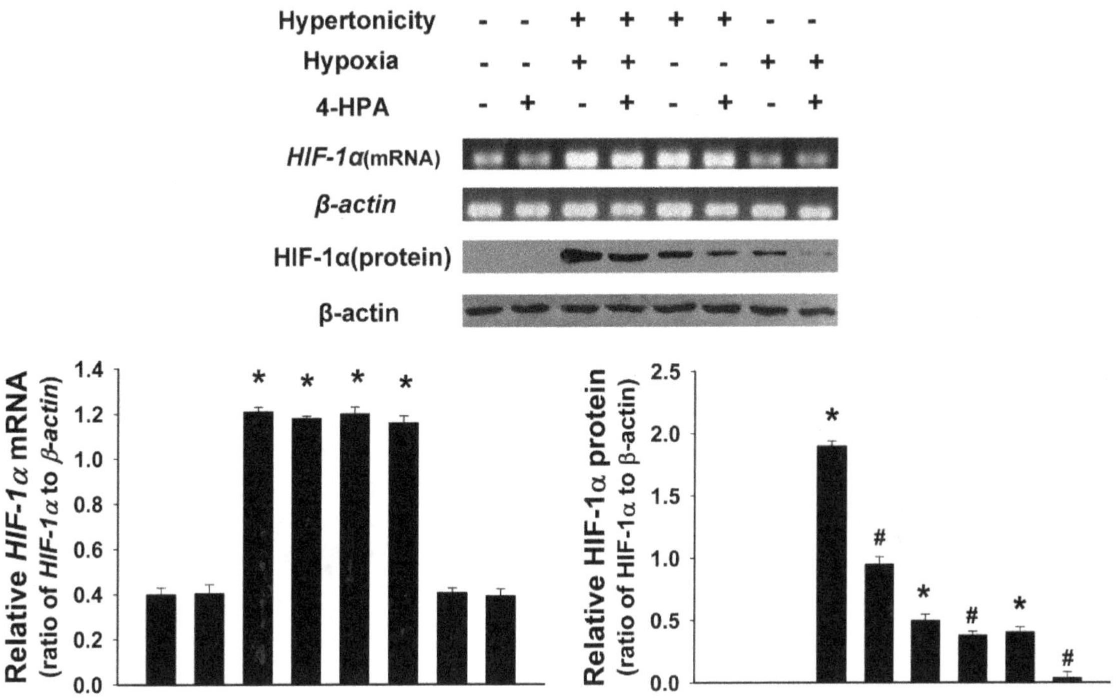

2.6. 4-HPA Decreased Hypertonicity and Hypoxia-Induced HIF-1α Protein Level through Inhibiting the Activations of Protein Translational Regulators, Including p70S6K1, S6 Ribosomal Protein, 4E-BP1, and eIF4E in Primary AEC

Since 4-HPA did not decrease hypertonicity and hypoxia-induced HIF-1α protein level via the inhibition of its mRNA expression (Figure 5), posttranscriptional mechanisms were likely involved. As shown in Figure 6, hypertonicity together with hypoxia promoted the phosphorylation but not the total protein levels of HIF-1α related translational regulators, including p70S6K1, S6 ribosomal protein, 4E-BP1, and eIF4E ($p < 0.05$), which were attenuated by 4-HPA treatment ($p < 0.05$) in AEC. Additionally, 4-HPA did not affect these translational regulators under normal condition. However, the activations of these translational regulators were not promoted by either hypertonicity or hypoxia alone and not affected by 4-HPA under hypertonic or hypoxic condition (data not shown).

Figure 6. Effects of 4-HPA on HIF-1α related protein translational regulators under hypertonicity and hypoxia conditions in primary AEC. Primary AEC were treated by hypertonicity and hypoxia in the absence or presence of 4-HPA for 4 h. Then, the cells were harvested for Western blotting and phosphorylation and total protein levels of HIF-1α related translational regulators, including p70S6K1 (**A**); S6 ribosomal protein (**B**); 4E-BP1 (**C**); and eIF4E (**D**) were detected. The ratios of HIF-1α related translational regulators to β-actin in protein levels from three independent experiments were obtained by density scanning of the Western blotting. Data are means ± SD, * $p < 0.05$ *vs.* control group, # $p < 0.05$ *vs.* hypertonicity + hypoxia group.

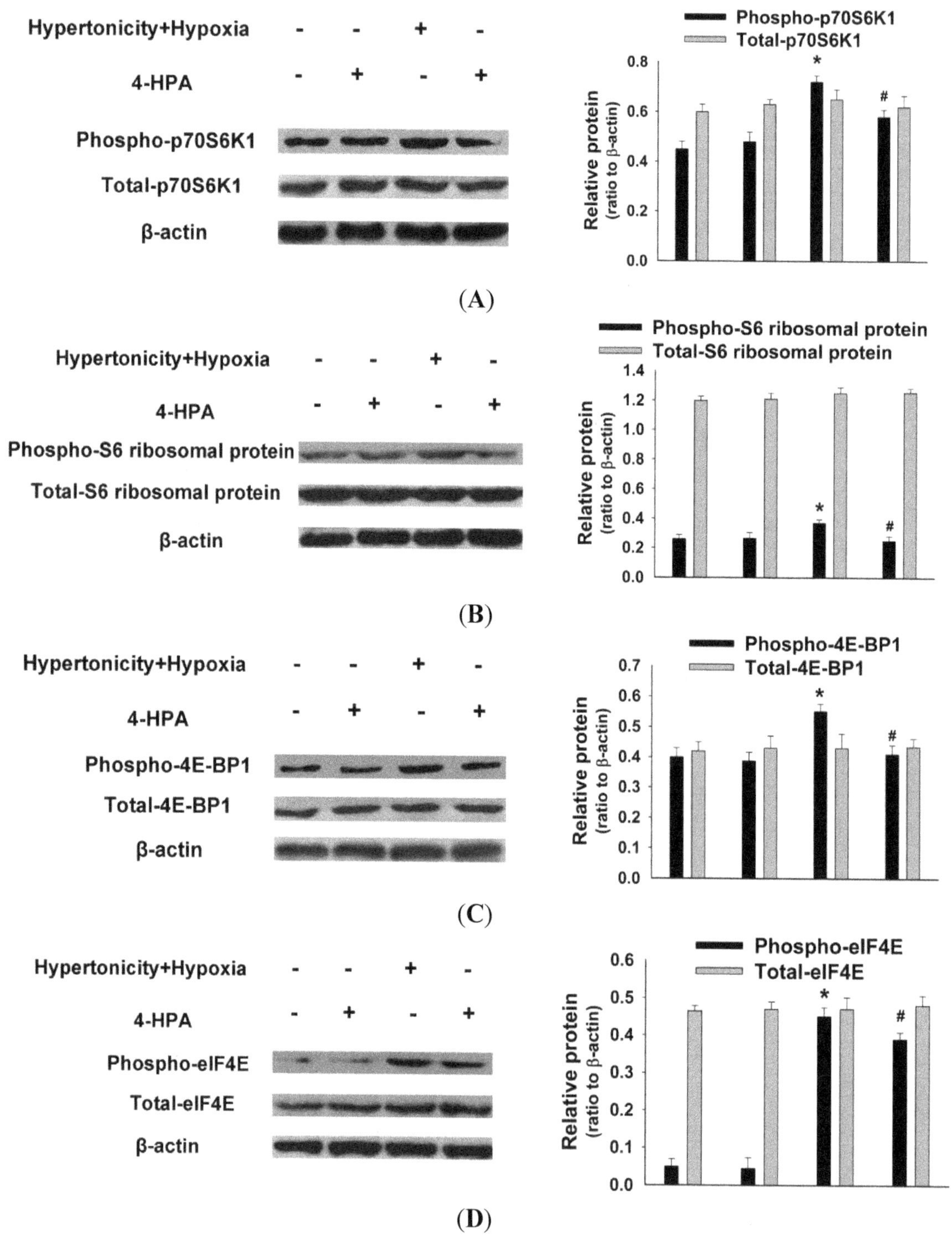

2.7. 4-HPA Decreased Hypertonicity and Hypoxia-Induced HIF-1α Protein Level through Promoting HIF-1α Protein Degradation, Which Was Associated with Prolyl Hydroxylase Domain Enzyme Isoform-2 (PHD2) Elevation in Primary AEC

In the presence of CHX (blocking ongoing protein synthesis), the half-life of HIF-1α protein was longer ($p < 0.05$) than that in the presence of 4-HPA treatment under hypertonic and hypoxic condition (Figure 7A) in primary AEC. Moreover, 4-HPA also increased the degradation of HIF-1α protein ($p < 0.05$) under hypoxic (Figure 7B) or hypertonic (Figure 7C) condition. As shown in Figure 7D, hypertonicity and hypoxia significantly decreased the protein level of prolyl hydroxylase domain enzyme isoform-2 (PHD2) which is an important enzyme isoform to regulate the stability of HIF-1α protein, and this effect was impaired by the treatment of 4-HPA. Our results provide the evidence that 4-HPA decreased hypertonicity and hypoxia-induced HIF-1α protein level through a mechanism that involves prolyl hydroxylase-dependent degradation.

Figure 7. Effects of 4-HPA on HIF-1α protein degradation under hypertonicty and hypoxia conditions in primary AEC. AEC were treated with hypertonicity (**C**); hypoxia (**B**); or both of the two (**A**) with or without 4-HPA treatment for 4 h, followed by incubation with 100 μM cycloheximide (CHX, blocking ongoing protein synthesis) from 0–30 min. Cell lysates were subjected to Western blotting using antibodies against HIF-1α and β-actin (the **left** panel) and the intensity of HIF-1α protein relative content was quantified (the **right** panel). The plot represented means ± SD from three independent experiments, * $p < 0.05$ *vs.* groups with 4-HPA treatment; and (**D**) prolyl hydroxylase domain enzyme isoform-2 (PHD2) protein of AEC which were treated with both hypertonicity and hypoxia in the presence and absence of 4-HPA was detected by Western blotting. Data are means ± SD, & $p < 0.01$ *vs.* control group, # $p < 0.05$ *vs.* hypertonicity + hypoxia group.

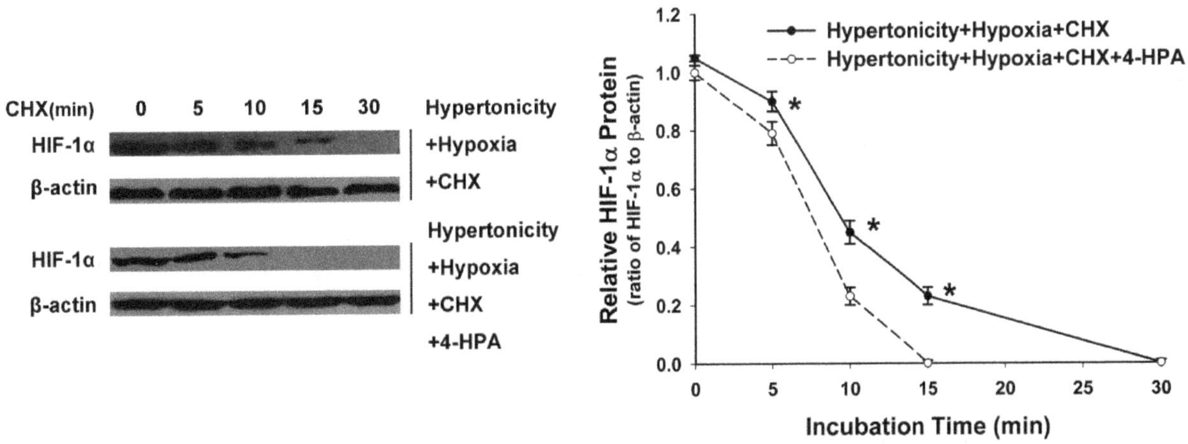

(A)

Figure 7. *Cont.*

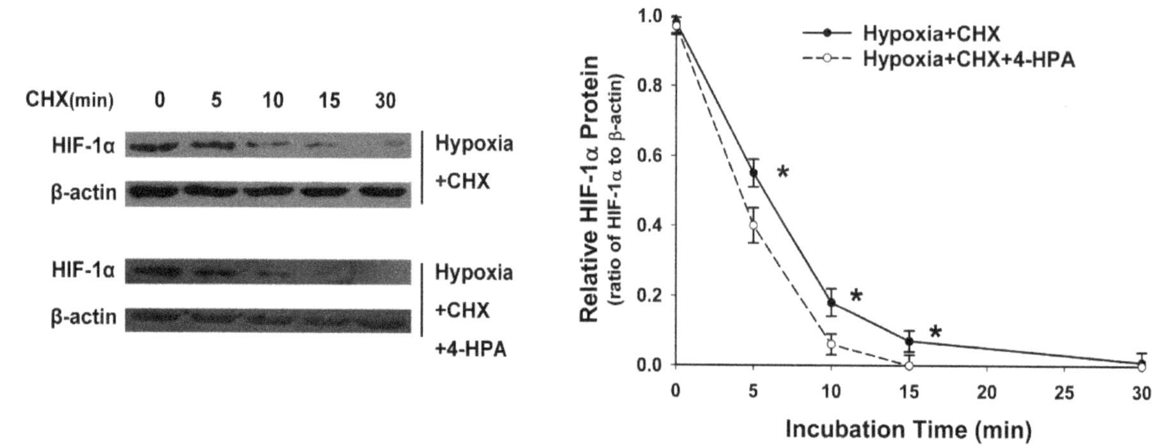

(B)

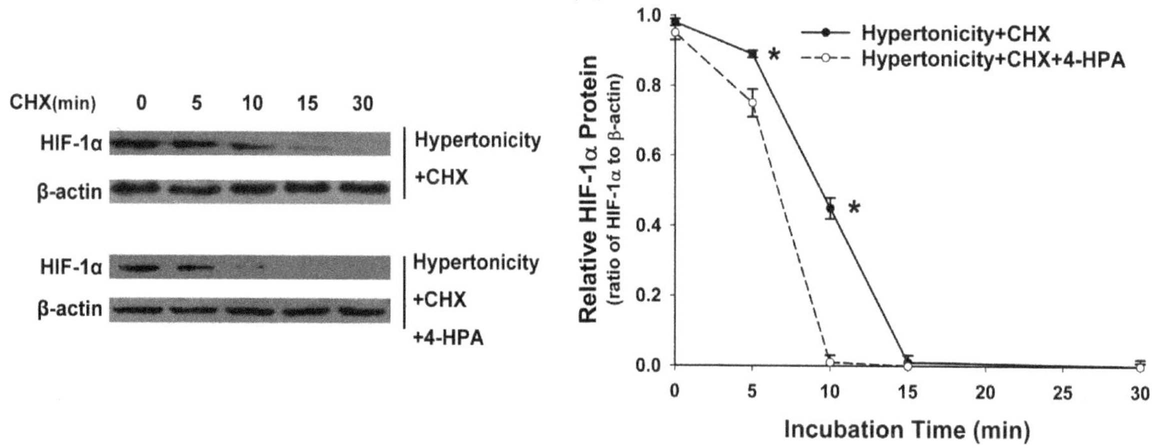

(C)

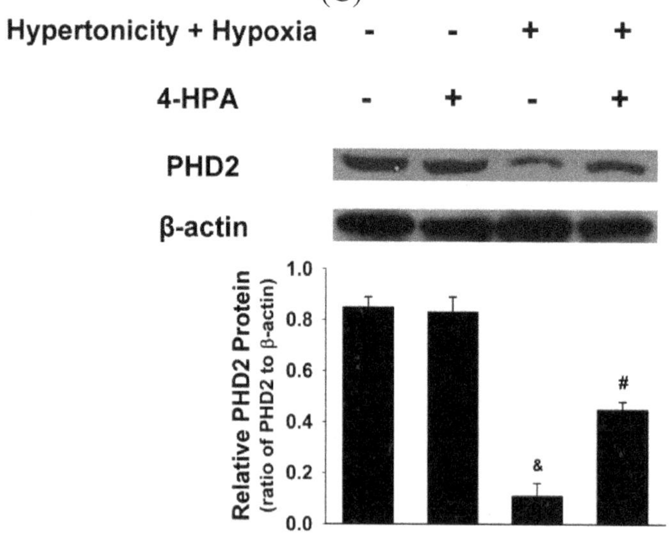

(D)

2.8. 4-HPA Decreased the Production of Inflammatory Cytokines through Suppressing Hypertonicity and Hypoxia-Induced HIF-1α in NR8383 Macrophages

Hypertonicity and hypoxia increased HIF-1α protein level ($p < 0.05$), which was markedly inhibited by HIF-1α siRNA or 4-HPA ($p < 0.05$) in NR8383 macrophages (Figure 8A). Meanwhile, TNF-α, IL-1β, and IL-6 contents in the supernatant from the cells stimulated with hypertonicity and hypoxia for 4 h were much more than those of control ($p < 0.05$) (Figure 8B–D). 4-HPA and HIF-1α siRNA similarly reduced the production of TNF-α, IL-1β, and IL-6. The scramble sequence exerted no significant impact on HIF-1α expression and the production of inflammatory cytokines in NR8383 macrophages.

2.9. 4-HPA Decreased Monolayer Permeability through Suppressing Hypertonicity and Hypoxia-Induced HIF-1α, Which Was Mediated by Inhibiting VEGF in Rat Lung Microvascular Endothelial Cell Line (RLMVEC)

As shown in Figure 9, hypertonicity and hypoxia increased rat lung microvascular endothelial cell line (RLMVEC) monolayer permeability ($p < 0.01$), and HIF-1α siRNA, sFlt-1 (*VEGF* antagonist), or 4-HPA did not affected it significantly during normal culture condition. Furthermore, hypertonicity and hypoxia-induced elevation of RLMVEC monolayer permeability was suppressed by HIF-1α siRNA, sFlt-1, and 4-HPA, respectively ($p < 0.05$) and there was no significant difference between these suppression effects. *VEGF* is a standard target gene of *HIF-1*. Therefore, 4-HPA decreased monolayer permeability through suppressing hypertonicity and hypoxia-induced HIF-1α, which was mediated by inhibiting *VEGF* in RLMVEC.

Figure 8. Effects of 4-HPA on inflammatory cytokines levels under hypertonicty and hypoxia conditions in NR8383 macrophages. (**A**) NR8383 cells were transfected with HIF-1α siRNA and a scramble sequence. Twenty-four hours after transfection, the cells with or without transfection were stimulated with hypertonicity and hypoxia in the absence or presence of 4-HPA for 4 h and then harvested for Western blotting; The supernatants of the cells were collected to detect the content of TNF-α (**B**); IL-1β (**C**); and IL-6 (**D**) by ELISA. Data are means ± SD from three independent experiments, * $p < 0.05$ *vs.* control group, # $p < 0.05$ *vs.* 2H group. 2H: hypertonicity and hypoxia, 2H + Scram: hypertonicity and hypoxia + scramble sequence, 2H + SiHIF: hypertonicity and hypoxia + HIF-1α siRNA.

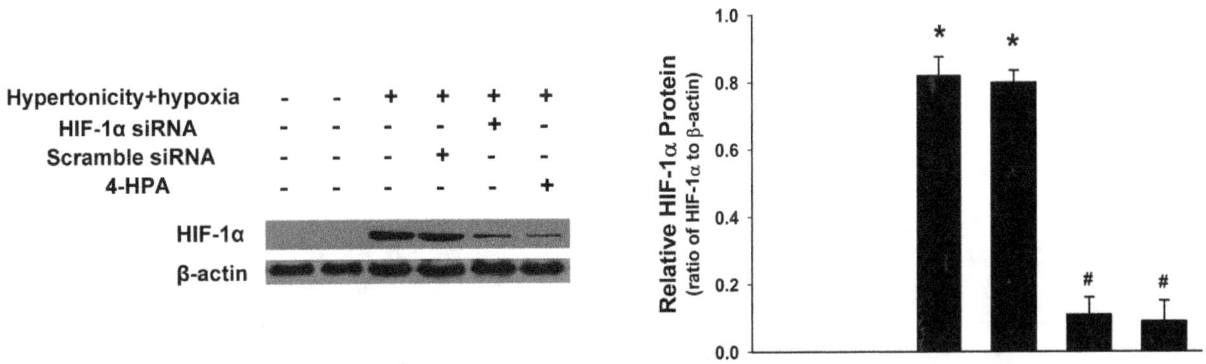

(**A**)

Figure 8. *Cont.*

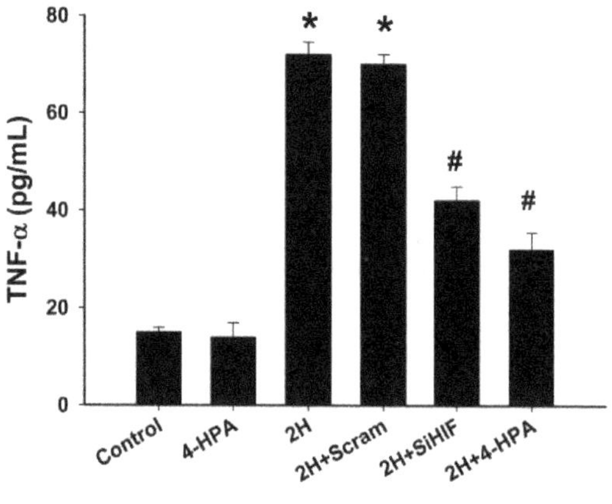

(B)

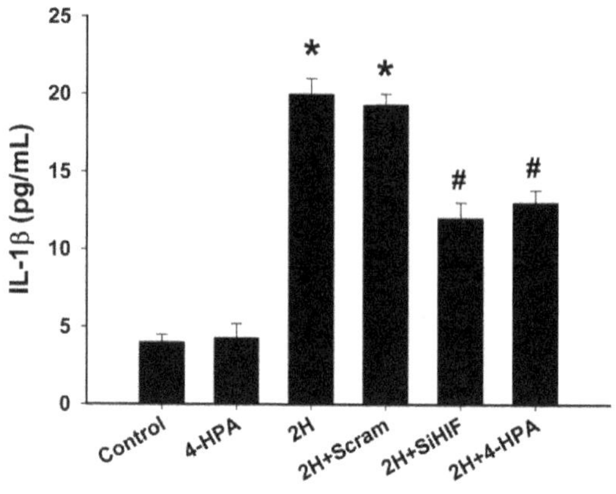

(C)

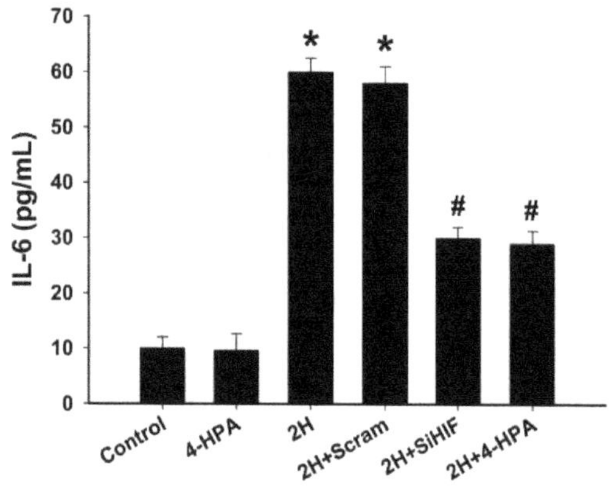

(D)

Figure 9. Effects of 4-HPA on monolayer permeability under hypertonicity and hypoxia conditions in rat lung microvascular endothelial cells (RLMVEC). RLMVEC were stimulated with HIF-1α siRNA, sFlt-1 (1 μM, vascular endothelial growth factor (*VEGF*)antagonist), 4-HPA, hypertonicity and hypoxia, hypertonicity and hypoxia + HIF-1α siRNA, hypertonicity and hypoxia + sFlt-1, hypertonicity and hypoxia + 4-HPA for 4 h, respectively. The RLMVEC monolayer permeability was measured with FITC-albumin (50 μM). Data are means ± SD, * $p < 0.01$ *vs.* control group, # $p < 0.05$ *vs.* hypertonicity and hypoxia group.

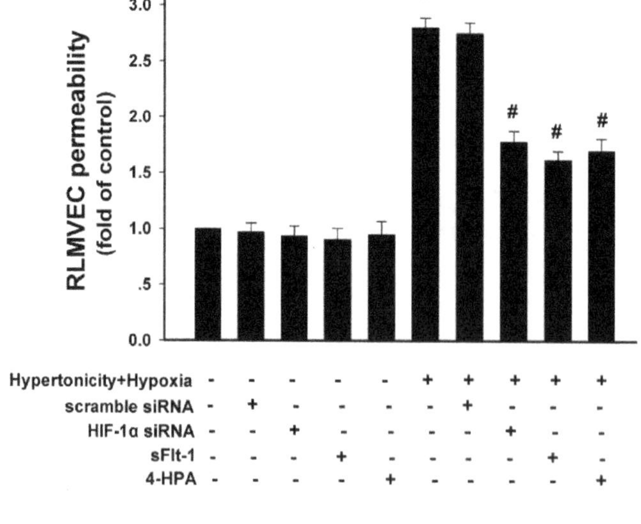

3. Discussion

The acute lung injury (ALI) induced by seawater aspiration had an acuter and rapider course than that induced by LPS [4,6–8]. The majority death induced by seawater aspiration happened within the first 6 h (Figure 2), which is greatly shorter than 40 h in LPS-induced ALI [29]. As Figures 2 and 3 shown, PaO_2 dropped precipitously to its minimum at 0.5 h and inflammation and edema in lungs were most serious at 4 h after seawater instillation in rats. These time points were also earlier than those of some other ALI [30,31]. Since the results (Figures 1–3) suggested that 4-HPA could attenuate the injuries in lungs rapidly after treatment, the agent should be used in the early stage of seawater aspiration-induced ALI.

The high level of $PaCO_2$ after seawater instillation suggested that there was pulmonary ventilatory insufficiency and local lung hypoxia. The treatment of 4-HPA increased PaO_2 and decreased $PaCO_2$ in seawater instillation rats (Figure 2). Since PaO_2 and $PaCO_2$ could indicate, at least partially, the degree of hypoxia within local lung tissue, 4-HPA might attenuate hypoxia in lung tissues in rats, which in turn inhibited HIF-1α indirectly. On the one hand, 4-HPA attenuated inflammation and edema within lung tissues to improve pulmonary membrane oxygenation, which could help to increase PaO_2. On the other hand, the Chinese traditional medicine used *Aster tataricus* of which 4-HPA is an active component to reduce and expel phlegm. Therefore, 4-HPA might have a similar function and decrease $PaCO_2$ through improving obstructive ventilatory disorder, which was not investigated in the current study.

Hypoxia increases HIF-1α protein by elevating its protein stability but not by prompting its mRNA expression [4,6–8]. However, instillation of seawater increased not only HIF-1α protein but also its mRNA expression (Figure 4). Therefore, hypertonicity induced by seawater instillation could be the factor which was accounted for the increase of *HIF-1α* mRNA expression. This hypothesis was demonstrated by our following experiments *in vitro* (Figure 5). Some previous studies reported that HIF-1α also responded to nonhypoxic stimuli such as hormones, growth factors, vasoactive peptides, cytokines, heat, hypertonicity, and LPS [13–16]. Our study demonstrated again that hypertonicity was a nonhypoxic stimulus of HIF-1α (Figures 4 and 5). In addition, a previous study reported that LPS induced HIF-1α synergistically with hypoxia [32]. Our results showed that hypertonicity could synergize with hypoxia to increase HIF-1α protein (Figure 5). Since our results showed that hypertonicity and hypoxia synergistically increased only HIF-1α protein but not mRNA level, posttranscriptional mechanisms were likely involved in this synergistic effect. We found hypertonicity together with hypoxia promoted the phosphorylation but not the total protein levels of HIF-1α related translational regulators, including p70S6K1, S6 ribosomal protein, 4E-BP1, and eIF4E, which were attenuated by 4-HPA treatment in AEC (Figure 6). 4-HPA inhibited the synergistic effect of hypertonicity and hypoxia on HIF-1α probably through suppressing synergistic protein translational process, which need further study to demonstrate. Although HIF-1α related protein translational regulators were not affected by hypertonicity or hypoxia alone (data not shown), HIF-1α protein degradation was suppressed by hypertonicity or hypoxia alone, which could be inhibited by 4-HPA (Figure 7). The HIF-1α protein levels which can be detected by Western blotting are mainly decided by three processes which are the transcription, translation, and degradation of HIF-1α protein. 4-HPA impacted HIF-1α protein levels following either hypertonicity or hypoxia through promoting HIF-1α protein degradation (Figure 7B,C) but not through impacting these translational regulators (data not shown). Moreover, 4-HPA decreased

HIF-1α protein levels following both hypertonicity and hypoxia through both inhibiting the activations of protein translational regulators (Figure 6) and promoting HIF-1α protein degradation (Figure 7A). In addition, hypertonicity or hypoxia alone did not impact these translational regulators but hypertonicity together with hypoxia synergistically increased them. Therefore, this synergistic effects might be impacted by 4-HPA which was not investigated in the current study. Taken all together, there are hypertonic and hypoxic factors in seawater aspiration-induced lung injury and these two main impact factors synergistically increased HIF-1α protein which was attenuated by 4-HPA. Therefore, our study focused on how the effects of the two factors together *in vitro* were affected by 4-HPA.

HIF-1 is a transcription factor which is essential for regulating oxygen homeostasis. It also regulates the expression of target genes important in angiogenesis, erythropoiesis, energy metabolism, and cell survival. However, there would be more detrimental effects of HIF-1α than beneficial ones when the injury factor such as LPS leads to HIF-1α overexpression, which needs an agent to inhibit [17]. In our study, the greatly increased HIF-1α protein induced synergistically by hypertonic and hypoxic factors contributed to the seawater aspiration-induced lung injury and we found that 4-HPA was a proper agent to attenuate the ALI by inhibiting HIF-1α.

4-HPA which can be secreted in saliva is a metabolite of aromatic amino acid catabolism. It is also an active component of some Chinese herb such as *Aster tataricus* and *Rhodiola rosea*, as well as an intermediate product of chemical synthesis of atenolol (β-receptor blocking agent) and puerarin (active component of *Lobed Kudzuvine Root*). Some previous studies reported that 4-HPA controlled the *NadA* gene expression and could become a potential hypopigmenting agent [23–25]. Our results suggested that 4-HPA was a good inhibitor of hypertonicity, hypoxia, or both of the two-induced HIF-1α expression. Additionally, 4-HPA, a water-soluble small molecular compound, could be a potential agent for the diseases with hypoxia-induced inflammation or edema and some carcinomas of which hypoxia-induced HIF-1α promoted the progress [33]. Moreover, HIF-1α played important roles in some diseases under hypertonic condition, such as diabetic eye disease [34] and some renal diseases [35]. Therefore, 4-HPA might be used in these fields.

4. Experimental Section

4.1. Animal Model and Grouping

Male Sprague–Dawley rats, weighing 180–220 g each, were obtained from the Animal Center (Fourth Military Medical University, Xi'an, China). These rats were kept in a temperature-controlled house with 12 h light-dark cycles and fed with standard laboratory diet and water *ad libitum*. All experiments approved by the Animal Care and Use Committee of the Fourth Military Medical University conformed to the Declaration of the National Institutes of Health Guide for Care and Use of Laboratory Animals (Publication No.85–23, revised in 1985).

Seawater Drowning Animal Model: the rats were anesthetized with 3% sodium pentobarbital (1.5 mL/kg, Sigma-Aldrich, St. Louis, MO, USA) intraperitoneally and maintained in the supine position during experiments with the head elevated 30°. A catheter was inserted into the right jugular artery to obtain blood samples. A 1 mL syringe was gently inserted into the trachea approximately 1.5 cm above the carina. Then, 4 mL/kg body weight of seawater was instilled within 4 min into both lungs. Seawater (osmolality 1300 mOsm/kgH_2O, pH 8.2, temperature 25 °C, specific weight (SW) 1.05, NaCl 26.518 g/L, $MgSO_4$ 3.305 g/L, $MgCl_2$ 2.447 g/L, $CaCl_2$ 1.141 g/L, KCl 0.725 g/L, $NaHCO_3$ 0.202 g/L, NaBr 0.083 g/L) was prepared according to the major composition of the East China Sea provided by Chinese Ocean Bureau (Beijing, China).

To assess mortality of rates, drowning rat models were prepared as mentioned before with or without different does of 4-HPA (50, 100 or 150 mg/kg body weight, i.p.) (solubility of 4-HPA, 150 mg/mL, pH 7.4). 4-HPA (Sigma-Aldrich, St. Louis, MO, USA, the chemical structure is showed in Figure 10) was administered after seawater instillation for 10 min. The mortality of rats were recorded every 2 h after seawater instillation in each group ($n = 20$).

Figure 10. The chemical structure of 4-HPA.

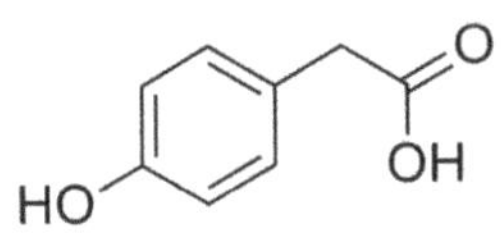

Rats were randomly divided into four groups ($n = 40$), (1) control; (2) 4-HPA (100 mg/kg) only; (3) seawater only; and (4) seawater + 4-HPA (100 mg/kg). In the seawater + 4-HPA group, rats were treated with 100 mg/kg 4-HPA after seawater instillation for 15 min. Rats were sacrificed at 2, 4, or 6 h after seawater instillation. Then, the thorax was opened rapidly and lungs were processed for studies in the manner described below.

4.2. PaO_2 and $PaCO_2$ Study

In each group, blood samples were obtained from a PE-50 catheter which was inserted in the right carotid artery at 0, 1, 2, 3, or 4 h after seawater instillation. Then, arterial oxygen tension (PaO_2) and arterial carbon dioxide tension ($PaCO_2$) of the blood samples was measured with a blood gas analyzer (Ymb-3100, Yima Opto-Electrical Technology Co., Ltd., Xi'an, China).

4.3. ELISA

The concentrations of TNF-α, IL-1β, and IL-6 were measured by using ELISA kits (R&D systems; Minneapolis, MN, USA). Lungs tissue and cells supernatant were processed according to the manufacturer's instructions for ELISA.

4.4. Bronchoalveolar Lavage Fluid (BALF) White Cell Count

After seawater instillation for 0, 2, 4, or 6 h, rats were anesthetized with intraperitoneal pentobarbital. The lungs were lavaged with 2.5 mL ice-cold phosphate buffered saline five times in all groups. The recovery ratio of the fluid was about 90%. The collected bronchoalveolar lavage fluid (BALF) was centrifuged at 520× *g* for 20 min at 4 °C. The cell pellet was then resuspended in 1 mL of red blood cell-lysis buffer to eliminate red cells. White cells were then re-pelleted by centrifugation at 520× *g* for 20 min at 4 °C. The cell pellet was again resuspended in phosphate buffer saline (PBS) and taken for cell counting using a hemocytometer.

4.5. Assessment of Pulmonary Vascular Leakage

Pulmonary vascular leakage was assessed as previously described [2] by quantitating extravasation of Evans blue into lung parenchyma. In brief, Evans blue dye (20 mg/kg, Sigma-Aldrich, St. Louis, MO, USA) was given intravenously to the rats 30 min before the animals were sacrificed. After the lung was rapidly removed from the thoracic cavity, normal saline was immediately injected into the right ventricle till there was effused clear fluid from the left atrium. The lung was removed and dried to a constant weight at 60 °C for 72 h. The dried lung was weighed and then incubated in formamide (3 mL/100 mg, Sigma-Aldrich, St. Louis, MO, USA) at 60 °C for 24 h. Then, the supernatant was separated by centrifugation at 5000× *g* for 30 min. The concentration of Evans blue in the supernatant was quantitated by the following formula: A620 (correction) = A620 − (1.426 × A740 + 0.030). The concentration of Evans blue in the lung tissue (ET) was determined from the generated Evans blue standard absorbance curves. At the same time, the concentration of Evans blue in blood (EB) was detected by the same method as described above. ELI = ET/(EB × dry lung weight) × 100%.

4.6. Wet-to-Dry Weight (W/D) Ratio

Wet-to-dry weight (W/D) ratio was used to represent the severity of lung edema. After lungs were separated from the thoracic cavity at the end of the experiment, the left lungs were weighed and then dried to constant weight at 50 °C for 72 h. The ratio of wet-to-dry was finally calculated by dividing the wet weight by the dry weight.

4.7. Histological Study

At the end of the experiments, the lung tissues were fixed with 4% paraformaldehyde for 24 h and embedded in paraffin. After deparaffinisation and dehydration, the lungs were cut into 5 μm sections and stained with hematoxylin and eosin.

4.8. Cell Culture and Treatment

Cell isolation and preparation of primary AEC (rat alveolar epithelial cells) monolayers: AT2 (alveolar epithelial type II) cells were isolated from adult male Sprague-Dawley rats (125–150 g) by disaggregation with elastate (2.0–2.5 U/mL; Worthington Biochemical, Freehold, NJ, USA), followed by differential adherence on IgG-coated bacteriological plates. All animals were treated in accordance with the guidelines and approval of the Fourth Military Medical University Institutional Animal Care and Use Committee. Freshly isolated AT2 cells were plated in minimal defined serum-free medium (MDSF) consisting of Dulbecco's modified Eagle's medium and Ham's F-12 nutrient mixture in a 1:1 ratio, supplemented with 1.25 mg/mL bovine serum albumin, 10 mM HEPES, 0.1 mM nonessential amino acids, 2.0 mM glutamine, 100 U/mL sodium penicillin G, and 100 μg/mL streptomycin. Cells were seeded onto tissue culture-treated polycarbonate filter cups (Nuclepore, Corning-Costar, Corning, NY, USA, 0.4 μm) at a density of 1.0×10^6 cells/cm^2 and grown to confluence for RNA and protein analyses. Media were changed on the second day after plating and every other day thereafter. Cultures were maintained in a humidified 5% CO_2 incubator at 37 °C. AT2 cell purity (>90%) was assessed by staining freshly isolated cells with tannic acid or an antibody

(Ab) to a lamellar membrane protein, p180 (Covance Research, Berkeley, CA, USA), followed by immunofluorescence visualization. Cell viability (>95%) was measured by trypan blue dye exclusion. Day of isolation is designated as day 0; cells were used on day 3 or 4.

Hypertonicity *in vitro*: Hypertonicity was induced by 25% seawater (seawater volume/(seawater volume + Ham's F12 medium volume) = 25%), osmolality 538.21 ± 0.99 mOsm/kgH_2O, pH 8.2, temperature 25 °C. In our preliminary experiment, HIF-1α protein level reached its maximum when AEC were stimulated by 25% seawater, compared with 12.5% or 37.5% seawater.

Hypoxia *in vitro*: AEC were cultured in a special humidified hypoxic chamber as previously described [19]. Use of an antechamber ensured that once cells became hypoxic, they were never re-exposed to a normoxic environment. The chamber utilized a positive pressure system and was supplied with a gas mixture of 3% O_2, 5% CO_2, and the balance nitrogen. Culture media and seawater (25%) used in the test were allowed to equilibrate to 3% O_2 before initiation of the test.

For effects of 4-HPA on HIF-1α expression induced by hypertonicity, hypoxia, or both of the two, primary AEC cells were stimulated with hypertonicity, hypoxia, or both of the two in the presence or absence of 4-HPA (100 μg/mL, Sigma-Aldrich, St. Louis, MO, USA) for 4 h. After being stimulated by diverse stimulus, HIF-1α protein, mRNA, HIF-1α related protein translational regulators (p70S6K1, S6 ribosomal protein, 4E-BP1, eIF4E), and HIF-prolyl hydroxylase domain enzyme isoform-2 (PHD2) protein levels of the cells were detected with Western blotting and RT-PCR. Additionally, stimulated AEC were incubated with 100 μM cycloheximide (CHX, blocking ongoing protein synthesis, obtained from EMD Biosciences, San Diego, CA, USA) from 0–30 min, then the cells were harvested at indicated time points for Western blotting.

4.9. Plasmid Construction and Transfection

The rat alveolar macrophage cell line NR8383 (endowed by Pharmacology Department, Fourth Military Medical University, Xi'an, China) was maintained in Ham's F12 medium (Sigma-Aldrich, St. Louis, MO, USA) supplemented with 10% fetal calf serum (FCS) (Sigma-Aldrich, St. Louis, MO, USA), 100 U/mL of penicillin (Sigma-Aldrich, St. Louis, MO, USA) and 100 μg/mL of streptomycin (Sigma-Aldrich, St. Louis, MO, USA) at 37 °C in a humidified atmosphere containing 5% CO_2 and 95% air.

HIF-1α siRNA was used to study the effect of 4-HPA on the production of inflammatory cytokines during hypertonic and hypoxic condition. The HIF-1α siRNA and the scramble sequence (Invitrogen, Grand Island, NY, USA) were kindly provided by Lili Liu (Department of Oncology, Tangdu Hospital, Fourth Military Medical University, Xi'an 710038, China), and the siRNA expression vector for HIF-1α was constructed as described previously [36]. NR8383 macrophages and rat lung microvascular endothelial cell line (RLMVEC) were transfected with HIF-1α siRNA or a scramble sequence by using Lipofectamine 2000 (Invitrogen, Carlsbad, CA, USA) according to the manufacturer's instructions. Twenty-four hours after transfection, NR8383 cells with or without transfection were stimulated with both of hypertonicity and hypoxia for 4 h and harvested for Western blotting to evaluate the changes of HIF-1α expression. Meanwhile, the supernatant was collected to detect the contents of TNF-α, IL-1β, and IL-6 by ELISA. In addition, RLMVEC with or without transfection were used in permeability assay below.

4.10. Permeability Assay

Rat lung microvascular endothelial cells (RLMVEC, VEC Technologies, Rensselaer, NY, USA) were cultured in high-glucose DMEM (Sigma-Aldrich, St. Louis, MO, USA) supplemented with 5% fetal bovine serum (FCS) (Sigma-Aldrich, St. Louis, MO, USA), 50 U/mL of penicillin (Sigma-Aldrich, St. Louis, MO, USA) and 50 μg/mL of streptomycin (Sigma-Aldrich, St. Louis, MO, USA) at 37 °C in a humidified atmosphere containing 5% CO_2 and 95% air. RLMVEC were seeded (~100,000 cells/insert) on polystyrene filters (No.3470, 6.5-mm diameter, 0.4-μm pore size; Costar Transwell, Cambridge, MA, USA). RLMVEC were grown to confluence over 48 h after which the cells were treated with (1) standard cell culture conditions; (2) HIF-1α siRNA; (3) 1 μM soluble VEGF receptor-1 (sFlt-1, provided by professor Lan Yang, No. 210 Hospital of PLA, Dalian, China); (4) 4-HPA (100 μg/mL); (5) hypertonicity + hypoxia; (6) hypertonicity + hypoxia + HIF-1α siRNA; (7) hypertonicity + hypoxia + sFlt-1; and (8) hypertonicity + hypoxia + 4-HPA for 4 h, respectively. Then, the RLMVEC were washed three times in serum-free medium, and FITC-labeled albumin (50 μM, Sigma-Aldrich, St. Louis, MO, USA) suspended in serum-free medium was added to the RLMVEC monolayers (100 μL, VEC Technologies, Rensselaer, NY, USA). The insert was placed in a new well of a 24-well plate containing serum-free medium (0.6 mL to ensure that the fluid volume on either side of the inserts was equalized to avoid a hydrostatic gradient that might alter the rate of albumin flux). Measuring the increase of fluoresceinisothiocyanate (FITC)-albumin in the lower well after 1 h assessed the transfer rate of albumin across the monolayer. FITC-albumin was quantified in a F4500 fluorimeter (Hitachi, Tokyo, Japan) and compared with a standard curve of fluorescence made with various dilutions of the FITC-albumin. The measurements of permeability were expressed as the fold of control.

4.11. Western Blotting

The lung tissues and cultured cells were prepared to extract proteins with lysis buffer (10 mM Tris pH 8.0, 1 mM EDTA, 400 mM NaCl, 10% glycerol, 0.5% NP-40, 5 mM sodium fluoride, 0.1 mM phenylmethylsulfonyl fluoride, 1 mM dithiothreitol). The lysates were centrifuged at 12,000 rpm for 30 min at 4 °C, and then supernatants were collected. Equal amounts (50 μg) of protein were separated by SDS-PAGE, transferred to nitrocellulose membrane at 100 V for 2.5 h at low temperature, and blocked with 5% skim milk for 2 h. Subsequently, anti-HIF-1α antibody (dilution 1:1000; Millipore, Bedford, MA, USA), anti-p70S6K1 (*M*r 70,000 ribosomal protein S6 kinase 1, 1:1000; Cell Signaling Technology, Danvers, MA, USA), anti-Phospho-p70S6K1 (Phosphorylated Thr-421/Ser-424) (1:500; Cell Signaling Technology, Danvers, MA, USA), anti-S6 ribosomal protein (1:100; Cell Signaling Technology, Danvers, MA, USA), anti-Phospho-S6 ribosomal protein (Ser-234/236) (1:500; Cell Signaling Technology, Danvers, MA, USA), anti-4E-BP1 (eukaryotic initiation factor 4E (eIF4E)-binding protein 1, 1:500, Cell Signaling Technology, Danvers, MA, USA), anti-Phospho-4E-BP1 (Ser-65) (1:500; Cell Signaling Technology, Danvers, MA, USA), anti-eIF4E (1:1000; Cell Signaling Technology, Danvers, MA, USA), anti-Phospho-eIF4E (Ser-209) (1:1000; Cell Signaling Technology), anti-PHD2 (1:1000, Sigma-Aldrich, St. Louis, MO, USA), and anti-β-actin (1:2000, Sigma-Aldrich, St. Louis, MO, USA) were respectively added and kept with the membranes at 4 °C overnight. After repeated washing, the membranes were incubated with horseradish peroxidase-conjugated anti-rabbit secondary antibody (1:2000, Sigma-Aldrich, St. Louis, MO, USA) and bands visualized by using the enhanced chemiluminescence (ECL) system (Amersham Pharmacia Biotech, Arlington Heights, IL, USA). The results were exprcssed as the ratio to β-actin level in the same protein samples.

4.12. Reverse Transcription-PCR

Total RNA was extracted respectively from lung tissues and cells with Trizol (Invitrogen, Grand Island, NY, USA) according to the manufacturer's instructions. The total RNA concentration was determined by spectrometric analysis. *HIF-1α* mRNA was examined by reverse transcription-PCR (RT-PCR) as per the manufacturer's instructions (Promeaga, Madison, WI, USA). A total of 1 μg of RNA was incubated with reverse transcriptase mixture at 50 °C for 30 min, followed by amplification with the specific primers (synthesized by Invitrogen). The primers for *HIF-1α* (575 bp) were (forward) 5'-GACACCGCGGGCACCGATT-3', and (reverse) 5'-GTTCATCGTCCTCCCCCGGC-3', and for *β-actin* (240 bp), were (forward) 5'-TAAAGACCTCTATGCCAACACAGT-3', and (reverse) 5'-CACGATGGAGGGCCGGACTCATC-3', respectively. Thirty-five amplification cycles consisting of 30 s of denaturation at 95 °C, 30 s of annealing at 55 °C, and 1 min of extension at 72 °C were performed. After amplification, the RT-PCR products were separated on 1% agarose gels (Invitrogen, Grand Island, NY, USA), and the bands were visualized by ethidium bromide (Invitrogen, Grand Island, NY, USA) staining. Quantitation was obtained by density scanning of the PCR bands using a Scion image analysis system (Beta 4.02, Scion Corporation, Colombo, Sri Lanka). The results were expressed as the ratio to β-actin mRNA level in the same RNA samples.

4.13. Statistical Analysis

Data are expressed as means ± SD Statistically significant differences between groups were determined by ANOVA followed by Student's test. Survival data were presented by the Kaplan Meier method [37] and comparisons were made by the log rank test. A statistical difference was accepted as significant if $p < 0.05$.

5. Conclusions

4-HPA attenuated inflammation and edema through the suppression of hypertonic and hypoxic induction of HIF-1α in seawater aspiration-induced lung injury in rats. It may be considered as a potential agent in treatment of seawater aspiration-induced lung injury.

Acknowledgments

This work was supported by grants from the National Research and Development of Important New drugs Foundation (No. 2009ZXJ09002-019) and the National Natural Science Foundation of China (No. 81270124).

Author Contributions

Z.L., R.X., F.J., and X.W. designed the research; Z.L., Z.Z., and W.L. conducted cell experiments; R.X., Z.Z., and Y.L. conducted animal experiments; Z.L. performed statistical analysis; X.W. and F.J. provided help with data interpretation; and Z.L. wrote the paper. All authors read and approved the final manuscript.

References

1. Van Beeck, E.F.; Branche, C.M.; Szpilman, D.; Modell, J.H.; Bierens, J.J. A new definition of drowning: Towards documentation and prevention of a global public health problem. *Bull. World Health Org.* **2005**, *83*, 853–856.
2. Li, J.; Xu, M.; Fan, Q.; Xie, X.; Zhang, Y.; Mu, D.; Zhao, P.; Zhang, B.; Cao, F.; Wang, Y.; *et al.* Tanshinone IIA ameliorates seawater exposure-induced lung injury by inhibiting aquaporins (AQP) 1 and AQP5 expression in lung. *Respir. Physiol. Neurobiol.* **2011**, *176*, 39–49.
3. Li, J.H.; Xu, M.; Xie, X.Y.; Fan, Q.X.; Mu, D.G.; Zhang, Y.; Cao, F.L.; Wang, Y.X.; Zhao, P.T.; Zhang, B.; *et al.* Tanshinone IIA suppresses lung injury and apoptosis, and modulates protein kinase B and extracellular signal-regulated protein kinase pathways in rats challenged with seawater exposure. *Clin. Exp. Pharmacol. Physiol.* **2011**, *38*, 269–277.
4. Fan, Q.; Zhao, P.; Li, J.; Xie, X.; Xu, M.; Zhang, Y.; Mu, D.; Li, W.; Sun, R.; Liu, W.; *et al.* 17β-Estradiol administration attenuates seawater aspiration-induced acute lung injury in rats. *Pulm. Pharmacol. Ther.* **2011**, *24*, 673–681.
5. Rui, M.; Duan, Y.Y.; Wang, H.L.; Zhang, X.H.; Wang, Y. Differences between seawater- and freshwater-induced lung injuries. *Chin. Crit. Care Med.* **2009**, *21*, 416–420.
6. Wang, Q.; Zheng, X.; Cheng, Y.; Zhang, Y.L.; Wen, H.X.; Tao, Z.; Li, H.; Hao, Y.; Gao, Y.; Yang, L.M.; *et al.* Resolvin D1 stimulates alveolar fluid clearance through alveolar epithelial sodium channel, Na,K-ATPase via ALX/cAMP/PI3K pathway in lipopolysaccharide-induced acute lung injury. *J. Immunol.* **2014**, *192*, 3765–3777.
7. He, J.; Zhao, Y.; Deng, W.; Wang, D.X. Netrin-1 promotes epithelial sodium channel-mediated alveolar fluid clearance via activation of the adenosine 2B receptor in lipopolysaccharide-induced acute lung injury. *Respiration* **2014**, 87, 394–407.
8. Xie, X.Y.; Zhang, B.; Li, J.H.; Fan, Q.X.; Zhang, Y.; Mu, D.G.; Li, W.P.; Xu, M.; Zhao, P.T.; Jin, F.G.; *et al.* Sodium tanshinone iia sulfonate attenuates seawater aspiration-induced acute pulmonary edema by up-regulating Na^+,K^+-ATPase activity. *Exp. Lung Res.* **2011**, *37*, 482–491.
9. Fan, Y.; Dong, W.; He, J.; Du, L.; Xu, G.; Liu, X.; Pei, Y.; Fu, G.; Ma, G. The effect of HJ-1 NO–HFJV respirator on treating pulmonary edema caused by seawater drowning. *J. Biomed. Eng.* **2002**, *19*, 526–528.
10. Zhao, X.W.; Zhang, J.P.; Huang, X.; Liu, Y.N. Effects of positive end expiratory pressure ventilation upon respiratory function and hydrophobic surfactants proteins in rabbit with seawater respiratory distress syndrome. *Zhonghua Yi Xue Za Zhi* **2009**, *89*, 3266–3270.
11. Sawada, S.; Ichiba, S.; Itano, H.; Shoga, K.; Shimizu, N. Experimental study of partial liquid ventilation in the setting of acute respiratory failure induced by sea water lung lavage in rabbits. *Acta Med. Okayama* **1998**, *52*, 131–137.

12. Wang, G.L.; Jiang, B.H.; Rue, E.A.; Semenza, G.L. Hypoxia-inducible factor 1 is a basic-helix-loop-helix-PAS heterodimer regulated by cellular O_2 tension. *Proc. Natl. Acad. Sci. USA* **1995**, *92*, 5510–5514.
13. Dery, M.A.; Michaud, M.D.; Richard, D.E. Hypoxia-inducible factor 1: Regulation by hypoxic and non-hypoxic activators. *Int. J. Biochem. Cell Biol.* **2005**, *37*, 535–540.
14. Oh, Y.T.; Lee, J.Y.; Yoon, H.; Lee, E.H.; Baik, H.H.; Kim, S.S.; Ha, J.; Yoon, K.S.; Choe, W.; Kang, I. Lipopolysaccharide induces hypoxia-inducible factor-1α mRNA expression and activation via NADPH oxidase and Sp1-dependent pathway in BV2 murine microglial cells. *Neurosci. Lett.* **2008**, *431*, 155–160.
15. Shein, N.A.; Horowitz, M.; Alexandrovich, A.G.; Tsenter, J.; Shohami, E. Heat acclimation increases hypoxia-inducible factor 1α and erythropoietin receptor expression: Implication for neuroprotection after closed head injury in mice. *J. Cereb. Blood Flow Metabol.* **2005**, *25*, 1456–1465.
16. Zhou, B.; Ann, D.K.; Li, X.; Kim, K.J.; Lin, H.; Minoo, P.; Crandall, E.D.; Borok, Z. Hypertonic induction of aquaporin-5: Novel role of hypoxia-inducible factor-1α. *Am. J. Physiol. Cell Physiol.* **2007**, *292*, C1280–C1290.
17. Yeh, C.H.; Cho, W.; So, E.C.; Chu, C.C.; Lin, M.C.; Wang, J.J.; Hsing, C.H. Propofol inhibits lipopolysaccharide-induced lung epithelial cell injury by reducing hypoxia-inducible factor-1α expression. *Br. J. Anaesth.* **2011**, *106*, 590–599.
18. Hellwig-Burgel, T.; Stiehl, D.P.; Wagner, A.E.; Metzen, E.; Jelkmann, W. Review: Hypoxia-inducible factor-1 (HIF-1): A novel transcription factor in immune reactions. *J. Interferon Cytokine Res.* **2005**, *25*, 297–310.
19. Irwin, D.C.; McCord, J.M.; Nozik-Grayck, E.; Beckly, G.; Foreman, B.; Sullivan, T.; White, M.; Crossno, J.T., Jr.; Bailey, D.; Flores, S.C.; *et al.* A potential role for reactive oxygen species and the HIF-1α-VEGF pathway in hypoxia-induced pulmonary vascular leak. *Free Radic. Biol. Med.* **2009**, *47*, 55–61.
20. Ng, T.B.; Liu, F.; Lu, Y.; Cheng, C.H.; Wang, Z. Antioxidant activity of compounds from the medicinal herb *Aster tataricus*. *Comp. Biochem. Physiol.* **2003**, *136*, 109–115.
21. Du, L.; Mei, H.F.; Yin, X.; Xing, Y.Q. Delayed growth of glioma by a polysaccharide from *Aster tataricus* involve upregulation of Bax/Bcl-2 ratio, activation of caspase-3/8/9, and downregulation of the Akt. *Tumour Biol.* **2014**, *35*, 1819–1825.
22. Yen, M.H.; Lee, J.J.; Yeh, C.F.; Wang, K.C.; Chiang, Y.W.; Chiang, L.C.; Chang, J.S. Yakammaoto inhibited human coxsackievirus B4 (CVB4)-induced airway and renal tubular injuries by preventing viral attachment, internalization, and replication. *J. Ethnopharmacol.* **2014**, *151*, 1056–1063.
23. Cloward, J.M.; Shafer, W.M. MtrR control of a transcriptional regulatory pathway in Neisseria meningitidis that influences expression of a gene (*NadA*) encoding a vaccine candidate. *PLoS One* **2013**, *8*, e56097.
24. Metruccio, M.M.; Pigozzi, E.; Roncarati, D.; Berlanda Scorza, F.; Norais, N.; Hill, S.A.; Scarlato, V.; Delany, I. A novel phase variation mechanism in the meningococcus driven by a ligand-responsive repressor and differential spacing of distal promoter elements. *PLoS Pathog.* **2009**, *5*, e1000710.
25. Wen, K.C.; Chang, C.S.; Chien, Y.C.; Wang, H.W.; Wu, W.C.; Wu, C.S.; Chiang, H.M.

Tyrosol and its analogues inhibit α-melanocyte-stimulating hormone induced melanogenesis. *Int. J. Mol. Sci.* **2013**, *14*, 23420–23440.

26. Lang, K.J.; Kappel, A.; Goodall, G.J. Hypoxia-inducible factor-1α mRNA contains an internal ribosome entry site that allows efficient translation during normoxia and hypoxia. *Mol. Biol. Cell* **2002**, *13*, 1792–1801.
27. Laughner, E.; Taghavi, P.; Chiles, K.; Mahon, P.C.; Semenza, G.L. HER2 (neu) signaling increases the rate of hypoxia-inducible factor 1α (HIF-1α) synthesis: Novel mechanism for HIF-1-mediated vascular endothelial growth factor expression. *Mol. Cell. Biol.* **2001**, *21*, 3995–4004.
28. Page, E.L.; Robitaille, G.A.; Pouyssegur, J.; Richard, D.E. Induction of hypoxia-inducible factor-1α by transcriptional and translational mechanisms. *J. Biol. Chem.* **2002**, *277*, 48403–48409.
29. Zhang, B.; Liu, Z.Y.; Li, Y.Y.; Luo, Y.; Liu, M.L.; Dong, H.Y.; Wang, Y.X.; Liu, Y.; Zhao, P.T.; Jin, F.G.; *et al.* Antiinflammatory effects of matrine in LPS-induced acute lung injury in mice. *Eur. J. Pharm. Sci.* **2011**, *44*, 573–579.
30. Iba, T.; Nagaoka, I.; Yamada, A.; Nagayama, M.; Miki, T. Effect of hemoperfusion using polymyxin B-immobilized fibers on acute lung injury in a rat sepsis model. *Int. J. Med. Sci.* **2014**, *11*, 255–261.
31. Gao, J.; Zhan, Y.; Chen, J.; Wang, L.; Yang, J. Triptolide ameliorates lipopolysaccharide-induced acute lung injury in rats. *Eur. J. Med. Res.* **2014**, doi:10.1186/2047-783X-18-58.
32. Mi, Z.; Rapisarda, A.; Taylor, L.; Brooks, A.; Creighton-Gutteridge, M.; Melillo, G.; Varesio, L. Synergystic induction of HIF-1α transcriptional activity by hypoxia and lipopolysaccharide in macrophages. *Cell Cycle* **2008**, *7*, 232–241.
33. Semenza, G.L. HIF-1 mediates metabolic responses to intratumoral hypoxia and oncogenic mutations. *J. Clin. Investig.* **2013**, *123*, 3664–3671.
34. Vadlapatla, R.K.; Vadlapudi, A.D.; Mitra, A.K. Hypoxia-inducible factor-1 (HIF-1): A potential target for intervention in ocular neovascular diseases. *Curr. Drug Targets* **2013**, *14*, 919–935.
35. Nangaku, M.; Rosenberger, C.; Heyman, S.N.; Eckardt, K.U. Regulation of hypoxia-inducible factor in kidney disease. *Clin. Exp. Pharmacol. Physiol.* **2013**, *40*, 148–157.
36. Liu, L.; Ning, X.; Sun, L.; Shi, Y.; Han, S.; Guo, C.; Chen, Y.; Sun, S.; Yin, F.; Wu, K.; *et al.* Involvement of MGr1-Ag/37LRP in the vincristine-induced HIF-1 expression in gastric cancer cells. *Mol. Cell. Biochem.* **2007**, *303*, 151–160.
37. Stel, V.S.; Dekker, F.W.; Tripepi, G.; Zoccali, C.; Jager, K.J. Survial analysis I: the Kaplan-Meier method. *Nephron. Clin. Pract.* **2011**, *119*, 83–88.

14

PSNO: Predicting Cysteine *S*-Nitrosylation Sites by Incorporating Various Sequence-Derived Features into the General Form of Chou's PseAAC

Jian Zhang [1], Xiaowei Zhao [1], Pingping Sun [1,2] and Zhiqiang Ma [1,*]

[1] School of Computer Science and Information Technology, Northeast Normal University, Changchun 130017, China; E-Mails: zhangj943@nenu.edu.cn (J.Z.); xwzhao_nenu@yeah.net (X.Z.); ppsun_nenu@yeah.net (P.S.)

[2] National Engineering Laboratory for Druggable Gene and Protein Screening, Northeast Normal University, Changchun 130024, China

* Author to whom correspondence should be addressed; E-Mail: zhiqiangma.nenu@gmail.com

---

Abstract: *S*-nitrosylation (SNO) is one of the most universal reversible post-translational modifications involved in many biological processes. Malfunction or dysregulation of SNO leads to a series of severe diseases, such as developmental abnormalities and various diseases. Therefore, the identification of SNO sites (SNOs) provides insights into disease progression and drug development. In this paper, a new bioinformatics tool, named PSNO, is proposed to identify SNOs from protein sequences. Firstly, we explore various promising sequence-derived discriminative features, including the evolutionary profile, the predicted secondary structure and the physicochemical properties. Secondly, rather than simply combining the features, which may bring about information redundancy and unwanted noise, we use the relative entropy selection and incremental feature selection approach to select the optimal feature subsets. Thirdly, we train our model by the technique of the *k*-nearest neighbor algorithm. Using both informative features and an elaborate feature selection scheme, our method, PSNO, achieves good prediction performance with a mean Mathews correlation coefficient (*MCC*) value of about 0.5119 on the training dataset using 10-fold cross-validation. These results indicate that PSNO can be used as a competitive predictor among the state-of-the-art SNOs prediction tools. A web-server, named PSNO, which implements the proposed method, is freely available at http://59.73.198.144:8088/PSNO/.

Keywords: cysteine *S*-nitrosylation sites; relative entropy selection; incremental feature selection; *k*-nearest neighbor

1. Introduction

S-nitrosylation (SNO) is one of the most ubiquitous post-translational modifications (PTMs) involving the covalent interaction of nitric oxide with the thiol group of cysteine residues [1]. Many lines of evidence have suggested that *S*-nitrosylation sites (SNOs) play key roles in providing proteins with structural and functional diversity, as well as in regulating cellular plasticity and dynamics. Malfunction or dysregulation of SNOs leads to a series of severe diseases [2], including developmental abnormalities and various diseases, such as cancer [3], Parkinson's [4], Alzheimer's [5] and amyotrophic lateral sclerosis [6]. Therefore, detecting possible SNO substrates and their corresponding exact sites is crucial for understanding the mechanisms of the biological processes of these diseases and promising great possibilities as effective therapeutic targets or diagnostic markers.

Several biochemical methodologies, including absorbance detection [7], colorimetric assays [8] and fluorescent assays [8,9], have been developed to identify SNOs. Compared with expensive and time-consuming biochemical experiments, computational methods are attracting more and more attention, due to their convenience and efficiency.

In 2001, Jaffrey made the first attempt to develop a biotin-switch technique (BST) for the large-scale detection of SNO substrates [10]. The BST includes three principal steps: (i) the methylthiolation of free protein thiols; (ii) the reduction of SNO bonds on Cys residues with ascorbate; and (iii) the ligation of thiols using *N*-[6-(Biotinamido)hexyl]-3'-(2'-pyridyldithio) propionamide (biotin-HPDP). Soon after that, Gross developed a predictor, named SNOSID [11]. This is a proteomic method, which identified endogenous and chemically-induced SNOs in proteins from tissues or cells. In 2009, Forrester explored a protein microarray-based approach using resin-assisted capture (RAC) to screen SNOs [12]. Compared with BST using a human embryonic kidney cell dataset, SNO-RAC outperformed it with higher sensitivity for proteins larger than ~100 kDa. Although these methods did make contributions to the development of the prediction of SNOs from different aspects, they were labor intensive and had a relatively low throughput.

Recent years have witnessed several computational methods that have been proposed in this field. Xue adopted a group-based prediction system for the prediction of kinase-specific SNOs and developed software named GPS-SNO (Group-based Prediction System) [13]. Li used a coupling pattern-based encoding scheme (CPR) and built a web server named CPR-SNO [14]. Xu introduced a position-specific amino acid propensity matrix to construct the predictor and built a free website, iSNO-pseudo-amino acid composition (PseAAC) [15]. As the iSNO-PseAAC treated all the proteins independently without taking into account any of their correlations, the following iSNO-AAPair incorporated some sequence correlation effects into the feature vector [16].

Each of the aforementioned methods has its own merit and does facilitate the development of this field. Although these computational models have been developed to predict SNOs, their accuracy is unsatisfactory, and they lack a detailed analysis of the features. Therefore, it is important to develop an efficient method for the site-specific detection of SNOs.

In this paper, we focus on the challenging problem of predicting SNOs based on primary sequence information. A novel method, PSNO, is proposed for differentiating SNOs from non-SNOs. Firstly, various informative sequence-derived features that effectively reflect the intrinsic characters of a given peptide are combined to construct informative features; Secondly, relative entropy selection and incremental feature selection are adopted to select the optimal feature subsets; Thirdly, we use *k*-nearest neighbor to identify SNOs based on the selected optimal feature subsets. In order to evaluate the proposed method with previous works fairly, 10-fold cross-validation is implemented on the widely-used low-similarity training dataset. The experimental results show that the proposed PSNO is a powerful computational tool for SNOs prediction. A web-server, named PSNO, that implements the proposed method is freely available at http://59.73.198.144:8088/PSNO/.

2. Results and Discussion

2.1. The Feature Selection Results

The output of the relative entropy selector was two lists: one was called the feature list, which sorted the features according to their importance to the class of samples; the other was called the coefficient list, which sorted the coefficient values in descending order (Table S1). In the coefficient value list, a feature with a larger index implied that it tended to play a more important role in identifying SNOs. Such a list of ranked features would be used in the following IFS procedure for searching the optimal feature subset.

Based on the results of the relative entropy selector, 458 individual classifiers were built by adding features one by one from the top of the feature list to the bottom (Table S2). As shown in Figure 1, the mean *MCC* values reached the maximum when 57 features were provided.

Figure 1. The IFS curve of 458 features for the training dataset. The *x*-axis and *y*-axis indicates the mean Mathews correlation coefficient (*MCC*) and number of features, respectively. When the number of selected features is 57, the mean *MCC* reaches the maximum, 0.51194.

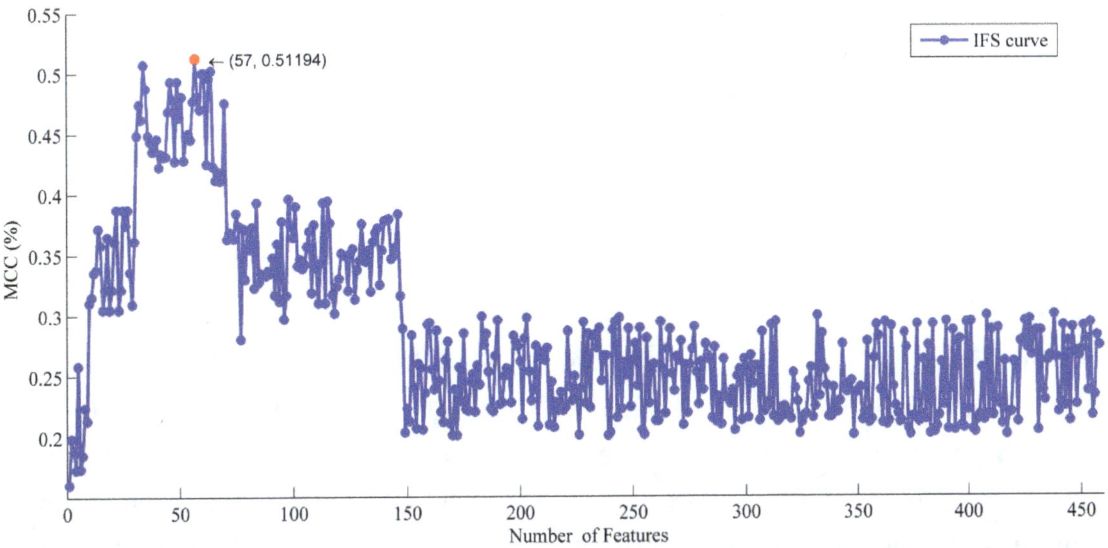

In this paper, 10-fold cross-validation was performed on the training dataset (731 SNOs and 810 non-SNOs). We obtained a mean accuracy of 68.85% using all the features with a sensitivity of 67.99%, a specificity of 69.63% and an *MCC* of 0.3759. Using 57 optimal features, our model produced 75.67% accuracy with 74.15% sensitivity, 77.04% specificity and an *MCC* of 0.5119. The results suggested that our feature selection approach successfully chose "good" features, as well as eliminated "bad" features.

2.2. Analysis of the Optimal Feature Set

To discover the different contributions of various types of features, we further investigated the distribution of each kind of feature in the final optimal feature subset. The results are shown in Figure 2. Of the 57 optimal features, 48 belonged to the evolutionary conservation score, three to the predicted secondary structure, six to the physicochemical properties, which indicated that all three types of features contribute to the prediction of protein SNOs. The detailed descriptions of the 57 optimal features are shown in the Table S3. In addition, evolutionary conservation scores accounted for the biggest part in differentiating SNOs from non-SNOs.

Figure 2. The distribution of each feature type in the final optimal feature subset. The *x*-axis and *y*-axis indicate the feature type and the number of selected features, respectively. Of the 57 optimal features, 48 belong to the evolutionary conservation score, three to the predicted secondary structure and six to the physicochemical properties.

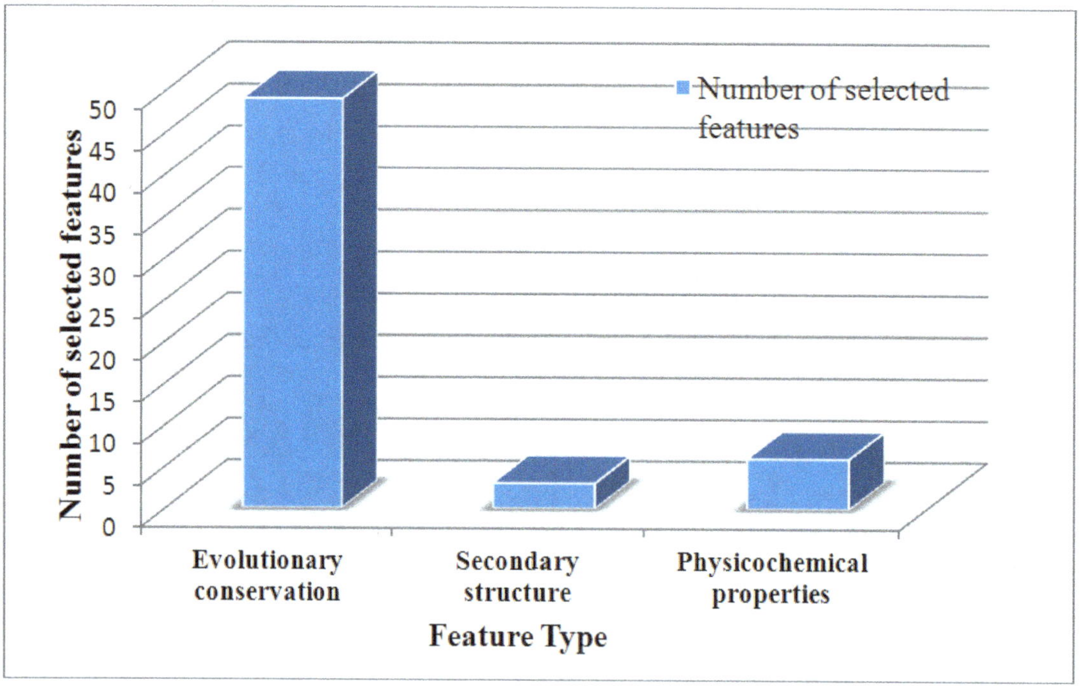

As is well known, all biological species were developed starting from a very limited number of ancestral species. Evolution was an eternal process that impenetrated the whole history of life. The evolution of protein sequences involved the changes, insertions and deletions of single residues or peptides along with the entire development of proteins [17]. Although some similarities may be eliminated after a long time of evolution, the corresponding protein zones may still share some common attributes, because the functional sites of a protein always locate in the conservation zone [18]. This explains why evolutionary conservation scores occupy the biggest part of the optimal subset. In addition, the features within the top 10 features in the final optimal feature subsets contained seven evolutional profile features.

We also calculated different kinds of features accounting for the various proportions of the optimal feature subset (Figure 3). The blue blocks represented the percentage of the selected features accounting for the whole optimal feature subsets, and the red ones represented the percentage of the selected features accounting for the corresponding feature type. Although, within the final optimal feature subset, a few secondary structure features are selected, we cannot say that the secondary structure features are not tightly related to SNOs. Among all nine secondary structure features, three features were selected in the optimal feature subsets.

Figure 3. The proportion of each type of feature in the optimal feature subset. The *x*-axis and *y*-axis indicate the feature type and the proportion of the selected features, respectively. The blue blocks represent the percentage of the selected features accounting for the whole optimal feature subsets, and the red ones represent the percentage of the selected features accounting for the corresponding feature type.

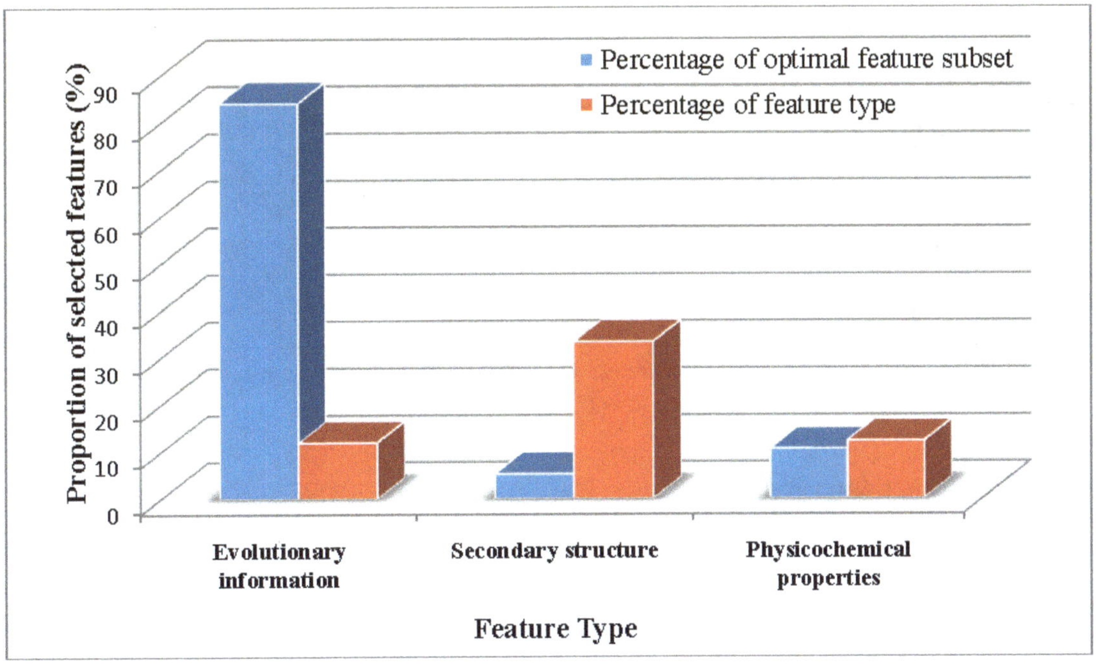

2.3. Comparison of PSNO with Other Methods

In this section, we compare PSNO with GPS-SNO [13], iSNO-PseAAC [15] and iSNO-AAPair [16], which were all sequence-based prediction methods. As the iSNO-AAPair was built on a different dataset (1530 human and mouse proteins), we adopted the independent dataset to compare our PSNO with iSNO-AAPair. In order to reach a consensus assessment with GPS-SNO and iSNO-PseAAC, a 10-fold cross-validation was adopted here to examine the prediction quality. Listed in Table 1 are the corresponding results obtained by the aforementioned two methods on the same training dataset. As can be seen, the *SN*, *ACC* and *MCC* rates achieved by PSNO were obviously higher than those by GPS-SNO with different thresholds and iSNO-PseAAC. Although the GPS-SNO [1] achieved the highest *SP* value, the *SN* and *MCC* value was relatively low. It may be that when the threshold parameter was set at "high", more non-SNOs tended to be correctly classified, while some SNOs were mistakenly identified as non-SNOs.

Listed in the Table S4 are the predicted results by PSNO for Xue's independent dataset. As we can see from Table S4, of the 2302 SNOs, 2188 were successfully identified. The overall success rate was about 95.05%.

In order to assess the ability of the proposed PSNO for practical applications, we adopted Xu's independent dataset containing 81 SNO and 100 non-SNO experimentally-verified peptides. Among the existing models for the prediction of the SNOs, the web server for the model proposed in [14] did not work, and the method in [19] had no web server at all. Therefore, the comparison was made among the following four methods: GPS-SNO, iSNO-PseAAC, iSNO-AAPair and ours, PSNO. Table 2 summarizes the results of PSNO with the existing prediction methods for the four different metrics. Using the optimal 57 features, the *SN*, *SP*, *ACC* and *MCC* values produced by PSNO are 87.7%, 85.0%, 86.2% and 0.72, respectively, which are about 8.1%~43.2%, 0.9%~9.8%, 5.5%~24.6% and 0.09~0.44 higher than previous studies.

Table 1. The performance comparison of PSNO with other existing prediction methods on the training dataset. GPS, group-based prediction system.

Predictor	*SN* (%)	*SP* (%)	*ACC* (%)	*MCC*
GPS-SNO [1]	18.88	**89.63**	56.07	0.1210
GPS-SNO [2]	28.04	81.98	56.39	0.1193
GPS-SNO [3]	45.01	73.33	59.90	0.1915
iSNO-PseAAC	67.01	68.15	67.62	0.3515
PSNO	**74.15**	77.04	**75.67**	**0.5119**

[1] The method proposed in [13] where the threshold parameter was set at "high"; [2] the method proposed in [13] where the threshold parameter was set at "medium"; [3] the method proposed in [13] where the threshold was set at "low". *SN*, *SP*, *ACC* and *MCC* represented the sensitivity, specificity, accuracy and the Mathews correlation coefficient, respectively.

Table 2. Comparison of PSNO with the existing prediction methods via Xu's independent dataset.

Predictor	*SN* (%)	*SP* (%)	*ACC* (%)	*MCC*
GPS-SNO [1]	44.5	81.0	64.7	0.28
iSNO-PseAAC	50.2	75.2	62.8	0.30
iSNO-AAPair	79.6	84.1	81.7	0.63
PSNO	**87.7**	**85.0**	**86.2**	**0.72**

[1] The method proposed in [13] where the threshold parameter was set at "medium". *SN*, *SP*, *ACC* and *MCC* represented the sensitivity, specificity, accuracy and the Mathews correlation coefficient, respectively.

In practical applications, the input should be entire protein sequences. To test the state-of-the-art web servers used for practical applications, our independent dataset (see Section 3.1) was used here. The predicted results are shown in Table 3. Our PSNO produced an *MCC* of 0.4475, which was about 14.22%~32.29% higher than previous studies.

Table 3. Comparison of PSNO with the existing prediction methods using our independent dataset. PseAAC, pseudo-amino acid composition.

Predictor	*SN* (%)	*SP* (%)	*ACC* (%)	*MCC*
GPS-SNO [1]	41.51	**70.87**	60.90	0.1244
iSNO-PseAAC	60.38	67.96	65.38	0.2722
iSNO-AAPair	66.04	66.02	66.03	0.3053
PSNO	**79.25**	67.96	**71.79**	**0.4475**

[1] The method proposed in [13] where the threshold parameter was set at "medium". SN, SP, ACC and MCC represented the sensitivity, specificity, accuracy and the Mathews correlation coefficient, respectively.

2.4. Implementation of PSNO Server

For the convenience of biology scientists, PSNO has been implemented as a free web server located at http://59.73.198.144:8088/PSNO/. Here, a step-by-step brief guide is given below to describe how to use it.

Step 1. Access the web server, and the home page is the default interface displayed (Figure 4). Click on the "Introduction" link to see a detailed description about the server, which includes the User's Guide, "Input", "Output", "Limitation" and "Requirement".

Step 2. You can either type or paste the query sequence into the text box in Figure 4. The query sequence should be in the FASTA format. The FASTA format sequence consists of a single initial line beginning with a symbol (">"), followed by lines of sequence data. You can click on the "Example" link to see the example sequences. You are also required to provide a valid email address in the text box.

Step 3. Click on the "Query" button to submit the computation request. PSNO begins processing and the predicted probabilities of a site being an SNOs or non-SNOs will be sent to you through the email provided.

Figure 4. The home page of the PSNO web server.

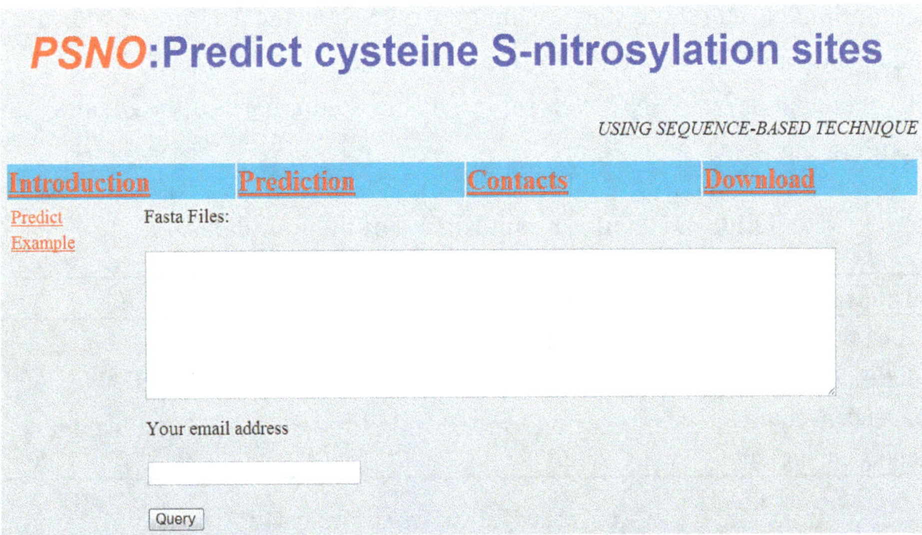

3. Materials and Methods

3.1. Benchmark Datasets

In order to reach a consensus assessment with previous studies [13,15,16], four datasets were used in this paper. The training dataset used in this paper was derived from dbSNO (http://dbsno.mbc.nctu.edu.tw), which integrated the experimentally verified cysteine SNOs from different species [20]. The training dataset contained 731 experimentally-verified SNOs and 810 experimentally verified non-SNOs from 438 randomly selected proteins, none of which had more than 40% similarity to any other. The peptide segments for SNOs and non-SNOs could be formulated by:

$$P = R_{-\xi} R_{-(\xi-1)} \dots R_{-2} R_{-1} C R_{+1} R_{+2} \dots R_{+(\xi-1)} R_{+\xi} \tag{1}$$

where $R_{-\xi}$ and R_{ξ} represented the ξ-th downstream and upstream residues from cysteine (C), respectively. *P* represented the peptide being either an SNO peptide or a non-SNO peptide. To test our method, as well as to reach a consensus assessment with previous investigators [13,15,16], ξ was set as 10 to compile the training dataset. If the upstream or downstream for a cysteine was less than 10, the lacking residues would be filled with dummy code X.

Xue's independent dataset [13,15] consisted of 461 experimentally-verified nitrosylated proteins from published literature or the UniProt database (http://www.uniprot.org/). All of these proteins are clustered with a threshold of less than 40% identity by CD-HIT (Cluster Database at High Identity with Tolerance) [21]. After using the same technique mentioned above, 2302 SNOs are compiled from the 461 nitrosylated proteins. None of these 2302 SNOs occurred in the training dataset. In [16], Xu developed a public independent dataset (81 SNOs and 100 non-SNOs). The corresponding nitrosylated proteins and sequences were taken from dbSNO and UniProt, respectively.

In practical applications, the input should be entire protein sequences. To test the state-of-the-art web servers used for practical applications, we collected a new independent dataset by extracting the experimental-verified 20 nitrosylated proteins from dbSNO. None of them occurred in the training dataset. After compiling based on the same technique, 53 SNOs and 103 non-SNOs are obtained from the 20 nitrosylated proteins. The sequences of these 20 proteins, as well as SNOs (red) and non-SNOs (blue) are freely available at our PSNO web server. Table 4 summarizes the detailed compositions of above-mentioned four datasets.

Table 4. Detailed compositions of the four datasets.

Dataset	Proteins	Peptides	SNOs	Non-SNOs
Training dataset	438	1541	731	810
Xue's independent dataset	461	2302	2302	0
Xu's independent dataset	-	181	81	100
Our independent dataset	20	156	53	103

"-" The paper [16] makes no mention.

3.2. Sample Formulation and Feature Construction

In order to build a powerful protein system, the first thing was to represent the sequences with proper and effective mathematical expressions, which can reflect the intrinsic correction with the target to be predicted. In this study, we incorporated sequence-derived features into pseudo-amino acid composition (PseAAC) to represent the sample of a target protein. The PseAAC method had been widely used in bioinformatics, such as identifying proteins attributes [22,23], predicting protein structures [24,25] and predicting protein classes [26,27]. According to a recent review [28], the general form of PseAAC for a protein could be formulated as:

$$P = [\psi_1, \psi_2 \cdots, \psi_u, \cdots, \psi_\Omega]^T \tag{2}$$

where T was a transpose operator and the ψ_1, ψ_2 ... depended on how to extract the desired information from the protein sequence of P. Here, several sequence-derived features were explored to distinguish the SNOs and non-SNOs. These features included evolutionary conservation scores, the predicted secondary structure and physicochemical properties.

3.2.1. Features of Evolutionary Conservation Scores

Evolutionary conservation scores had been widely used by the investigators to predict various attributes of proteins, such as predicting the protein subcellular location [29], identifying the subnuclear protein location [30] and identifying the protease family [31]. To incorporate evolutionary conservation scores, PSSM (Position-specific Scoring Matrix) was generated by the program "blastpgp" (PSIBLAST) [32], which was used to search the Swiss-Prot database (released on 15 May 2011; http://www.ebi.ac.uk/swissprot/) through 3 iterations (−j 3) and an *e*-value threshold of 0.0001 (−h 0.0001) for multiple sequence alignment against the protein, P. According to [33], the sequence evolution information of protein P with L amino acid residues could be expressed by a $20 \times L$ matrix, as given by:

$$P_{PSSM} = \begin{bmatrix} E_{1,1} & E_{1,2} & \cdots & E_{1,20} \\ E_{2,1} & E_{2,2} & \cdots & E_{2,20} \\ \vdots & \vdots & \vdots & \vdots \\ E_{L,1} & E_{L,2} & \cdots & E_{L,20} \end{bmatrix} \tag{3}$$

where $E_{i,j}$ represented the score of the amino acid in the i-th position of the sequence that was being changed to amino acid type j ($j = 1, 2, \ldots, 20$) during the evolutionary process.

PSSM scores were generally displayed as positive or negative integers. Positive scores (ratio > 0) indicated that the given amino acid substitution exceeded the expected frequency, suggesting that this substitution was surprisingly favored in the alignment than expected by chance, while negative scores (ratio < 0) indicated the opposite; that the frequency occurred less than the expected frequency, suggesting that the substitution was not favored.

The preference of evolutionary conservation in SNOs and non-SNOs were calculated and displayed in a heat map (Figure 5). In this figure, amino acids were sorted in both the x-axis and y-axis. The color palette from black to yellow indicated a growing preference for evolutionary conservation in SNOs and non-SNOs. The yellow color indicated the higher probability of the appearance of evolutionary conservation, while the black color meant less appearance. For instance, the substitution of C/H (*x*-axis/*y*-axis) was black, while the H/C (*x*-axis/*y*-axis) was yellow in SNOs, which suggested that the mean probabilities (or tendency) for His being substituted by Cys was higher than that for Cys being substituted by His in the SNOs. In addition, the H/C of non-SNOs was red. This determined the mean probabilities (or tendency) for His being substituted by Cys in SNOs being higher than those in non-SNOs. Generally speaking, compared with non-SNOs, evolutionary-conserved sets were preferred to aggregate in SNOs, which indicated critical active sites or functional residues that may be required for other intermolecular interactions being abundant in these peptides.

Figure 5. The heat maps of the preference of evolutionary conservation in *S*-nitrosylation sites (SNOs) and non-SNOs. The yellow color indicates the higher probability of appearance of evolutionary conservation, while the black color indicates less appearance.

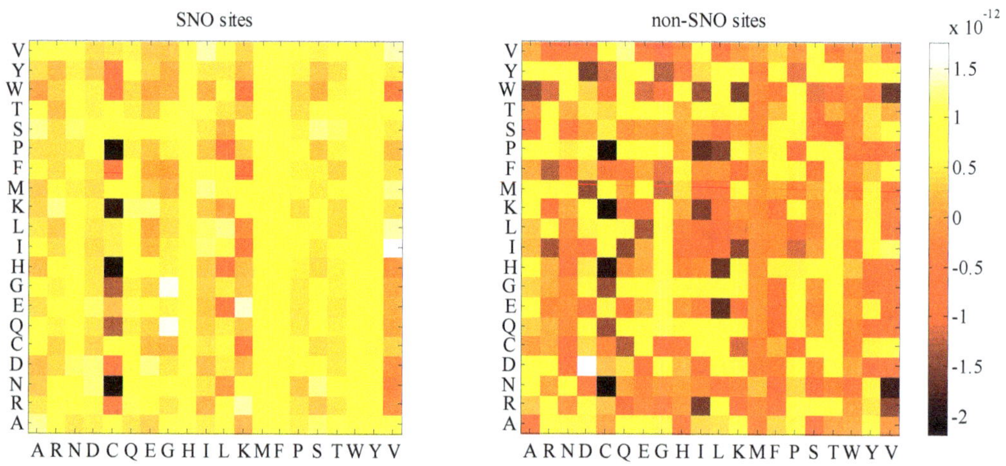

In order to make the descriptor uniformly cover the peptide, we used the elements in the above equation for PSSM (Equation (3)) to define a new matrix, M_{PSSM}, as formulated by:

$$M_{PSSM} = \begin{bmatrix} \sum E_{1,1} & \sum E_{2,1} & \cdots & \sum E_{20,1} \\ \sum E_{1,2} & \sum E_{2,2} & \cdots & \sum E_{20,2} \\ \vdots & \vdots & \vdots & \vdots \\ \sum E_{1,20} & \sum E_{2,20} & \cdots & \sum E_{20,20} \end{bmatrix} \quad (4)$$

where the value of $\sum E_{i,j}$ equaled the sum of amino acid type *i* being changed to amino acid type *j* in above-mentioned matrix P_{PSSM}. In summary, 400 features were obtained to construct features of evolutionary conservation scores.

3.2.2. Features of Predicted Secondary Structure

Consider the fact that proteins with low sequence similarity, but in the same structural class, are likely to share high similarity in their corresponding secondary structural elements. Therefore, it would be useful to encode the protein sequences by taking into account the secondary structure information. In this study, several predicted secondary structure-based features were introduced to further improve low-similarity protein prediction accuracy. In this work, PSIPRED [34] was adopted to explore the secondary structure of a query protein sequence. The outputs of PSIPRED were encoded in terms of "C" for coil, "H" for helix and "E" for strand. The total number, average length and composition percent of C, H and E segments were calculated and constructed for the predicted secondary structure features. These features were defined as follows:

$$Total\_number_{\alpha} = \sum \alpha \tag{5}$$

$$Average\_length_{\alpha} = \frac{\sum \alpha}{\sum segment_{\alpha}} \tag{6}$$

$$Composition\_percent_{\alpha} = \frac{\sum \alpha}{\sum H + \sum E + \sum C} \tag{7}$$

where $\alpha = \{H,E,C\}$, $\sum \alpha$ is the sum of the secondary structure of type α in the peptide. $\sum segment_{\alpha}$ is the sum of segments of type α in the peptide. As a result, 3 + 3 + 3 = 9 features were obtained to construct the predicted secondary structure features.

3.2.3. Features of Physicochemical Properties

Forty nine selected physical chemical, energetic and conformational properties, which have been observed to be widely used in pre-works [29,35,36], were used here. More detailed descriptions can be found at http://www.cbrc.jp/~gromiha/fold_rate/property.html. For each sequence, 49 properties values were firstly calculated by taking the sum of each property value over the whole residues and then divided by the length of the sequence. In this encoding scheme, a peptide was encoded by a 49-dimensional vector.

3.3. The Relative Entropy Selection

Commonly, the combination of various features would bring more informative features to the classifier. Nevertheless, some "bad" features were also added and became the unwanted noise. This noise, which was redundant with other features, may deteriorate the performance of learning algorithms and decrease the generalization power of the learned classifiers [37]. In order to get rid of the related or noisy feature, the feature selection approach for the optimal subset of features from a high-dimensional feature space was a critical job in machine learning. Relative entropy selection (*i.e.*, Kullback–Leibler divergence) [38] was proven to be a powerful method to identify those features that were the most useful in describing the essential differences among the possible classes. In this algorithm, relative entropy can be defined the as:

$$D_{KL}(P||Q) + D_{KL}(Q||P) \tag{8}$$

where P and Q are the conditional probability density function of a feature under two different classes; $D_{KL}(P||Q)$ is the *K–L* divergence of Q from P and $D_{KL}(Q||P)$ was the *K–L* divergence of P from Q. After the calculation, we got a feature list, L:

$$L = \{f_1, f_2, f_3, \ldots, f_i, \ldots\} \text{and } i = \{1,2,3\ldots N\} \tag{9}$$

In this feature list, L, the index, i, of each feature indicated the importance of f_i to the class of the sample.

3.4. Incremental Feature Selection

Through the relative entropy selection, we obtained the ranked feature list. In order to determine which features should be selected for the optimal feature set for our model, the incremental feature selection (IFS) procedure [19] was adopted here to search for a good feature subset involving finding those features that were highly correlated with the decision features, but that are uncorrelated with each other.

During the IFS procedure, we added the feature in the ranked feature list one by one from the top to the bottom. After a feature had been added, a new feature subset was composed. For each new feature subset, a classifier was built based on the new feature subset using 10-fold cross-validation on the training dataset. As a result, 458 individual classifiers were constructed for the 458 feature subsets. By doing so, a table named IFS, with one column for the feature index and the other column for the prediction performance of each individual classifier, was obtained. An IFS curve was drawn to identify the best prediction performance, as well as the corresponding optimal feature subsets.

3.5. K-Nearest Neighbor Algorithm

The *k*-nearest neighbor algorithm (KNN) is quite popular in pattern recognition and machine learning. According to the KNN algorithm [39], the query sample would be assigned to the subset represented by its *k*-nearest neighbors. In this study, if the majority of the *k*-nearest neighbors of the query sample is a positive sample, this means that it is an SNO site. Otherwise, the query sample is regarded as a negative one. There are many different distances to measure the nearest neighbors for the KNN algorithm, such as the Hamming distance [40], Euclidean distance [40] and the Mahalanobis distance [41]. In order to build a KNN model, we tested different *k*-values from 3 to 19, as well as various different definitions. The best performance was achieved with $K = 9$ using the Euclidean distance.

3.6. Assessment of Prediction Accuracy

Four routinely used evaluation indexes were adopted in this paper, *i.e.*, sensitivity (*SN*), specificity (*SP*), accuracy (*ACC*) and the Mathews correlation coefficient (*MCC*).

$$ACC = \frac{TP + TN}{TP + TN + FP + FN} \tag{10}$$

$$SN = \frac{TP}{TP + FN} \tag{11}$$

$$SP = \frac{TN}{TN + FP} \tag{12}$$

$$MCC = \frac{TP \times TN - FP \times FN}{\sqrt{(TP + FN)(TP + FP)(TN + FP)(TN + FN)}} \tag{13}$$

where *TP*, *TN*, *FP* and *FN* were the abbreviations of true positives, true negatives, false positives and false negatives. In this paper, *MCC* was used as the major evaluation criteria to evaluate the performance of the proposed approach as the positive and negative samples in the training dataset were imbalanced.

3.7. Cross-Validation Test

In statistical prediction, the independent dataset, sub-sampling (*k*-fold cross-validation) and jackknife analysis (leave-one-out) are the three cross-validation methods that are often used to assess a prediction tool for its effectiveness in practical application. In order to reach a consensus assessment with previous studies [13,15,16], we used the same 10-fold cross-validation to examine the prediction performance as done by many studies for SNOs prediction. Firstly, the dataset was randomly divided into ten equal subsets; then, nine subsets were used for training and the remaining one for testing. The procedure was repeated 10 times, and the final performance was calculated by averaging over 10 testing sets. The system architecture of the proposed model is illustrated in Figure 6.

Figure 6. The system architecture of the proposed model. Three different types of sequence-derived features, *i.e.*, evolutionary conservation, secondary structure and physicochemical properties, are generated and constructed as the feature space. Relative entropy selection and the incremental feature selection (IFS) procedure are adopted to select the optimal feature subset. The final results are obtained by using 10-fold cross-validation based on the *k*-nearest neighbor (KNN) and the selected optimal feature subsets.

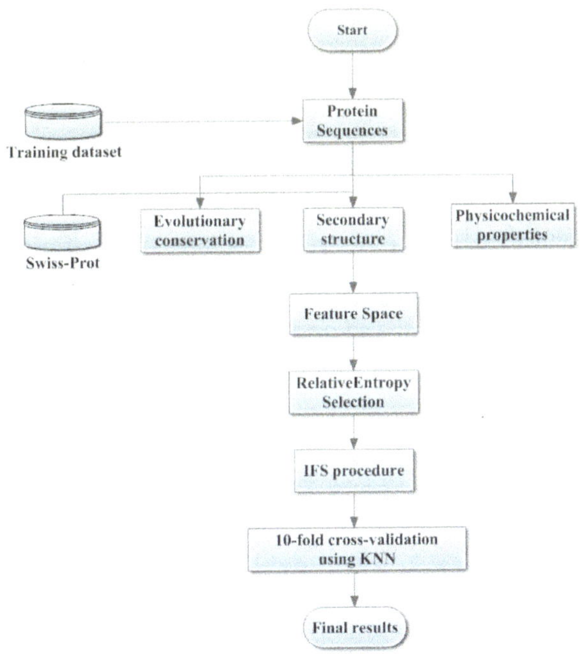

4. Conclusions

In this paper, we present a novel method named PSNO based on sequence-derived features and effective feature selection techniques to identify SNOs. The PSNO model achieves a promising performance and outperforms many other prediction tools. We ascribe the excellent performance of our predictor PSNO to two aspects. The first aspect is the informativeness of the feature vector in our model in representing proteins. The feature vector in this study includes an evolutionary profile, a secondary structure and physicochemical properties. However, rich information also brings the enlargement of the dimension and worsening of the predictor, which needs a proper feature selection strategy. Therefore, the second aspect is the effectiveness of relative entropy selection, followed by the IFS procedure. By means of powerful feature selection, an optimal set of 57 features, which contribute significantly to the prediction of SNOs, are selected. With the 57 optimal features selected, our predictor achieves an overall accuracy of 75.67% and an *MCC* of 0.5119 on a training dataset using 10-fold cross-validation. Theoretically, the protein structures can bring rich information to construct powerful prediction models compared to simple sequences. However, the sequence-based prediction is an alternative to the structure-based prediction in the absence of structures. As a result of the completion of whole-genome sequencing projects, the sequence-structure gap is rapidly increasing. Thus, it would be a powerful prediction tool to identify SNOs for newfound proteins without structure information. For the convenience of biology scientists, the proposed PSNO has been implemented as a web server and is freely available.

Acknowledgments

This work was supported by the Fundamental Research Funds for the Central Universities (Grant No. 12QNJJ005, 14QNJJ029), the Postdoctoral Science Foundation of China (Grant No. 2014M550166, 111900166), and the Research Fund for the Doctoral Program of Higher Education of China (Grant No. 20130043110016).

Author Contributions

J.Z. conceived the idea of this research and was in charge of the PSNO implementation. X.W.Z. and P.P.S. performed the research including data collection, test and analysis. P.P.S. and Z.Q.M. optimized the research and participated in the development and validation of the Web server. X.W.Z. suggested extension and modifications to the research. Z.Q.M. supervised the whole research and revised the manuscript critically. All authors have read and approved the final manuscript.

References

1. Foster, M.W.; Douglas, T.H.; Jonathan, S.S. Protein *S*-nitrosylation in health and disease: A current perspective. *Trends Mol. Med.* **2009**, *15*, 391–404.
2. Foster, M.W.; Timothy, J.M.; Jonathan, S.S. *S*-nitrosylation in health and disease. *Trends Mol. Med.* **2003**, *9*, 160–168.
3. Aranda, E.; López-Pedrera, C.; de La Haba-Rodriguez, R.J.; Rodriguez-Ariza, A. Nitric oxide and cancer: The emerging role of *S*-nitrosylation. *Curr. Mol. Med.* **2012**, *12*, 50–67.
4. Uehara, T.; Nakamura, T.; Yao, D.; Shi, Z.Q.; Gu, Z.; Ma, Y.; Lipton, S.A. *S*-nitrosylated protein-disulphide isomerase links protein misfolding to neurodegeneration. *Nature* **2006**, *441*, 513–517.
5. Nakamura, T.; Cieplak, P.; Cho, D.H.; Godzik, A.; Lipton, S.A. *S*-nitrosylation of Drp1 links excessive mitochondrial fission to neuronal injury in neurodegeneration. *Mitochondrion* **2006**, *10*, 573–578.
6. Schonhoff, C.M.; Matsuoka, M.; Tummala, H.; Johnson, M.A.; Estevéz, A.G.; Wu, R.; Mannick, J.B. *S*-nitrosothiol depletion in amyotrophic lateral sclerosis. *Proc. Natl. Acad. Sci. USA* **2006**, *103*, 2404–2409.

7. Lindermayr, C.; Saalbach, G.; Durner, J. Proteomic identification of *S*-nitrosylated proteins in Arabidopsis. *Plant Physiol.* **2005**, *137*, 921–930.
8. Cook, J.A.; Kim, S.Y.; Teague, D.; Krishna, M.C.; Pacelli, R.; Mitchell, J.B.; Wink, D.A. Convenient colorimetric and fluorometric assays for *S*-nitrosothiols. *Anal. Biochem.* **1996**, *238*, 150–158.
9. Gaston, B. Nitric oxide and thiol groups. *Biochim. Biophys. Acta* **1999**, *1411*, 323–333.
10. Jaffrey, S.R.; Snyder, S.H. The biotin switch method for the detection of *S*-nitrosylated proteins. *Sci. Signal.* **2001**, *2001*, doi:10.1126/stke.2001.86.pl1.
11. Hao, G.; Derakhshan, B.; Shi, L.; Campagne, F.; Gross, S.S. SNOSID, a proteomic method for identification of cysteine *S*-nitrosylation sites in complex protein mixtures. *Proc. Natl. Acad. Sci. USA* **2006**, *103*, 1012–1017.
12. Forrester, M.T.; Thompson, J.W.; Foster, M.W.; Nogueira, L.; Moseley, M.A.; Stamler, J.S. Proteomic analysis of *S*-nitrosylation and denitrosylation by resin-assisted capture. *Nat. Biotechnol.* **2009**, *27*, 557–559.
13. Xue, Y.; Liu, Z.; Gao, X.; Jin, C.; Wen, L.; Yao, X.; Ren, J. GPS-SNO: Computational prediction of protein *S*-nitrosylation sites with a modified GPS algorithm. *PLoS One* **2010**, *5*, e11290.
14. Li, Y.X.; Yuan, H.S.; Ling, J.; Nai, Y.D. An efficient support vector machine approach for identifying protein *S*-nitrosylation sites. *Protein Pept. Lett.* **2011**, *18*, 573–587.
15. Xu, Y.; Ding, J.; Wu, L.Y.; Chou, K.C. iSNO-PseAAC: Predict cysteine *S*-nitrosylation sites in proteins by incorporating position specific amino acid propensity into pseudo amino acid composition. *PLoS One* **2013**, *8*, e55844.
16. Xu, Y.; Shao, X.J.; Wu, L.Y.; Deng, N.Y.; Chou, K.C. iSNO-AAPair: Incorporating amino acid pairwise coupling into PseAAC for predicting cysteine *S*-nitrosylation sites in proteins. *PeerJ* **2013**, *1*, e171.
17. Chou, K.C.; Shen, H.B. Large-Scale plant protein subcellular location prediction. *J. Cell. Biochem.* **2007**, *100*, 665–678.
18. Chou, K.C.; Chun, T.Z. Prediction of protein structural classes. *Crit. Rev. Biochem. Mol. Biol.* **1995**, *30*, 275–349.
19. Li, B.Q.; Hu, L.L.; Niu, S.; Cai, Y.D.; Chou, K.C. Predict and analyze *S*-nitrosylation modification sites with the mRMR and IFS approaches. *J. Proteomics* **2012**, *75*, 1654–1665.
20. Chen, Y.J.; Ku, W.C.; Lin, P.Y.; Chou, H.C.; Khoo, K.H.; Chen, Y.J. *S*-alkylating labeling strategy for site-specific identification of the *S*-nitrosoproteome. *J. Proteome Res.* **2010**, *9*, 6417–6439.
21. Li, W.; Godzik, A. Cd-hit: A fast program for clustering and comparing large sets of protein or nucleotide sequences. *Bioinformatics* **2006**, *22*, 1658–1659.
22. Lin, H.; Ding, H.; Guo, F.B.; Zhang, A.Y.; Huang, J. Predicting subcellular localization of mycobacterial proteins by using Chou's pseudo amino acid composition. *Protein Pept. Lett.* **2008**, *15*, 739–744.
23. Nanni, L.; Lumini, A.; Gupta, D.; Garg, A. Identifying bacterial virulent proteins by fusing a set of classifiers based on variants of Chou's pseudo amino acid composition and on evolutionary information. *IEEE/ACM Trans. Comput. Biol. Bioinform. (TCBB)* **2012**, *9*, 467–475.
24. Zou, D.; He, Z.; He, J.; Xia, Y. Supersecondary structure prediction using Chou's pseudo amino acid composition. *J. Comput. Chem.* **2011**, *32*, 271–278.

25. Sahu, S.S.; Panda, G. A novel feature representation method based on Chou's pseudo amino acid composition for protein structural class prediction. *Comput. Biol. Chem.* **2010**, *34*, 320–327.
26. Qiu, J.D.; Huang, J.H.; Shi, S.P.; Liang, R.P. Using the concept of chous pseudo amino acid composition to predict enzyme family classes: An approach with support vector machine based on discrete wavelet transform. *Protein Pept. Lett.* **2010**, *17*, 715–722.
27. Zhou, X.B.; Chen, C.; Li, Z.C.; Zou, X.Y. Using Chou's amphiphilic pseudo-amino acid composition and support vector machine for prediction of enzyme subfamily classes. *J. Theor. Biol.* **2007**, *248*, 546–551.
28. Chou, K.C. Some remarks on protein attribute prediction and pseudo amino acid composition. *J. Theor. Biol.* **2011**, *273*, 236–247.
29. Xie, D.; Li, A.; Wang, M.; Fan, Z.; Feng, H. LOCSVMPSI: A web server for subcellular localization of eukaryotic proteins using SVM and profile of PSI-BLAST. *Nucleic Acids Res.* **2005**, *33*, W105–W110.
30. Mundra, P.; Kumar, M.; Kumar, K.K.; Jayaraman, V.K.; Kulkarni, B.D. Using pseudo amino acid composition to predict protein subnuclear localization: Approached with PSSM. *Pattern Recognit. Lett.* **2007**, *28*, 1610–1615.
31. Chou, K.C.; Shen, H.B. ProtIdent: A web server for identifying proteases and their types by fusing functional domain and sequential evolution information. *Biochem. Biophys. Res. Commun.* **2008**, *376*, 321–325.
32. Qiu, W.R.; Xiao, X.; Chou, K.C. iRSpot-TNCPseAAC: Identify recombination spots with trinucleotide composition and pseudo amino acid components. *Int. J. Mol. Sci.* **2014**, *15*, 1746–1766.
33. Altschul, S.F. Evaluating the statistical significance of multiple distinct local alignments. In *Theoretical and Computational Methods in Genome Research*; Springer US: New York, NY, USA, 1997; pp. 1–14.
34. McGuffin, L.J.; Bryson, K.; Jones, D.T. The PSIPRED protein structure prediction server. *Bioinformatics* **2000**, *16*, 404–405.
35. Gromiha, M.M.; Selvaraj, S. Importance of long-range interactions in protein folding. *Biophys. Chem.* **1999**, *77*, 49–68.
36. Gromiha, M.M. A statistical model for predicting protein folding rates from amino acid sequence with structural class information. *J. Chem. Inf. Model.* **2005**, *45*, 494–501.
37. Qian, J.; Miao, D.Q.; Zhang, Z.H.; Li, W. Hybrid approaches to attribute reduction based on indiscernibility and discernibility relation. *Int. J. Approx. Reason.* **2011**, *52*, 212–230.
38. Johnson, D.H.; Sinanovic, S. *Symmetrizing the Kullback-Leibler Distance*; Technical Report for Computer and Information Technology; Rice University: Houston, TX, USA, 2001.
39. Keller, J.M.; Michael, R.G.; James, A.G. A fuzzy *k*-nearest neighbor algorithm. *Syst. Man Cybern. IEEE Trans.* **1985**, *4*, 580–585.
40. Mardia, K.V.; John, T.K.; John, M.B. *Multivariate Analysis*; Academic Press: London, UK, 1980.
41. Read, C.B.; Samuel, K.; Norman, L.J. *Encyclopedia of Statistical Sciences*; Wiley: Hoboken, NJ, USA, 1982.

Permissions

All chapters in this book were first published by MDPI; hereby published with permission under the Creative Commons Attribution License or equivalent. Every chapter published in this book has been scrutinized by our experts. Their significance has been extensively debated. The topics covered herein carry significant findings which will fuel the growth of the discipline. They may even be implemented as practical applications or may be referred to as a beginning point for another development.

The contributors of this book come from diverse backgrounds, making this book a truly international effort. This book will bring forth new frontiers with its revolutionizing research information and detailed analysis of the nascent developments around the world.

We would like to thank all the contributing authors for lending their expertise to make the book truly unique. They have played a crucial role in the development of this book. Without their invaluable contributions this book wouldn't have been possible. They have made vital efforts to compile up to date information on the varied aspects of this subject to make this book a valuable addition to the collection of many professionals and students.

This book was conceptualized with the vision of imparting up-to-date information and advanced data in this field. To ensure the same, a matchless editorial board was set up. Every individual on the board went through rigorous rounds of assessment to prove their worth. After which they invested a large part of their time researching and compiling the most relevant data for our readers.

The editorial board has been involved in producing this book since its inception. They have spent rigorous hours researching and exploring the diverse topics which have resulted in the successful publishing of this book. They have passed on their knowledge of decades through this book. To expedite this challenging task, the publisher supported the team at every step. A small team of assistant editors was also appointed to further simplify the editing procedure and attain best results for the readers.

Apart from the editorial board, the designing team has also invested a significant amount of their time in understanding the subject and creating the most relevant covers. They scrutinized every image to scout for the most suitable representation of the subject and create an appropriate cover for the book.

The publishing team has been an ardent support to the editorial, designing and production team. Their endless efforts to recruit the best for this project, has resulted in the accomplishment of this book. They are a veteran in the field of academics and their pool of knowledge is as vast as their experience in printing. Their expertise and guidance has proved useful at every step. Their uncompromising quality standards have made this book an exceptional effort. Their encouragement from time to time has been an inspiration for everyone.

The publisher and the editorial board hope that this book will prove to be a valuable piece of knowledge for researchers, students, practitioners and scholars across the globe.

List of Contributors

Zeenat Mirza
Proteomics and Structural Biology Unit, Fundamental and Applied Biology Group, King Fahd Medical Research Center, King Abdulaziz University, Jeddah 21589, Saudi Arabia
Department of Biophysics, All India Institute of Medical Sciences, New Delhi 110029, India

Vikram Gopalakrishna Pillai
Department of Biophysics, All India Institute of Medical Sciences, New Delhi 110029, India
Hospital of Philadelphia, Philadelphia, PA 19104, USA

Wei-Zhu Zhong
Gordon Life Science Institute, Boston, MA 02478, USA

Shuwang Gu and Yasen Jiao
School of Computer Science and Technology, Tianjin University, Tianjin 300072, China
Tianjin Key Laboratory of Cognitive Computing and Application, Tianjin University, Tianjin 300072, China

Pufeng Du
School of Computer Science and Technology, Tianjin University, Tianjin 300072, China
Tianjin Key Laboratory of Cognitive Computing and Application, Tianjin University, Tianjin 300072, China
Department of Computer Science, City University of Hong Kong, Kowloon, Hong Kong

Wang-Ren Qiu
Computer Department, Jing-De-Zhen Ceramic Institute, Jingdezhen 333046, China

Xuan Xiao
Computer Department, Jing-De-Zhen Ceramic Institute, Jingdezhen 333046, China
Information School, ZheJiang Textile & Fashion College, Ningbo 315211, China
Gordon Life Science Institute, Belmont, MA 02478, USA

Kuo-Chen Chou
Center of Excellence in Genomic Medicine Research (CEGMR), King Abdulaziz University, Jeddah 21589, Saudi Arabia
Gordon Life Science Institute, Belmont, MA 02478, USA

Jung Sik Huh
Department of Urology, School of Medicine, Jeju National University, Jeju 690-756, Korea

Yoongho Lim
Division of Bioscience and Biotechnology, Konkuk University, Seoul 143-701, Korea

Zhiqian Liu, Lei Shan, Qingyan Sun and Weidong Zhang
Department of Phytochemistry, School of Pharmacy, School of Pharmacy, Second Military Medical University, 325 Guo He Road, Shanghai 200433, China

Jianjun Fu
Shanghai Key Laboratory of New Drug Design, School of Pharmacy, East China University of Science and Technology, 130 Mei Long Road, Shanghai 200237, China

Stefania-Felicia Barbuceanu, Diana Carolina Ilies and Valeria Radulescu
Organic Chemistry Department, Faculty of Pharmacy, "Carol Davila" University of Medicine and Pharmacy, 6 Traian Vuia, 020956 Bucharest, Romania

Gabriel Saramet
Pharmaceutical Technology Department, Faculty of Pharmacy, "Carol Davila" University of Medicine and Pharmacy, 6 Traian Vuia, 020956 Bucharest, Romania

Valentina Uivarosi
General and Inorganic Chemistry Department, Faculty of Pharmacy, "Carol Davila" University of Medicine and Pharmacy, 6 Traian Vuia, 020956 Bucharest, Romania

Constantin Draghici
"C.D. Nenitescu" Institute of Organic Chemistry, Romanian Academy, 202B Splaiul Independenței, 060023 Bucharest, Romania

Mostafa M. Ghorab and Mansour S. Alsaid
Department of Pharmacognosy, College of Pharmacy, King Saud University, Riyadh 11451, Saudi Arabia

Marwa G. El-Gazzar
Department of Drug Radiation Research, National Center for Radiation Research and Technology, Nasr City, Cairo 113701, Egypt

Guanhong Xu, Yue Chen, Kun Shen and Fei Li
School of Pharmacy, Nanjing Medical University, Nanjing 210029, China

Yan He
Department of Internal Neurology, Nanjing Children's Hospital Affiliated to Nanjing Medical University, Nanjing 210008, China

Xiuzhen Wang
School of Pharmacy, Nanjing Medical University, Nanjing 210029, China
School of Pharmacy, China Pharmaceutical University, Nanjing 210009, China

Yan Huang, Yi Lu, Lei Zhang, Jia Yan, Jue Jiang and Hong Jiang
Department of Anesthesiology, School of Medicine, Shanghai Ninth People's Hospital Affiliated to Shanghai Jiao Tong University, Shanghai 200011, China

Xiaoran Yin, Xiaoning Li, Xinghuan Xue, Xijing Wang, Xinlian Liu and Hongbing Ma
Department of Oncology, the Second Affiliated Hospital of Xi'an Jiaotong University, Xi'an 710004, China

Jun Zhang, Dong Liu, Cheng Feng and Chenlei Cai
Department of Digestion, the Second Affiliated Hospital of Xi'an Jiaotong University, Xi'an 710004, China

Rongrui Liang
Department of Oncology, the First Affiliated Hospital of Soochow University, No. 188, Shizi Street, Suzhou 215006, China

Kun Zhuang
Department of Digestion, Xi'an Central Hospital, Xi'an 710003, China

Fuchun Jing
Department of Digestive Diseases, Baoji People's Hospital, Baoji 721000, China

Jun Wang
Department of Gastroenterology, Xi'an Hospital of Traditional Chinese Medicine, Xi'an 710001, China

Manh Tin Ho and Young Mee Kim
Department of Biochemistry, School of Medicine, Jeju National University, Jeju 690-756, Korea

Hyun Sik Kang
Department of Pediatrics, School of Medicine, Jeju National University, Jeju 690-756, Korea

Moonjae Cho
Department of Biochemistry, School of Medicine, Jeju National University, Jeju 690-756, Korea
Institute of Medical Science, Jeju National University, Jeju 690-756, Korea

You-Chang Oh, Yun Hee Jeong, Won-Kyung Cho, Min-Jung Gu and Jin Yeul Ma
Korean Medicine (KM)-Based Herbal Drug Development Group, Korea Institute of Oriental Medicine, 461-24, Jeonmin-dong, Yuseong, Daejeon 305-811, Korea

Sunhyo Ryu, Hyeonsook Cheong and Yoonkyung Park
Department of Biotechnology, Chosun University, Gwangju 501-759, Korea

Peter I. Song
Department of Dermatology, University of Arkansas for Medical Sciences, Little Rock, AR 72205, USA

Chang Ho Seo
Department of Bioinformatics, Kongju National University, Kongju 314-701, Korea

Ronggang Xi, Zhiran Zhang, Yan Liu and Xiaobo Wang
Department of Pharmacological and Toxicological Research Centre, No. 210 Hospital of Chinese People's Liberation Army, Dalian 116021, China

Faguang Jin and Wangping Li
Department of Respiration, Tangdu Hospital, Fourth Military Medical University, Xi'an 710038, China

Zhongyang Liu
Department of Pharmacological and Toxicological Research Centre, No. 210 Hospital of Chinese People's Liberation Army, Dalian 116021, China
Department of Respiration, Tangdu Hospital, Fourth Military Medical University, Xi'an 710038, China

Pingping Sun
School of Computer Science and Information Technology, Northeast Normal University, Changchun 130017, China
National Engineering Laboratory for Druggable Gene and Protein Screening, Northeast Normal University, Changchun 130024, China

Jian Zhang, Xiaowei Zhao and Zhiqiang Ma
School of Computer Science and Information Technology, Northeast Normal University, Changchun 130017, China

Index

www.ingramcontent.com/pod-product-compliance
Lightning Source LLC
LaVergne TN
LVHW081020210926
848485LV00004B/909
9781639877812